PHYSICAL THERAPY *of the* LOW BACK

THIRD EDITION

Edited by

Lance T. Twomey, AM, PhD, BSc(Hon)
President and Vice-Chancellor
Curtin University of Technology
Perth, Western Australia
Australia

James R. Taylor, MD, PhD, FAFRM(Sci)
Adjunct Professor
School of Health Sciences
Curtin University of Technology
Visiting Professor
Australian Neuromuscular Research Institute
QEII Medical Center
Perth, Western Australia
Australia

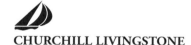

CHURCHILL LIVINGSTONE
A Harcourt Health Sciences Company

New York   Edinburgh   London   Philadelphia

CHURCHILL LIVINGSTONE

A Harcourt Health Sciences Company

The Curtis Center
Independence Square West
Philadelphia, Pennsylvania 19106

NOTICE

Physical Therapy is an ever-changing field. Standard safety precautions must be followed, but as new research and clinical experience broaden our knowledge, changes in treatment and drug therapy become necessary or appropriate. Readers are advised to check the product information currently provided by the manufacturer of each drug to be administered to verify the recommended dose, the method and duration of administration, and contraindications. It is the responsibility of the treating physician relying on experience and knowledge of the patient to determine dosages and the best treatment for the patient. Neither the Publisher nor the editor assumes any responsibility for any injury and/or damage to persons or property.

The Publisher

Library of Congress Cataloging-in-Publication Data

Physical therapy of the low back / [edited by] Lance T. Twomey, James R. Taylor.–3rd ed.
    p.   cm.
    Includes bibliographical references and index.
    ISBN 0-443-06552-7
    1. Backache—Physical therapy.   2. Backache.   I. Twomey, Lance T.   II. Taylor, James R., Ph. D.
    [DNLM: 1. Back Pain—rehabilitation.   2. Physical Therapy.   WE 755 P578 2000]
RD771.B217 P49 2000
617.5'64062—dc21

00-022470

Acquisitions Editor: Andrew Allen
Senior Editorial Assistant: Suzanne Hontscharik

PHYSICAL THERAPY OF THE LOW BACK   ISBN 0-443-06552-7

Printed in the United States of America.

Last digit is the print number: 9   8   7   6   5   4   3   2   1

To our wives,
Meg and Mamie

CONTRIBUTORS

Nikolai Bogduk, MD, PhD, DSc, DipAnat, DipPainMed, FAFRM, FFPM(ANZCA)
Professor of Anatomy and Musculoskeletal Medicine, University of Newcastle; Director, Newcastle Bone and Joint Institute, University of Newcastle, Royal Newcastle Hospital, Newcastle, New South Wales, Australia

Margaret I. Bullock, PhD, BAppSc
Professor, School of Health and Rehabilitation Sciences, The University of Queensland, Brisbane, Queensland, Australia

Joanne E. Bullock-Saxton, PhD, MPhtySt(Man), BPhty(Hon)
Senior Lecturer, Department of Physiotherapy, The University of Queensland, Brisbane, Queensland, Australia

Caroline Drye Taylor, MS, PT
Faculty, Kaiser Permanente Hayward Physical Therapy Residency Program in Advanced Orthopaedic Manual Therapy, Hayward, California; Physical Therapist, Redwood Orthopaedic Physical Therapy, Inc., Castro Valley, California

Joseph P. Farrell, MS, PT
Consultant, Kaiser Permanente Hayward Physical Therapy Residency Program in Advanced Orthopaedic Manual Therapy, Hayward, California; Physical Therapist, Redwood Orthopaedic Physical Therapy, Inc., Castro Valley, California

Ruth Grant, MAppSc, BPT
Professor of Physiotherapy and Pro Vice Chancellor, Division of Health Sciences, University of South Australia, Adelaide, South Australia, Australia

Julie A. Hides, PhD, MPhtySt, BPhty
Clinical Supervisor, Department of Physiotherapy, The University of Queensland, Mater Hospitals Back Stability Clinic, Brisbane, Queensland, Australia; Physiotherapy Research Coordinator, Mater Misericordiae Hospitals, South Brisbane, Queensland, Australia

Gwendolen A. Jull, MPhty, GradDipManTher, FACP
Associate Professor, Department of Physiotherapy, The University of Queensland, Brisbane, Queensland, Australia

Michael Koury, MS, PT
Faculty, Kaiser Permanente Hayward Physical Therapy Residency Program in Advanced Orthopaedic Manual Therapy, Hayward, California; Physical Therapist, Redwood Orthopaedic Physical Therapy, Inc., Castro Valley, California

Robin A. McKenzie, DipPhTh, DMT, DMDT
President, McKenzie Institute International, Waikanae, New Zealand

Akiko Okifuji, PhD
Assistant Professor, Department of Anesthesiology, University of Washington, Seattle, Washington

Peter O'Sullivan, PhD, GradDipManipPhysio, DipPhysio
Private Practitioner; Lecturer, Curtin University of Technology, Perth, Western Australia, Australia

Carolyn A. Richardson, PhD, BPhty(Hon)
Reader and Associate Professor, Department of Physiotherapy, The University of Queensland, Brisbane, Queensland, Australia

Nils Schönström, MD, PhD
Consultant, Department of Orthopaedics, Ryhov Hospital, Jönköping, Sweden

Jeffrey J. Sherman, PhD
Acting Assistant Professor, Department of Anesthesiology, University of Washington, Seattle, Washington

James R. Taylor, MD, PhD, FAFRM(Sci)
Adjunct Professor, School of Health Sciences, Curtin University of Technology; Visiting Professor, Australian Neuromuscular Research Institute, QEII Medical Center, Perth, Western Australia, Australia

Patricia H. Trott, MSc, GradDipAdvManTher, FACP
Associate Professor, School of Physiotherapy, University of South Australia, Adelaide, South Australia, Australia

Dennis C. Turk, PhD
John and Emma Bonica Professor of Anesthesiology and Pain Research, Department of Anesthesiology, University of Washington, Seattle, Washington

Lance T. Twomey, AM, PhD, BSc(Hon)
President and Vice-Chancellor, Curtin University of Technology, Perth, Western Australia, Australia

PREFACE

The third edition of *Physical Therapy of the Low Back* demonstrates just how far knowledge of the structure and function of the lumbar spine and of the clinical management of low back pain has progressed since 1987, when the first edition was published.

The format of the book remains similar to that of past editions. The first four chapters consider contemporary knowledge of morphology, pathology, biomechanics, and function. The next nine chapters provide information important to physical management and understanding, while the new final chapter synthesizes current knowledge, provides a rationale for physical therapy, and looks confidently toward the future. In this regard, the first chapter "The Lumbar Spine from Infancy to Old Age" has been completely rewritten and updated. Two new chapters have been included. These are Chapter 13, written by Dr. Dennis Turk and colleagues on the psychological aspects of lumbar spinal pain, and Chapter 7, written by Professor Jim Taylor and Dr. Peter O'Sullivan, on lumbar segmental instability. All other chapters have been thoroughly revised, updated, and, in some instances, largely rewritten. This third edition preserves the philosophy evident in earlier editions by combining contemporary science with clinical practice.

In part, this book provides a forum that welcomes differences of opinion and allows their expression. The editors do not necessarily agree with all points of view expressed, but in the absence of clear proof, believe they should be presented. We ask the reader to look critically at the views presented and to distinguish among the science (which is clearly identified) and the clinical hypotheses, which are based on that science and may not as yet have been subject to thorough clinical research. Thus the reader will note the emphasis on lumbar segmental instability in this volume, especially in Chapters 1, 7, and 8, and that the views so expressed are in marked distinction to those in Chapter 5 by the eminent clinician, Robin McKenzie. Contemporary information is provided, and the intelligent therapist will make up her/his mind on the issue involved in the light of personal experience and by continuing to be involved in the considerable amount of new published material, which is progressively clarifying the issue.

Low back pain remains an almost universal condition in all countries and societies. The improvements in public health and in the quality and accuracy of the information available to the general public have ensured a better understanding of how this disabling condition can be effectively managed and treated. Physical treatment involves a judicious mix of limited rest, back education, and mobility and exercise and an intelligent approach to work and to leisure. Under some clearly defined circumstances, it also includes manipulation, a procedure in which physical therapists with appropriate training can clearly make a difference. In view of the debate presently occurring in the United States, this issue needs to be reinforced and emphasized.

The workload of this third edition has largely fallen on the broad shoulders of Jim Taylor. This is due to my current role as President of Curtin University and needs to be clearly acknowledged.

Lance T. Twomey

CONTENTS

1

The Natural History of the Lumbar Spine

James R. Taylor
Lance T. Twomey

The human lumbar spine, balanced on the pelvis by its muscles and ligaments, supports the whole length of the spine above it in the erect posture. The human lumbar spine is unique in its fully erect posture. In four-footed animals the tasks of weightbearing and locomotion are shared by four limbs, and the thoracolumbar spine forms an upwardly convex bridge between the forelimbs and the hindlimbs. In humans, the thoracic spine maintains its primary kyphosis but the lumbar spine develops a lordosis on adoption of upright posture in infancy; this lordotic posture is generally maintained throughout life.

In this erect column, the lowest parts bear the highest loads. This is reflected in the large size of the lumbar vertebrae and in the thickness and high proteoglycan content of lumbar intervertebral discs. In addition, the lumbar spine has wide ranges of flexion, extension, and lateral bending. These dual functions of loadbearing and movement in this strong, dynamic organ should be maintained over a life span of 70 to 80 years or more. There are variations in the structure and function of the spine according to familial characteristics, age, gender, and life-style influences on wear and tear. The flexibility and bounce of youth usually give place to the stiffness and slow movement of old age, but degenerate discs, vertebral osteophytes, and a stiff back are not inevitable accompaniments of aging.

The spine is the central skeletal axis of the body. The musculoskeletal and visceral structures of the head, neck, upper limbs, and torso are supported by it, or hung from it. This skeletal axis is strong but not static. The contrary requirements of strength and mobility are met by combining strong individual intervertebral joints allowing limited movement with a large number of motion segments, which collectively provide large ranges of movement.

Considering the lumbosacral spine in particular, its strength, resilience, and mobility are all essential to normal human activity. Lumbopelvic posture affects the posture of the whole spine and head. Pelvic obliquity from unequal leg lengths results in compensatory scoliosis[1, 2]; variation in pelvic tilt results in increased lumbar lordosis, or a "flat back."[3] Lumbar stiffness restricts locomotion, bending and lifting, and many other normal, everyday activities. Lumbar spinal osteoporosis leads to shortening with aging and may allow the rib cage to abut on the pelvis, further restricting movements. Thorough knowledge of normal development, normal adult anatomy, and age changes in the lumbar lumbar spine is essential to a proper understanding of spinal biomechanics and to accurate diagnostic skills.

This chapter describes how the complex structure of the lumbar spine varies throughout life and how it is designed to cope with its diverse functions. Descriptions of development, adult anatomy, aging, and injuries are based on our own studies of large series of lumbar spines[4–13] and on other authorities as referenced.

DEVELOPMENT AND GROWTH OF THE LUMBAR SPINE

General Principles

The processes of development and growth determine the normal adult structure and function of the lumbar vertebral column. Malformations result from abnormal genetic, chemical, or mechanical influences on growth.

By growth we mean increase in size by increase in cell numbers, cell size, and cell products such as proteoglycans and collagen fibers. Most cell multiplication takes place in the prenatal phase, and postnatal growth is achieved more by increases in cell size and cell products. Development also involves cell differentiation; cells become more specialized and less versatile as they multiply. Cells differentiate as their genetic program is influenced by their position in the embryo and their contact and interaction with other cells, and by mechanical and hormonal factors. Some cells produce diffusible chemicals that influence the development of neighboring tissues, but many control mechanisms are incompletely understood.[14]

Summary of Early Development

In the third week of embryonic life, before development of a vertebral column, the axis of the flat embryonic disc is determined by the appearance and longitudinal growth of the rod-like notochord between the ectoderm and the endoderm. The embryonic disc can now be described as having headward and tailward ends. Soon mesoderm, the third primary layer of the embryo, develops on each side of the notochord, between the ectoderm and the endoderm.

The cells of the rod-like notochord influence the development of other cells around them. They induce thickening of the adjacent dorsal ectoderm to form a neural plate, which then folds along its length to form the neural tube, parallel to and behind the notochord. The notochord and neural tube together induce the formation of the original mesodermal vertebral column around them. At this stage the paraxial mesoderm on each side of the notochord is segmented into a large number of somites, or blocks of mesoderm. The medial parts of these blocks of mesoderm are called sclerotomes and

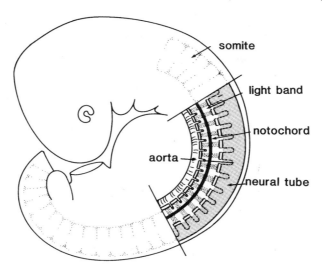

Fig. 1-1 A diagram of a 7 mm crown-rump length human embryo shows the outlines of somites on the external surface. The center section shows median plane structures. The intersegmental branches of the aorta are at the levels of the light bands (primitive vertebral bodies). Vertebral arch processes are growing around the neural tube. The notochord (black) passes through the centers of the light bands and dark bands (primitive intervertebral discs). (From Taylor and Twomey[17] with permission.)

they are the building material from which the primitive spinal column is formed around the notochord.

As the embryo grows, it folds and bends; the sides of the embryonic disc fold ventrally to enclose the primitive gut tube; the cylindric embryo also curls up, the head and tail curving ventrally to form the primary curve of the vertebral column. Anterior to the primitive spine is the primitive aorta with its regular paired branches (Fig. 1-1).

Three Developmental Stages

Three developmental stages of the vertebral column can be identified—the mesodermal stage, the cartilaginous stage, and the osseous stage.

Mesodermal Stage

The mesodermal (blastemal) column is formed around the notochord from the sclerotome portions of the somites.[15–18] Although it is formed from segmented mesoderm, this original mesodermal condensation around the notochord is continuous. It resegments into alternate light and dark bands along its length. Vertebral arch processes grow around the neural tube from each light band, and the aorta sends branches around the middle of each light band. The light bands grow in height four times more rapidly than the adjacent dark bands.

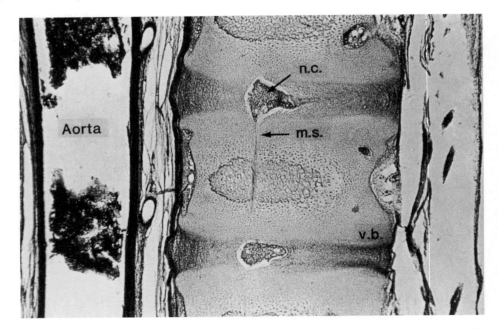

Fig. 1-2   A median sagittal section of the thoracic spine of a 75 mm (11th week) human fetus shows the cartilage stage of vertebral development. At the center of each cartilage model of a vertebra, calcified zones with hypertrophied chondrocytes herald the formation of centers of ossification (centra). The dark anterior rim around the calcified zone represents the first bone formation within the vertebral body (vb). The notochord has segmented to form a primitive nucleus pulposus (nc) in each disc. The mucoid streak (ms) is all that remains of the notochordal track through the vertebra.

Cartilaginous Stage

Each light band differentiates into a cartilage model of a vertebra at the beginning of the fetal stage (2 months' gestation).[18] The rapid differentiation and growth of the fetal cartilage models of vertebrae are accompanied by notochordal segmentation where the notochord disappears from the centers of vertebral bodies and aggregates in the developing discs (Fig. 1-2). Each notochordal segment forms a nucleus pulposus at the center of a dark band or developing disc.[19] At the periphery of this primitive intervertebral disc, fibroblasts and collagen bundles form a lamellar pattern. Soon, blood vessels grow into the cartilaginous vertebra, and centers of ossification appear.

Osseous Stage

Three primary centers of ossification appear in each vertebra. Bilateral vertebral arch centers appear first. The earliest vertebral arch centers are in the cervicothoracic region, but the process rapidly extends up and down the column, the sacrococcygeal centers appearing last, although the mid-thoracic centers are the last presacral centers to appear.[20] A single primary center for each vertebral body forms the centrum (Fig. 1-2). These single centers may have a bilobed appearance in vertical sections through the plane of the notochord as a result of a temporary inhibition of ossification around the notochordal track.[19,21] The first centra appear near the thoracolumbar junction; then the others appear in sequence up and down the column.

The process of ossification extends through the cartilage model of each vertebra, but cartilage growth plates persist to ensure growth. The cartilage plates on the upper and lower vertebral surfaces remain cartilaginous throughout life.

Dorsal-Midline Growth Plate.   A single growth plate in the midline of the vertebral arch (Fig. 1-3) persists until 1 year postnatally.

Neurocentral Growth Plates.   These persist on each side, between the arch and the centrum, until 3 to 7 years, ensuring growth of the spinal canal to accommodate growth of the spinal cord and cauda equina.

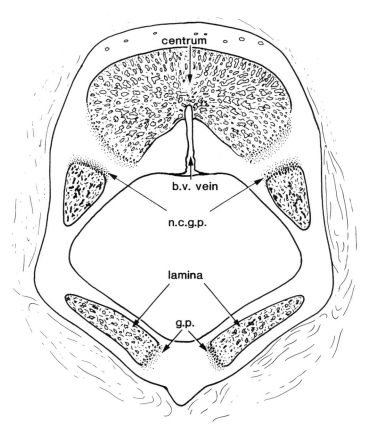

Fig. 1-3 Growth plates: this tracing of a horizontal section of a fetal lumbar vertebra (32nd week) shows the neurocentral growth plates *(ncgp)* and the vertebral arch growth plate *(gp)*. There is only one center of ossification for each side of the vertebral arch, but the plane of the section has missed the bone of the middle part of each half arch.

Cartilage–Plate Growth Plates. Growth plates at the upper and lower vertebral end-plates ensure growth in height of the vertebra. These are parts of the cartilage plates capping the cephalic and caudal surfaces of the vertebral body (Fig. 1-4). A rim of bone appears around the periphery of each cartilage plate between 9 and 12 years.[8,16] This "ring apophysis" fuses with the vertebral body at 18 to 20 years in males[22] and 2 years earlier in females (Fig. 1-5). The rim sometimes fails to fuse with the centrum, appearing as a "limbus vertebra" on radiographs (see Fig. 1-9).

Growth and Development of Intervertebral Discs

The annulus fibrosus of each disc is recognizable from a very early stage of development when the fibroblasts of the dark bands align themselves in a lamellar pattern and begin to form collagenous lamellae. A central nucleus pulposus appears when the notochord segments. The notochordal segments grow and expand rapidly at the center of each disc, particularly in the lumbar region. At the cartilage plates the disc structure interlocks with the cartilage models of the vertebral bodies (see Fig. 1-5). This enables the growing nucleus to be entirely enclosed in an envelope formed by the annulus and the cartilage plates. The growing fetal and infant discs are very vascular, both in their annulus and in their cartilage plates, but during the first few years of childhood these vessels gradually disappear so that the disc of the adult is avascular. The nucleus is avascular at all stages of development. The outer annulus retains some small blood vessels in later childhood and adolescence. In infants, where small blood vessels enter the posterolateral sur-

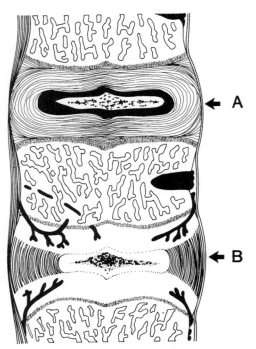

Fig. 1-4 **(A)** The intervertebral disc of a full-term fetus, viewed by polarized light, showing the continuity of the inner two thirds of the anulus with the lamellar structure of the cartilage plates. **(B)** The lower disc as seen by normal transmitted light, showing the outlines of blood vessels supplying the disc. Central indentations of the cartilage plates from the nucleus pulposus indicate where the notochordal track originally passed through the column. The growth plates of the vertebral endplates are seen. The posterocentral black area in the vertebra is the basivertebral vein. (From Taylor and Twomey[17] with permission.)

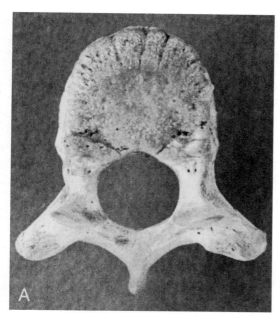

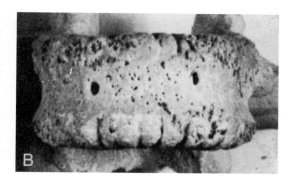

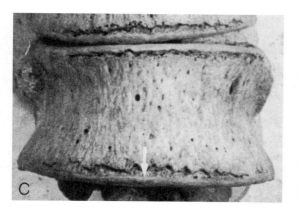

Fig. 1-5 **(A)** The superior surface of a juvenile thoracic vertebra shows radial grooves due to the inhibition of ossification by vascular canals. The lines of neurocentral fusion can also be seen. **(B)** The anterior surface of the same vertebra shows the same deep grooves where the vessels enter the cartilage plates from the periosteum. **(C)** A fully grown but skeletally immature vertebral body shows the upper and lower ring apophyses fusing with the centrum. Small vascular foramina pass between each apophysis and the centrum. (From Taylor and Twomey[17] with permission.)

faces of each disc, small nerves accompany them. These nerve fibers remain in the outer annulus when the blood vessels disappear.

There are regional variations in the development of intervertebral discs. The discs are thickest with the largest nucleus in the lumbar region, where they form one third to one half of the length of the growing lumbar spine.

The notochordal cells disappear from the center of each disc in later childhood, when the disc becomes avascular and the cell population of the adult nucleus is composed of fibroblasts and chondrocytes. These cells survive better in an avascular environment.[8, 19]

Growth in Length of the Vertebral Column as a Whole

Growth is most rapid prenatally. The rate of growth decreases throughout infancy and childhood, with a growth spurt in adolescence. The spine contributes 60 percent of sitting height. Measurements of sitting height can be used to chart postnatal growth in spinal length.[23] Sitting height growth rate declines from 5 cm per year in the second year of life, to 2.5 cm per year between 4 and 7 years and to 1.5 cm per year just before adolescence. The adolescent growth spurt for the spine begins at 9 years in females, lasting until 14 years, and peaking at 12 years, with a sitting height growth velocity of 4 cm per year. In males the growth spurt lasts from 12 to 17 years with a peak growth velocity of 4 cm per year at 14 years.

The thoracolumbar spine matures earlier than the cervical or sacral spine. The thoracolumbar spine grows rapidly just before and after puberty. Its growth in length is 60 percent more rapid in the female than in the male between the ages of 9 and 13 years, but after 13 years the male spine grows more rapidly (Fig. 1-6). Spine length is 99 percent complete, on average, by

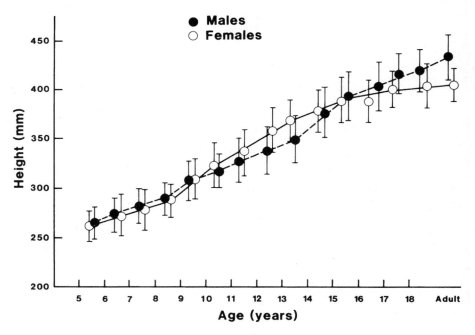

Fig. 1-6 Cross-sectional data for male and female growth in thoracolumbar spine length based on measurements in 1500 subjects. This shows how pre-adolescent and adolescent growth spurts in females make the female spine longer than the male spine from 11 years to 15 years. The effect of the later male adolescent growth spurt at about 14 years then becomes evident.

15 years in girls and 17 years in boys, but there is wide variation. Risser's sign (the lateral appearance, medial excursion, and fusion of the iliac crest apophyses) coincides with individual completion of spinal growth.[23] The mature spine length usually forms a greater proportion of total stature in females than in males.

Control Mechanisms in Normal and Abnormal Development

A Synopsis of Notochordal, Neural, Vascular, and Mechanical Influences

1. The notochord and neural tube induce the sclerotomes to form the original vertebral column around them.[8, 19]
2. Resegmentation of the original continuous column is related to the regular arrangement of the intersegmental arteries.[24]
3. The notochord forms the nucleus pulposus, which grows rapidly in fetuses and infants; notochordal cells atrophy and disappear during childhood.[8, 19]
4. Chordomas, which are rare, malignant tumors usually seen in a retropharyngeal or sacrococcygeal situation, may result from long-term persistence of notochordal cells in adults.[19]
5. Congenital block vertebrae, butterfly vertebra, or hemivertebra may result from abnormal notochordal segmentation, persistence of the notochordal track, or primary absence of segmental blood vessels.[23]
6. Weak areas in the cartilage plates, along the original notochordal track, or at former vascular canals, are sites of disc prolapse into vertebral bodies, forming Schmorl's nodes.[8, 17]
7. Growth of the spinal cord and cauda equina controls growth of the vertebral arches and spinal canal, just as brain growth influences skull-vault growth.[25] Spina bifida is a developmental anomaly that varies from simple splitting of the vertebral arch (spina bifida occulta), which is common and innocuous, to complete splitting of skin, vertebral arch, and underlying neural tube (rachischisis) with associated neurologic deficits.[25] Adequate folate intake during pregnancy may prevent this anomaly.
8. Mild asymmetry of the right and left halves of the vertebral arches is common and is determined by normal growth patterns. It produces slight rotation of the anterior elements to the left in infancy and to the right in adolescence. This may determine the direction of curvature of scoliosis in both its physiologic and progressive forms.[20]
9. Lumbar zygapophyseal joint facets are coronally oriented in infants; they grow backward from their lateral margins and change from planar to biplanar facets with coronal and sagittal components in children with different functions in controlling spinal movements.[7, 23, 26]
10. When infants begin to stand and walk, there is an increase in the lumbosacral angle, increased lordosis, and changes in the shape of the intervertebral discs and in the position of the nucleus pulposus. The vertebral

bodies increase their anteroposterior growth rate. The vertebral end-plates change their shape from convex in infants to concave in children. The end-plate concavity is opposite the maximum bulge of the nucleus pulposus.[1, 27] Pelvic obliquity and lumbar scoliosis are associated with asymmetric end-plate concavities.

11.   Sexual dimorphism in vertebral-body shape and spinal posture develops in childhood and adolescence in association with different hormonal influences and differences in muscle development.[28] These differences probably contribute to the greater prevalence of progressive scoliosis in females than in males.[28, 29]

12.   Scheuermann's disease, with irregularity of the vertebral end-plates in adolescence, is associated with abnormal vascular development and the development of multiple Schmorl's nodes.[23, 30] Some of these topics are now discussed in more detail.

Vertebral Column Segmentation and Segmental Anomalies

The original vertebral column can be distinguished as a condensation of mesenchyme around the notochord in embryos of 2 mm crown–rump length at about 3 weeks' gestation. It is formed by the medial migration of cells from the sclerotomes, and it is originally continuous and unsegmented. It resegments into alternate light and dark bands, with the light bands at the level of the intersegmental branches of the aorta (see Fig. 1-1). When the light bands form cartilaginous vertebrae and the dark bands form the intervertebral disc, the muscles, derived from the myotomes of the somites, bridge over the discs and are attached to the vertebrae. This vertebral resegmentation allows the alternation of muscle and bone that is essential for movement.[18]

The intersegmental branches of the dorsal aorta influence vertebral column resegmentation by virtue of their placement around the centers of the light bands, where they provide nutrition for the more rapid growth of the primitive vertebrae.[23] Anomalies of these paired, regularly spaced aortic branches may result in anomalies of segmentation.[24] A unilateral hemivertebra results if one side of the vertebral body fails to develop. As there is only one primary center of ossification for the centrum, the anomaly originates during a preosseous stage of development. Absence of an intersegmental vessel on one side may give rise to a unilateral hemivertebra, which will be associated with a sharply angled congenital scoliosis (Fig. 1-7).

As the light bands grow rapidly, they appear to expel notochordal tissue into the slowly growing intervertebral discs. Each notochordal segment forms a nucleus pulposus. Notochordal tissue grows rapidly by cell multiplication and production of mucoid matrix at the center of the fetal disc. Absence of a notochordal segment allows two centra to fuse, forming congenital block vertebrae as no nucleus pulposus forms to separate them.

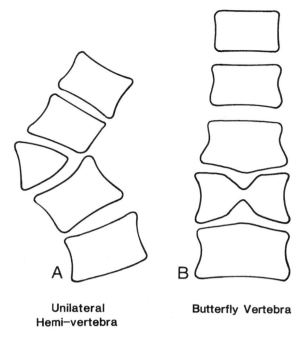

A   Unilateral
Hemi–vertebra

B   Butterfly Vertebra

Fig. 1-7   Tracings from anteroposterior radiographs of juveniles showing congenital anomalies. **(A)** shows the appearance of a unilateral hemivertebra, with an angled scoliosis. **(B)** shows a butterfly vertebra, due to late persistence of the notochordal track through the vertebral body. This contrasts with the different effect on ossification shown in Fig. 1-8.

Later Notochordal Development and "Butterfly Vertebra"

The notochordal nucleus pulposus grows rapidly in the fetus and infant.[8,31] The notochordal cells produce enzymes that loosen and digest the inner margins of the surrounding annulus and cartilage plates, incorporating these tissues into the expanding nucleus. The annulus and cartilage plates grow rapidly to keep pace with the "erosion" of their inner margins by the notochordal nucleus. Notochordal cells do not normally survive beyond childhood, except perhaps in Schmorl's nodes, or in the disc remnants of the sacrum. Their demise is associated with the dramatic decrease in vascularity of the surrounding tissues during childhood.

The mucoid streak persists for a while in the cartilage models of the vertebrae as an acellular notochordal track, but when ossification of the centrum commences, it is usually obliterated. Persistence of parts of the notochordal track through the centrum is quite common in infancy[19,21] but is rare after infancy. If a complete notochordal track persists, a butterfly vertebra is the result (Fig. 1-7). Persistence of the notochordal track in infancy produces a misshapen vertebra (Fig. 1-8) at the vertebral end-plates. This may be responsible for the "Cupid's bow" appearance frequently seen in lower lumbar vertebral bodies in adults.[21,32]

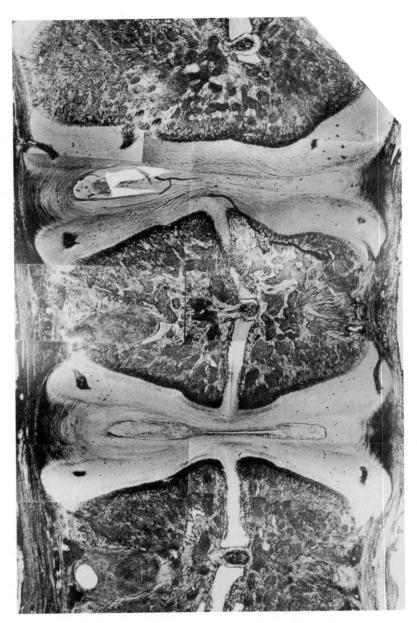

Fig. 1-8 A median sagittal section of thoracic vertebrae and discs in a 1-month-old infant demonstrates persistence of the notochord track through the thoracic vertebral bodies. The mucoid streak normally disappears from the vertebrae at about 20 weeks gestation. The deformities of the vertebral end-plates appear to result from attempts by the bone to "grow around" the persisting mucoid streak. The nucleus pulposus is bilocular because of the bony deformities. (From Taylor[21] with permission.)

Other Vascular and Notochordal Influences

Disappearance of Notochordal Cells from the Nucleus Pulposus

The cartilage plates of fetuses and infants have an excellent blood supply, which brings nutrition to the rapidly growing intervertebral disc.[8, 19] The vascular arcades approach close to the growing notochordal nucleus pulposus (see Fig. 1-4, *B*). When the disc mass increases and its vessels disappear during childhood, the notochordal cells die, to be replaced by chondrocytes, cells better adapted to an avascular environment.

Schmorl's Nodes.   The cartilage plates have a consistently situated, funnel-shaped defect on their nuclear aspect, where the notochordal track formerly penetrated the column, just behind the center of each vertebral end-plate (see Fig. 1-4). These weak points are the sites of central Schmorl's nodes. This common form of Schmorl's nodes occurs almost as frequently in adolescents and young adults as in older adults,[33] indicating their association with this developmental weakness.

When the vascular channels of the cartilage plates disappear in childhood, the canals are plugged by loose connective tissue, leaving channels of reduced resistance from the nucleus to the peripheral vertebral spongiosa.[17] These channels, arching around the advancing ossification front of the centrum, inhibit ossification locally, causing a toothed or grooved surface on the growing vertebral end plates of adolescents (see Figs. 1-4,*B* and 1-5,*A* and *B*). The vascular channels are pathways for "peripheral disc prolapses" into the anterior spongiosa or between the ring apophysis and the centrum, forming a limbus vertebra (Fig. 1-9).

Schmorl's nodes occur in lower thoracic and upper lumbar vertebrae of 38 percent of adult spines, more often in males than females. Central nodes are probably asymptomatic; anterior nodes may be associated with trauma and a complaint of localized somatic back pain.[23]

Scheuermann's Disease.   Multiple Schmorl's nodes, both large and small, are seen in Scheuermann's juvenile kyphosis, together with a radiologic appearance of irregularity of the vertebral end-plates. Large anterior nodes are sometimes associated with anterior vertebral body collapse and wedging. Multiple Schmorl's nodes may be associated with juvenile osteoporosis predisposing to vertebral end-plate weakness.[34] Alternatively, an abnormally vascular end-plate may contribute to end-plate weakness. We have noted increased vascularity of vertebral end-plates around Schmorl's nodes.[30]

Scoliosis and Growth

Normal growth factors in fetuses and children contribute to common forms of physiologic scoliosis in infants and adolescents. Asynchronous appearance of right and left ossification centers in fetal thoracic vertebral arches is

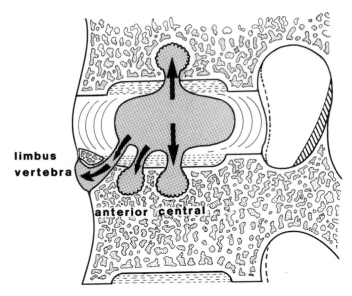

Fig. 1-9 Varieties of Schmorl's nodes (intravertebral disc herniation). The common central nodes occur through cartilage plate weaknesses left by the notochordal track (see Fig. 1-4). Peripheral herniations along weak channels left by vascular canals are less frequent (see Fig. 1-5). Anterior disc herniation between the centrum and the ring apophysis is termed a *limbus vertebra*. "Central nodes" are slightly posterior of center in adults, due to the predominant growth at the anterior vertebral body surface. (From Twomey and Taylor[17] with permission.)

quite common; those on the right often appear before the corresponding left centers. The better-oxygenated blood from the left ventricle may supply the right midthoracic vertebral arches, while the less-well-oxygenated blood from the right ventricle, through the ductus arteriosus, supplies the left vertebral arches.[20,35] The asynchronous appearance of vertebral arch centers correlates with measured asymmetry in infant vertebral arches (R > L), and with the observation that infantile thoracic scoliosis tends to be convex to the left (Fig. 1-10).

There is evidence that the asynchronous growth of vertebral arches (R > L) in fetuses and infants may persist until asynchronous closure of the neurocentral growth plates at 6 to 7 years, which leads to reversal of the infantile asymmetry in thoracic vertebral arches of older children (L > R) due to the later closure of the left neurocentral growth plates (see Fig. 1-10).

In adolescents the left arches are often larger than the corresponding right arches.[20] The twist to the right of the midthoracic anterior elements from 7 years onward is associated with a predominantly right convexity of thoracic scoliotic curvatures in adolescents. A left-sided flattening of the anterior surfaces of midthoracic vertebrae also appears in older children, where the vertebrae are in contact with the aorta. Aortic pressure flattens the anterior left surfaces of thoracic vertebral bodies and may also twist these vertebral bodies to the right.[20,23,35] The different position of the lumbar aorta on the anterior surfaces of L2–4 and the different shape of the lumbar

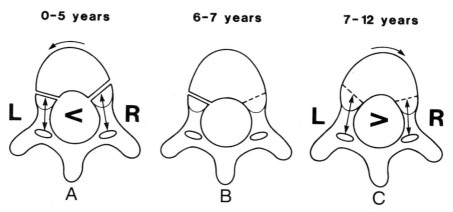

Fig 1-10   Diagram of three stages of growth in midthoracic vertebrae, showing minor asymmetries due to asynchronous growth. **(A)** In the fetus, infant, and young child the right neural arch is generally slightly larger than the corresponding left arch, possibly from a better blood supply to the right side in the fetus. **(B)** At neurocentral closure there is often earlier closure on the right than on the left. **(C)** After the age of 7 years the left arch is often slightly larger than the right arch, with the appearance of vertebral body rotation to the right, from asymmetric pressure by the aorta. (From Taylor and Twomey[23] with permission.)

vertebral bodies may relate to a slight twist to the left in some lumbar vertebral bodies.[35,36] These asymmetries are minor. They accompany normal growth and probably determine the side of scoliosis, but they are not the cause of progressive scoliosis. Other causes operate in the multifactorial etiology of structural scolioses.

Growth of Lumbar Zygapophyseal Joints

Lumbar zygapophyseal facets, like thoracic facets, are flat and coronally oriented in fetuses and infants. When infants walk upright, the lumbar articular facets begin to grow in a posterior direction from their lateral margins, changing their shape and orientation. The original coronally oriented part remains, but a sagittally oriented component is added to the joint (Fig. 1-11). In adult joints, from Ll–2 to L3–4, the posterior two thirds of the joint is approximately sagittal and the anterior third is approximately coronal (see Fig. 1-19). Remodelling at the junction of the two parts makes the joints surfaces curved. In transverse sections or CT scans the concave superior articular facet is seen to "embrace" the smaller convex inferior facet (see Fig. 1-20). Both curved articular surfaces are inclined approximately parallel to the long axis of the spine. The lower lumbar facets are more coronally oriented and flatter than the upper facets.[7,37,38]

The coronal and sagittal components of the articular surfaces relate to different functions of control of movement in flexion and axial rotation, respectively. The subchondral bone plate (SCP) of the superior articular facet becomes much thicker in its anterior coronal part than in the sagittal part, developing a wedge shape in transverse section, which reflects greater com-

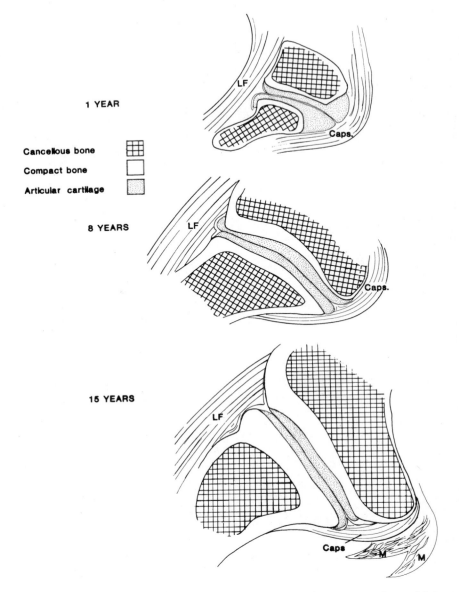

1 YEAR

Cancellous bone
Compact bone
Articular cartilage

8 YEARS

15 YEARS

Fig. 1-11 Tracings from horizontal sections of three L4–5 zygopophyseal joints at 1 year, 8 years, and 15 years show "rotation" of the joint plane from the coronal plane toward the sagittal plane during growth, due to posterior growth from the joint's lateral margins, with remodeling. The ligamentum flavum *(LF)*, fibers of multifidus *(M)* and the posterior fibrous capsule *(Caps)* are also shown. The subchondral bone plate, deep to the articular cartilage, becomes thicker with growth, especially anteriorly.

pressive loading in the coronal part of the joint.[7] The SCP and articular cartilage reach their maximum thickness in young adult life. The adult hyaline cartilage is about 1 mm thick on each facet. It has a very smooth surface, and the matrix and cells stain lightly and evenly in the healthy joint. It is joined to the underlying SCP by a thin, regular, calcified layer. In the growing joint the subchondral bone is vascular, but with maturation this vascularity declines.

Growth of Vertebral Bodies and Intervertebral Discs

Changes on Assumption of Erect Posture

There are changes in the shape of lumbar vertebral bodies after infancy, due to the mechanical forces on the spine in erect posture. These changes result from loadbearing in erect posture and from a change in the position of the growing nucleus pulposus as lordosis is established.[39] Infant lumbar vertebrae have convex upper and lower end-plates, and the main part of each nucleus pulposus is situated posterior to the center of the disc. As the infant stands and learns to walk, the lumbar curvature changes from kyphosis to lordosis, the disc changes its shape, and the nucleus pulposus moves with growth to a central position. The convex vertebral endplates of infants become concave during childhood, the concavities appearing opposite the maximum bulge of the nucleus pulposus.[6,8,19]

The other important changes in vertebral shape due to erect posture loadbearing are the relative increases in the anteroposterior and transverse dimensions of vertebral bodies and discs. These changes in the predominant direction of growth give the lumbar spine more stability in the sagittal and coronal planes. They also reflect the ready response of growing bones to mechanical forces at this age. In nonambulatory children, these normal changes in vertebral and disc shape do not appear. Such children have very square vertebrae with a slender spinal column on lateral radiographs, without the normal concavities in the endplates (Fig. 1-12). This abnormal shape is due to decreased horizontal growth rather than to any increase in vertical growth.[6,8] A similar square shape, from a different cause, is seen when the posterior surfaces of vertebral bodies are scalloped by resorption in the presence of a tumor in the vertebral canal.

Sexual Dimorphism in Vertebral Body Shape

From the age of 8 or 9 years onward, gender differences appear in thoracic and lumbar vertebral shape.[28] Female vertebrae grow in height more rapidly than male vertebrae, giving a more slender vertebral column. Male vertebrae grow more in both transverse and anteroposterior dimensions than female vertebrae, throughout the whole adolescent growth period, and appear wider and more squat than female vertebrae on radiographs (Fig. 1-13).[28]

Fig. 1-12 Tracings from lateral radiographs of ambulant and nonambulant subjects show the effect of weightbearing on growth. In the absence of weightbearing in erect posture, no end-plate concavity appears, and anteroposterior vertebral body growth is severely retarded. (From Taylor[27] with permission.)

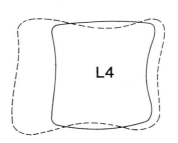

—— non-ambulant (14 year female)

- - - ambulant (15 year female)

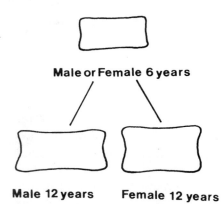

Male or Female 6 years

Male 12 years   **Female 12 years**

Fig. 1-13 Gender difference in vertebral-body shape is shown in tracings from anteroposterior radiographs. At the age of 6 years there is no gender difference but by 12 years, male vertebral bodies are broader and female vertebral bodies tend to be taller. (From Taylor and Twomey[17] with permission.)

Measurements in a growing population showed that the thoracolumbar spine grows in height 1.7 times more rapidly in females than males between the ages of 9 and 13 years.[40] After the age of 14 years, the male spine grows in length more rapidly than the female spine, but the greater transverse growth of male vertebrae maintains the shape difference described. These vertebral shape differences in males and females are accompanied by differences in muscular support because the effect of testosterone on muscle is to increase both its bulk and its strength-per-unit cross-sectional area. The thicker male vertebral column has better muscular support than the slender female column. When axially loaded, an average female column would buckle more easily than an average male column, with a greater tendency to progression of scoliosis in females than in males.[28]

It is interesting to note that these growth-related gender differences in vertebral shape are diminished by age changes in vertebral shape in elderly adults, where there is "thickening of the waist" of vertebral bodies, and vertebral shortening due to increased endplate concavity.[10,41]

ADULT ANATOMY

Correlation of Vertebral Structure and Function

Weightbearing in the Lumbar Spine

The vertebral bodies and intervertebral discs bear over 80 percent of the static compressive load in erect posture.[42] The progressive increase in the surface area of the vertebral end plates from C2 to the lower lumbar spine reflects the progressive increase in loading from above down. According to Davis,[43] vertebral body end surface area is maximal at L4. The end surface of L5 can be smaller because its forward tilt transfers a larger part of its load to the vertebral arches through the very thick pedicles and transverse processes that characterize L5.

Except for the bony rim a few millimeters wide, each vertebral end plate is covered by a plate of hyaline cartilage about 1 mm thick (Figs. 1-14 and 1-15). The outer fibrous annulus is attached to the bony rim, and the inner

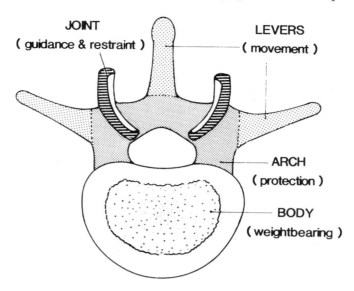

Fig. 1-14   Diagram relating basic structure to principal functions.

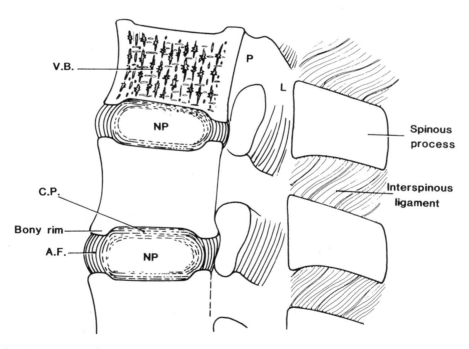

Fig. 1-15   A median sagittal section shows the internal "architecture" of a vertebral body *(VB)* and an intervertebral disc. In the vertebral body, vertical trabeculae form weightbearing beams, which are stiffened by transverse trabecular cross ties to prevent them buckling under load. In the disc, the annulus fibrosus *(AF)* has two parts: the ligamentous outer annulus attaches to the vertebral rims; the fibro-cartilaginous lamellae of the inner annulus are continuous with the lamellar structure of the cartilage plates *(CP)* as revealed by polarized light. The *AF* and *CPs* form an envelope that encloses the nucleus pulposus *(NP)*. *P* = pedicle; *L* = lamina.

fibrocartilaginous annulus is attached to the peripheral parts of the cartilage plate,[19] forming an elliptical envelope for the incompressible "fluid" nucleus pulposus. The average height of adult male lumbar vertebral bodies is about 25 mm and the discs are from 10 to 12 mm thick at their centers. Their average anteroposterior diameter is from 30 to 35 mm. Their transverse dimensions increase from about 40 mm at L1 to about 50 mm at L5. Female vertebral dimensions are on average about 15 percent smaller.[10, 19] The girth of the column is dependent in part on the effect of muscular forces during growth, and the female vertebral column is more slender than the male column.

Each vertebral body is kidney shaped and covered by a thin shell of compact bone. Its internal bony architecture reflects its weightbearing function (see Fig. 1-15). Sagittal section shows the predominantly vertical orientation of its trabeculae, with cross ties particularly numerous near the upper and lower end-plates. The vertical bony trabeculae are quite rigid but can bend slightly when loaded. Unsupported vertical columns would bend beyond their elastic capacity and fracture if they did not have the support of the transverse cross ties, which increase their rigidity. Red hemopoetic marrow fills the honeycombed interstices of this trabecular scaffolding. This composite structure provides both strength and resilience with a small amount of "give" in response to loading, but the main shock absorbers are the intervertebral discs, whose structure and function will be described in detail later.

Protection of Neural Structures

The vertebral arches, formed by the pedicles and laminae, protect the structures in the spinal canal and intervertebral foramina (Fig. 1-16). The arches do not form a continuous column like the discs and vertebral bodies. They form zyagapophyseal joints (Z joints) through their articular processes, but the gaps between the laminae, medial to the Z joints, are bridged by the elastic ligamenta flava. The rounded pedicles project backward from the upper outer margins of a vertebral body, and the flat laminae meet in the midline behind the spinal canal. The pedicles are oval in section with a thick cortex (surgeons use them as points of fixation for screws and plates). The laminae are flat plates of bone that cover the posterior aspect of the spinal canal, containing the conus of the spinal cord and the cauda equina within the dural sac (see Fig. 1-14). In spinal stenosis, parts of the laminae may be removed (laminectomy) to "decompress" the cauda equina. The canal can be entered by a needle inserted in the gap between the adjacent laminae of lower lumbar vertebrae, below the level of the spinal cord. The epidural space is entered first by passing the needle through the ligamentum flavum into the epidural fat. When the needle is passed through the fibrous dura and its membranous inner lining of arachnoid, it enters the subarachnoid space containing the cerebrospinal fluid and the cauda equina (see Figs. 1-16 and 1-17).

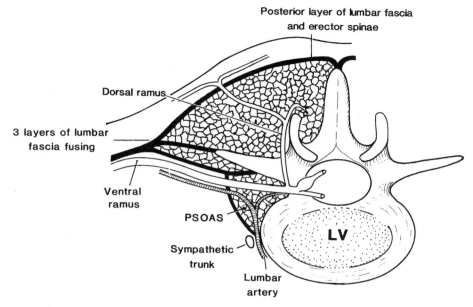

Posterior layer of lumbar fascia
and erector spinae

Dorsal ramus

3 layers of lumbar
fascia fusing

Ventral
ramus

PSOAS

Sympathetic
trunk

Lumbar
artery

LV

Fig. 1-16 Diagram illustrating the three layers of the lumbar fascia, attached to the spinous and transverse processes and enclosing the quadratus lumborum and the erector spinae. The psoas major is enclosed in its own fascial envelope. The formation of a spinal nerve and its division into ventral and dorsal rami is shown. (Modified from Last S: Anatomy: Regional and Applied (2nd ed.). Churchill Livingstone, Edinburgh, 1959.).

Control of Movements: Levers and Joints

Each vertebral arch has a number of processes that act as levers for movement and as guides and restraints for movements (see Fig. 1-14). Each arch has two transverse processes and one spinous process to which muscles and ligaments are attached; they act like levers. Two superior articular processes project upward from the arch, and two inferior articular processes project downward. The articular facets on these processes form zygapophyseal joints, which act as guide rails for movement in flexion, extension, and side bending; the facets resist axial rotary movements and partly restrain flexion and extension.

The transverse processes are mostly long, flat, and "spatulate"; those of L3 are longest, those of L1 shortest, but those of L5 are thick, rounded, and strong. Occasionally the transverse processes of L1 are enlarged with joints, forming lumbar ribs. Their anterior surfaces give attachment to the psoas major and quadratus lumborum (see Fig. 1-16). The tips of the L5 transverse processes are attached to the iliac crests by iliolumbar ligaments, which contribute to the stability of the lumbosacral junction.

On the back of the base of each transverse process is an "accessory tubercle." A small mamillo-accessory ligament bridges over from this tubercle to the adjacent mamillary process of the superior articular process, forming

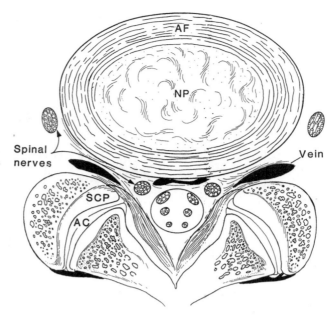

Fig. 1-17   The motion segment has three joints, the disc consisting of the annulus fibrosus *(AF)* and nucleus pulposus *(NP)* and two zygapophyseal joints with concave superior articular facets receiving the convex facets of the vertebra above. The facets are lined by articular cartilages *(AC)* supported by subchondral plates *(SCP)* of compact bone. The anterior capsule is formed by the ligamentum flavum, and the posterior fibrous capsule bridges from the posterior margin of the superior articular process to the posterior surface of the lamina of the vertebra above. The triangular spinal canal contains the cauda equina in the dural sac, and in its lateral corners the spinal nerves are passing down toward the next pair of intervertebral foramina. Those spinal nerves, which passed out of the upper part of the intervertebral foramina, lie close to the lateral surfaces of the disc. There are large veins in the anterior epidural space that connect through the intervertebral foramina with segmental veins.

a tunnel for the descending medial branch of the dorsal ramus. This nerve supplies the inferior part of a zygapophyseal joint and the superior recess of the next zygapophyseal joint.

The lumbar spinous processes are large and hatchet shaped, projecting straight backward from the junction of the right and left laminae at a level 1 cm or more below the corresponding vertebral bodies. The wide gutter-shaped hollow on each side, between the spinous and transverse processes, is filled by the post-spinal muscles, the more superficial and laterally placed longitudinal fibers of erector spinae and the deep, medially placed obliquely oriented multifidus. These are enclosed in a strong "corset-like" envelope formed by the posterior and middle layers of the lumbodorsal fascia, which take attachment from the tips of the spinous and transverse processes (see Fig. 1-17). These muscles cover the backwardly projecting lumbar zygapophyseal joints, the laminae, and the ligamenta flava. All these muscles are extensors, but the deepest fascicles of the lumbar multifidus muscles also play an important role as stabilizers of the zygapophyseal joints. The three layers of the lumbar fascia join together laterally, giving attachment to the transversus and internal oblique muscles, which are also important stabilizers of the lumbar motion segments. Detailed descriptions of all the muscles appear in chapter 4.

The Lumbar Articular Triad: Mobility with Stability

The multisegmental construction of the spine combines strength with stability. The lumbar vertebral column is required to provide stability in loadbearing and a wide range of mobility. Mobility and stability are usually in inverse proportion to each other, but these two contradictory requirements are achieved in the lumbar spine by virtue of its multisegmental construction. Each mobile segment consists of one intervertebral disc and two zygapophyseal joints, with their ligaments, muscles, and nerves. Each intact individual segment has only a limited range of movement and therefore remains stable. However, the five lumbar mobile segments collectively provide large ranges of sagittal and coronal plane movement. True axial rotation is very restricted, but some limited axial rotary movement is provided by coupling of coronal and sagittal plane movements, as the facets are not quite "vertical" but have a slight forward slope of about 8 degrees.

The combination of a strong intervertebral disc with two synovial Z joints forms a lumbar articular triad, with great strength and stability, which at the same time provides adequate mobility. The interdependence of the disc and zygapophyseal joints will become clear as each is described.

The Intervertebral Disc

The disc provides the main strength and stiffness of the motion segment, but its slight compliance and its considerable thickness ensure a useful movement range. It is a structure of unique simplicity in concept, but with a complexity of fine structure in its parts. It is generally described as formed by an annulus fibrosus and a nucleus pulposus, but the cartilage plates are integral parts of the disc, which bind and unite it to the vertebral bodies above and below.[8, 19] The cartilage plates and the inner annulus fibrosus form a continuous envelope enclosing the nucleus pulposus (Fig. 1-18).

Annulus Fibrosus. The annulus fibrosus consists of 12 to 16 concentric lamellae. The annular lamellae are arranged in spiralling sheets around the circumference of the nucleus. The lamellae of the outer part follow an almost straight course from the vertebral rim above to the vertebral rim below. The inner lamellae are curved with an outward convexity passing around the nucleus from one cartilage plate to the other. The parallel fibers of each successive sheet of collagen bundles cross the fibers of the next sheet at an interstriation angle of about 57 degrees.[44] The arrangement is not unlike that of the layering of an onion. This arrangement gives the annulus great strength.

The annulus shows two distinguishable parts, which have different structures and functions. The thin, outer fibrous annulus is like a ligament,

**Sagittal section of lower lumbar disc from
18 year old male subject**

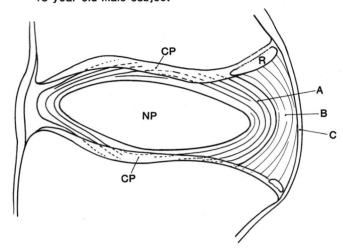

Fig. 1-18 A diagram based on accurate tracing from a sagittal section of a normal 18-year-old lumbar disc showing the parts of the disc, including the large central nucleus pulposus *(NP)* enclosed by the cartilage plates *(CP)* and the annulus fibrosus, which has two parts: **(A)** the fibrocartilaginous inner annulus, which is continuous with the cartilage plates above and below, and **(B)** the ligamentous outer annulus, which attaches to the vertebral rim or, in the immature, to the ring apophysis *(R)*. The longitudinal ligaments cover the anterior and posterior surfaces of the annulus. *C* = anterior longitudinal ligament.

attached to the vertebral rims above and below. Its collagenous fibers are not enclosed in proteoglycan matrix. They are designed to withstand tensile forces, and their ends are firmly embedded in the bony vertebral rims all around their circumferences. The inner fibrocartilaginous annulus is rich in proteoglycans and is continuous with the cartilage plates above and below, forming an envelope for the nucleus. Polarized light studies[8, 19] can trace a direct continuity from the inner fibrocartilaginous lamellae of the annulus into the horizontal lamellae of the "hyaline" cartilage plates above and below the nucleus. This forms an inextensible but deformable annulus–cartilage plates envelope enclosing the nucleus pulposus.

Cartilage Plates. The "hyaline" cartilage plates were developmentally parts of the cartilage model of the vertebral body before it ossified, and are sometimes described as its unossified epiphyses. In growing individuals, there are growth plates at the junction of the bony vertebral body and the cartilage plate that ensure growth in vertebral height. Only the peripheral rims of the cartilage plates ossify, when the ring apophyses appear at puberty and fuse with the centrum at maturity. In adults, each cartilage plate is "cemented" to the end-surface of the vertebral body by a layer of calcified cartilage that is penetrated by a number of vascular buds from the vertebral spongiosa. These do not penetrate far into the cartilage plates, but they are essential to the nutrition of the avascular disc. Injury in young people may cleave the disc from the vertebra along the line of the bone cartilage junction (epiphyseal separation), showing that the cartilage plates are more firmly attached to the disc than to the vertebra.[4,5]

Nucleus Pulposus.   The infant nucleus pulposus is a viscous, fluid structure with a clear, watery matrix.[8,19] Its appearance and consistency change with maturation as many collagen bundles are produced in the nucleus and its water content decreases. As this happens the clear-cut boundary between the nucleus and annulus, characteristic of infancy and childhood, becomes blurred. However, the healthy young adult nucleus still behaves hydrostatically as a proteoglycan-rich, viscous fluid[45] with a high water content, which is incompressible, but it can change shape.[46] By changing shape as the lumbar spine bends, the disc acts as a joint. The nucleus acts as a shock absorber by receiving axial loads and redistributing them centripetally to the surrounding envelope, dissipating the vertical forces in horizontal directions. The enclosure of this proteoglycan-rich nucleus by the annulus and cartilage plates is an important loadbearing mechanism, but the elliptic envelope itself, formed by the inner annulus and cartilage plates, also plays an important role in axial loadbearing. It also has a high proteoglycan content, each collagen fibril being surrounded by a long cylindric collar of proteoglycan with its associated water. The "inflation" of this cylindric collar resists deformation under axial loading, as the effect of the collar is to attempt to straighten the collagen fibrils. The envelope would thus tend to form a sphere rather than an ellipse, resisting axial compressive loads and reinforcing the shock-absorbing and loadbearing functions of the nucleus.[45]

The nucleus is held under tension within the envelope formed by the annulus and cartilage plates. This tension, or turgor, is produced by the chemical force resulting from the water-attracting capacity of the proteoglycan macromolecules acting against the inextensibility of the envelope. These macromolecules make space for, or "imbibe," water. In recumbent posture, at night, the discs imbibe water to the limit of their envelopes' capacity and during the course of each day, axial compression, from erect posture loading, squeezes out water, so that the discs become slightly thinner. On average, adults lose about 17 mm of height during the day and regain it when recumbent at night.[19] At autopsy, discs that are cut open swell quite soon by absorbing water from the atmosphere. At discography, healthy adult discs show an enclosed nucleus where the contrast adopts a "hamburger" shape as seen in lateral projections. Healthy discs actively resist the injection of contrast, while degenerate discs allow the contrast to enter with relatively little resistance. Forcible injection into an intact disc in a fresh autopsy specimen causes the lordotic spine to straighten.

It is clear from the structural description of a fibrocartilaginous envelope formed by annulus and cartilage plates containing a softer, proteoglycan and water-rich nucleus, and from the consistency of this structural arrangement in normal lumbar discs (as opposed to cervical discs, where posterior annular fissuring is an early event), that the nucleus can deform readily as the disc moves but it cannot change its position. In the fetus, during antenatal growth, the nucleus does change position, slowly over a period of weeks and months as a function of differential growth, but once growth is complete the nucleus, as a relatively soft pulpy center, simply changes shape in response to bending and compression forces. However, prolonged application of these forces results in creep, with redistribution of the water component of the disc, as explained under age changes in this chapter and also in Chapter 2.

Nerves and Vessels.   The outer third of the lumbar annulus is innervated, and the nerve fibers usually penetrate about six lamellae deep in the normal annulus.[52] No nerves have been demonstrated in the cartilage plates[47,48] but they may penetrate via age-related or traumatic fissures into the inner parts of a degenerate disc.[49] Discogenic pain usually results from extension of fissuring into the outer innervated part of the annulus[50] or from inflammatory changes in the torn outer annulus. The outer annulus and cartilage plates are vascular in the fetus and infant, where vessels enter all around the disc from the vertebral periosteum and also into the posterolateral part of the disc, but disc vascularity is progressively reduced with maturation, especially in early chidhood.[8,19,45]

Nutrition of the Adult Disc.   Lumbar discs are said to be the largest avascular structures in the adult body. The disc receives nutrition by diffusion from its surfaces. Small vascular buds enter the cartilage plates from the vertebral spongiosa by penetrating the calcified cartilage layer binding the cartilage plate to the bony centrum; a few small blood vessels also persist in the longitudinal ligaments and in the surface layers of the annulus under these ligaments.[8,51] The avascular disc contains a population of chondrocytes and fibroblasts, which become more sparse as one passes from the annulus to the nucleus; the cells in the disc receive their nutrition by diffusion from the few vessels in the outer annulus and from the more numerous vascular buds in the cartilage plates.[53] Buckwalter[54] suggests that decreased nutrition with aging is a major factor in disc degeneration. It is also suggested that cigarette smoking decreases disc nutrition, whereas regular motion can improve disc nutrition.[55,56]

Zygapophyseal (Facet) Joints

These paired, synovial joints are the principal guiding and restraining mechanism of the mobile segment. The disc is very strong, but without the zygapophyseal joints it would suffer damage from repeated shearing and axial rotary strains. The zygapophyseal joints are essential to protect the lumbar discs from these rotational and translational strains, which would overstretch or shear the annular collagen fibers so that the mobile segment would become unstable. The zygapophyseal joints permit movement to occur in the sagittal and coronal planes, but they restrain axial rotation, and as the other movements, especially flexion, approach end range, they bring these movements to a halt.[23,57,58] They also widen the axial loadbearing base. In normal, erect posture they bear 15 to 20 percent of axial loading.[42] This load-bearing function is small in erect posture but larger in the extended spine and also in the flexed spine, particularly when the flexed spine is loaded, as when lifting weights from ground level. The zygapophyseal joints can be sources of back pain when their fibrous capsules or synovial folds are injured or irritated. Their articular cartilages have no nerve supply, so the joints surfaces cannot be sources of pain in a healthy joint. However, the subchondral bone is innervated, so that in advanced osteoarthritis, when the cartilage is worn away and bone bears on bone, the bony surfaces may be pain sources.

Joint Anatomy

Articular Facets. The articular surfaces of the zygapophyseal joints[7,37] are formed between the medially facing superior articular processes (SAP) and the laterally facing inferior articular processes (IAP) of the vertebra above (Fig. 1-19). They are described as having plane or flat articular surfaces, but as a rule, only the lumbosacral facets have flat articular surfaces. The superior articular facets at other levels are usually concave as seen in transverse section in the horizontal plane, as in CT scans (Fig. 1-20). The concave SAP encloses the smaller convex IAP. In the vertical plane both facets are flat and both articular surfaces are oriented, approximately parallel to the long axis of the spine, though they show a slight forward slope of about 8° (or slightly more at L5-S1).

Facet Orientation and Function. From the functional point of view, one may consider the facets as biplanar in the horizontal plane (see Fig. 1-19). The anterior third of a superior articular process is oriented close to the coronal plane and this may be called its coronal component. This part limits forward translation of the upper vertebra in flexion and helps to control flexion. The posterior third is oriented close to the sagittal plane and may be regarded as the sagittal component; it restrains axial rotation (see Fig. 1-19). The articular surfaces of the superior articular process may be curved in a regular concavity, or the two parts may meet at a rounded angle, the joint resembling a boomerang in transverse section. The five lumbar zygapophyseal joints show a progressive change in orientation from L1 down to L5: the sagittal component is largest in Ll–2 and the coronal component is largest in L5-SI. The angle each joint makes with the midline increases from above down, the largest change being between L3–4 and L4–5. The more coronal orientation at the lower two levels reflects their function in protecting the discs from shearing forces in the more lordotic lower lumbar spine (Fig. 1-21). The sagittal component of the joints appears designed to block axial rotation around the usual midline axis of rotation near the posterior surface of the intervertebral disc, but some coupled axial twisting is possible, as measurement studies in whole lumbar columns in vitro and in vivo show.[61] This twisting movement is severely limited when individual mobile segments are tested in rigid experimental conditions that only permit true

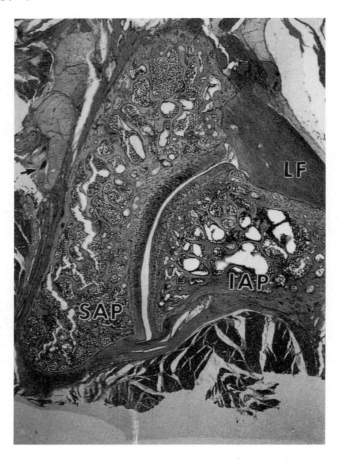

Fig. 1-19   A stained 100 micron transverse section of an L3–4 zygapophyseal joint from a young adult (compare with Fig. 1-29, *A*). The convex articular surface of the inferior articular process *(IAP)* fits neatly into the concave articular surface of the superior articular process *(SAP)*. The articular cartilages, containing plentiful chondrocytes, are supported by subchondral bone plates where the bone is more dense than in the underlying cancellous bone, which contains bone marrow. The joint is enclosed in front by the thick ligamentum flavum *(LF)* and behind by a thin fibrous capsule, which is covered by fibers of multifidus. A small arrow lateral to the SAP indicated the medial branch of the dorsal ramus of the spinal nerve. (From Taylor and Twomey, Reprinted with permission from Boyling and Palastanga: Grieves Modern Manual Therapy (2nd ed.). Churchill Livingstone, New York, 1994, p. 101.)

axial rotation, but when torque is applied to the whole, unrestrained lumbar spine, there is a coupled sagittal and coronal plane movement that mimics axial rotation. Nevertheless, axial rotation is mainly a movement of the thoracic spine and not of the lumbar spine.

The function of the coronal components of the joints in limiting flexion is less well known. Posterior-release studies show that loading of the zygapophyseal facets, by the forward translational force that accompanies flexion, is the single most important restraint to flexion at end-range, more important than tension in the posterior ligaments in bringing flexion to a

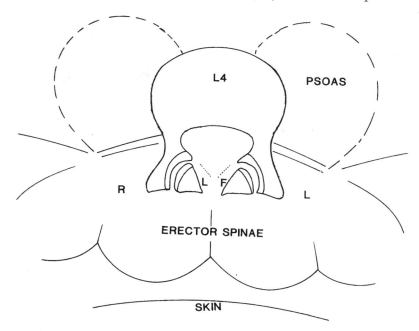

Fig. 1-20   This tracing from a CT scan shows soft-tissue outlines of psoas, lateral, and medial parts of erector spinae, and the outlines of the L3–4 zygapophyseal joints. The "joint space" (articular cartilage) and the compact bone of the subchondral bone plate with its coronal and sagittal components are distinguished. *LF* = ligamentum flavum.

halt.[37,57] The chondrocyte swelling and chondromalacia that selectively occur in the coronal components of the joints in young adults indicate that these parts are subject to greater compressive loads than the sagittal components.[7]

Joint Capsule and Synovium.   Each joint is enclosed by a fibrous capsule posteriorly, and the elastic ligamentum flavum forms its anteromedial capsule (see Fig. 1-19). The posterior capsule is frequently directly continuous with the posterior margin of the articular cartilage lining the superior articular facet. This capsular attachment gives the appearance of extending the concave socket for the convex inferior facet. The anterior capsule, being elastic, is tight in all joint positions. The slightly oblique posterior capsule is tight in extension, but in flexion it is relatively slack and depends on the deep fascicles of multifidus for "tensioning" (Figs. 1-19 and 1-22). The fibrous capsule is quite loose above and below at the superior and inferior or "polar" joint recesses.[7,37,63] A neurovascular bundle supplies each joint recess and large, vascular, synovial folds extend from the polar recesses into the joint, projecting for a short distance between the upper and lower articular surfaces. In healthy, young joints, these vascular fat-pads adapt easily to the changing shape of the joint as it moves.[64] With aging or after injury, the synovial folds become more fibrous and rigid at their tips, and the vascular, fat-filled folds are less able to adapt their shape to different joint positions.[64] The vascular folds may be caught between the joint surfaces in very rapid

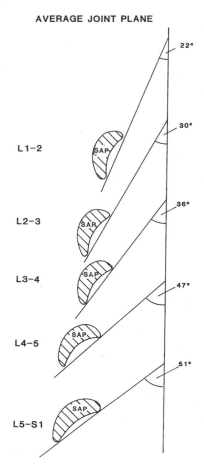

AVERAGE JOINT PLANE

22°

L1-2

30°

L2-3

36°

L3-4

47°

L4-5

51°

L5-S1

Fig. 1-21   The segmental variation in the orientation of lumbar zygapophyseal joint planes is shown based on measurement of joint angles in over 200 CT scans. The average joint angles of the superior articular processes *(SAP)* with the mid-sagittal plane are shown. It should be noted that there is a good deal of variation in shape and orientation between individuals. The upper two joints tend to be sagittally oriented, while lowest two joints are generally more coronally oriented.

movements and they are readily bruised in spinal injuries. Small fibrofatty synovial fringes also extend around the posterior margin of each joint as space fillers, from a base on the posterior fibrous capsule to an apex projecting between the rounded articular margins. The fat pads in the inferior recesses of the lower lumbar joints are particularly large.[63] They have been shown to be innervated by small nerves,[65] some of which contain substance P and probably are nociceptive nerves.[66]

The inferior recess fat pads are largely extracapsular and occupy small hollows in the laminae below the joints, but each communicates with the intra-articular vascular synovial fold through a hole in the inferior capsule. The fluid fat flows freely in and out of the intra-articular synovial fold during upward and downward gliding movements of the joint.

Deep Muscle Attachments.   There are small vertical ridges or tubercles on the posterior edge of each SAP, close to their posterior articular margins. These are the mamillary tubercles. The deep lumbar fascicles of multifidus are attached to them. A deep lumbar fascicle of multifidus descends obliquely from the lamina at the base of a spinous process, two segments above, to the lateral margin of each joint (see Fig. 1-22). It uses this

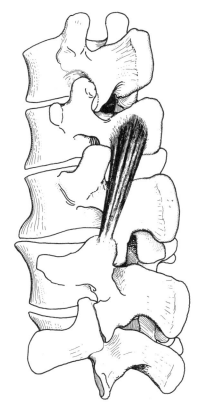

Fig. 1-22   Based on dissection studies, a single fascicle of the lumbar multifidus is shown descending obliquely from the spinous process of L2 to the mamillary tubercle on the superior articular process of L4, with some capsular insertion at the superior part of the L3–4 joint. This is one deep unit of a larger, more complex muscle. The obliquity of this deep fascicle would allow it to extend the joints and also to exert a small rotary force at the two mobile segments it crosses. Its principal function is probably as a stabilizer at the L3–4 zygapophyseal joint. This view contrasts with most textbook descriptions.[7,67] (From Taylor and Twomey[7] with permission.)

attachment to control joint posture and maintain close apposition between the posterior zygapophyseal joint surfaces.[7,67] This action is somewhat analogous to the rotator-cuff function at the shoulder joint. Like the rotator-cuff muscles, multifidus is also partly inserted into the joint capsule. Observations on transverse sections of postmortem lumbar zygapophyseal joints suggest that multifidus helps to maintain joint congruity, because without muscle activity, the posterior capsule appears to be slack and the posterior joint surfaces separate slightly when the muscle is removed.[67,23,7] Appearances on computed tomography (CT) scans of some chronic low back pain patients and patients with segmental instability suggest atrophy or fatty replacement of these deep muscles.

Articular Cartilage.   The smooth zygapophyseal joint articular cartilages covering each surface are about 1 mm thick. These smooth surfaces, bathed in the viscous synovial fluid, provide almost friction-free gliding movements. Zygapophyseal articular cartilage, like all articular cartilage, is avascular and has no nerve supply, so that it is insensitive, though the subchondral bone contains nerves. The well-innervated posterior joint capsule is partly attached to the posterior margin of the articular cartilage as well as to the adjoining bone. Articular cartilage receives its nutrition from the synovial fluid that bathes it, circulation of the fluid being aided by movements of the joint. From the fourth decade onward, changes in the staining characteristics of the articular cartilage of the coronal component of the joint include hypertrophy of chondrocytes with intense staining of the surrounding matrix, especially in the mid zone. This suggests a response to high compressive loading in these parts of the joints.[7,37] These cellular changes progress to splitting of the cartilage in the coronal component of the superior articular process, along lines parallel to the collagen framework (see Fig. 1-29, *B* and *C*). This is characteristic of chondromalacia.

Lumbosacral Joints

The unique configuration of the human lumbosacral angle imposes unique biomechanical loading conditions, which may result in failure of the components that support the high loads in this area. The anterior surface of the sacrum is normally inclined at an angle of about 60 degrees to the vertical plane, giving a sharp change in direction at the lumbosacral angle. This angulation involves a division of vertical weight-bearing loads through the lumbar spine into two vectors, a major vector (65 percent) downward and backward through the sacrum, and a lesser vector (35 percent) downward and forward, parallel to the upper surface of Sl. The anteriorly directed vector exerts a shearing force on the lumbosacral joints.[43] This shearing force is resisted by (1) the two lumbosacral zygapophyseal joints; (2) the lumbosacral intervertebral disc; and (3) the iliolumbar ligaments. The lumbosacral facets, as the most rigid structures, bear most of the shearing stress.

This loading is transmitted upward from the inferior articular process of L5, through the pars interarticularis of L5, a narrow isthmus of bone between its superior and inferior articular facets. This bridge of bone is the weakest link in the chain and is the part most likely to fail under repetitive loading.[68] A fracture of the pars interarticularis is termed *spondylolysis*. Deprived of this bony support, the shearing force is now supported by the iliolumbar ligaments and the lumbosacral disc. These may be stretched and deformed so that the L5 vertebral body may separate from its arch and slip forward on S1 (olisthesis), with fissuring in the tissues of the disc. This anterior slip is termed *spondylolisthesis*. Spondylolysis, mostly at L5, is seen frequently in sports involving sudden loading of the lumbosacral joints in extension, or in repetitive lumbosacral flexion and extension.[69] There may be a developmental component in its etiology, e.g., a developmentally narrow isthmus in the pars interarticularis, but the condition is not congenital because it is not found in fetuses and infants; it may be seen from childhood and adolescence onward. It may then be asymptomatic but it is a painful condition when it occurs as a stress fracture in athletes. A previously asymptomatic spondylolysis may become symptomatic after injury. Where it has been present for some months or years in athletes, it may be asymptomatic at rest but become painful when stressed by repetitive physical activity.[70]

Spondylolisthesis is more likely to follow spondylolysis in young people with compliant discs and less likely in old people with stiff discs, but there is no hard-and-fast rule linking age to slip. Spondylolysis is not the only possible result of the particular stresses at the lumbosacral joints and in the lower lumbar spine. Degenerative changes in the lumbosacral articular triad and in the L4–5 articular triad are also common. Internal disc disruption and intervertebral disc rupture with nuclear extrusion are most common in the lowest two intervertebral discs.[71] Zygapophyseal joint arthritis is also most common in the lower lumbar and lumbosacral joints.[72] Wear-and-tear changes, with remodeling of the lumbosacral facets, may render them incompetent, and accompanying degeneration in the lumbosacral disc may result in a degenerative form of spondylolisthesis.

Internal disc disruption, with extension of fissures into the outer third of the annulus, is a far more common cause of discogenic pain than nuclear herniation.[50,73] When there are injuries or degenerative changes that weaken the motion segment to the point of segmental instability, it may manifest as a retrolisthesis of L4 on L5[74] (see chapter 7).

Spinal Ligaments

The anterior and posterior longitudinal ligaments form long ribbonlike ligaments that line the anterior and posterior surfaces of the vertebral bodies and intervertebral discs of the whole vertebral column. Their fibers are longer than those of the annulus and cross several segments. They form contrasting shapes: the broad ribbon of the anterior longitudinal ligament has parallel margins, and the posterior longitudinal ligament is dentate in outline, widest at the discs and narrowest at the middle of each vertebral body. The anterior ligament interchanges fibers with the anterior vertebral periosteum and the anterior annulus of each disc, but the posterior ligament is only attached at the discs. Its narrow part bridges over a concavity behind each vertebral body, which contains the anterior epidural veins where they drain the basivertebral veins from each vertebral body. These relatively thin longitudinal ligaments are, nevertheless, important structures as many of their fibers bridge over several segments, giving them a greater capacity for stretch than the annulus fibrosus. The posterior ligament may form the last line of defense against herniation of an intervertebral disc into the spinal canal.

The laminae are joined together by the ligamenta flava, which pass from the upper margin of the lamina below to the inner margin of the lamina above. They also extend laterally to form the anterior capsules of the zygapophyseal joints. The spinous processes are connected by oblique interspinous and supraspinous ligaments (see Fig. 1-15). The intertransverse ligaments are parts of the middle layer of the lumbar fascia.

Ligamenta Flava

These yellow, elastic ligaments are thickest in the lumbar region, where they are 2 to 3 mm thick. Medial to the zygapophyseal joints their elastic fibers pass vertically between adjacent laminae; with the laminae they form the posterior boundary of the spinal canal. There may be a narrow midline cleft between the right and left halves of each ligamentum flavum. Their lateral fibers spread over the anterior aspect of each zygapophyseal joint. These lateral fibers are directed obliquely upward and laterally to form the anterior capsules of the joints. The elasticity of the ligamenta flava maintains the smooth regular contour of the spinal canal in all postures of the spine, and they add strength to the anterior parts of the zygapophyseal joints by holding the articular surfaces together. They are stretched by flexion and thicken without buckling during extension in the healthy spine. If an intervertebral disc loses its normal thickness or a vertebral body loses height with aging, the more fibrous ligamentum flavum of the older person may thicken and bulge into the canal.[75,76] This bulging or buckling would narrow the spinal canal, particularly in extended posture. Apparent thickening of the ligamentum flavum may be due to underlying bony hypertrophy in the zygapophyseal joints. The ligamenta flava help to resist spinal flexion, but their restraint to excessive flexion is less than the restraining force due to the buildup of pressure between the zygapophyseal articular facets.[57]

Supraspinous and Interspinous Ligaments

The supraspinous ligaments and most of the interspinous ligaments are fibrous or collagenous structures, reinforced by the most medial fibers of the erector spinae and by the interspinales. They extend down to L5 but not below L5, except as fibrous muscle insertions. The fibers of each interspinous ligament run upward and backward from one spinous process to the next one (see Fig. 1-15), as a double layer with a narrow interval between them.[77] Anteriorly they are continuous with the ligamentum flavum on each side. These ligaments also appear designed to limit flexion,[77] but posterior release experiments[57] suggest that their role is less than that of other posterior element structures.

The Spinal Canal and Its Contents

The Spinal Cord, Cauda Equina, and Meninges

The lumbar spine doubles as a mobile supporting structure and as a conduit for the lower end of the spinal cord and the cauda equina. The lower part of the spinal cord is a vital part of the central nervous system containing control centers for reflex activity in the lower limbs, bladder, bowel, and reproductive organs. It is also a relay for motor and sensory communication between the brain and the lower parts of the body. The lumbar enlargement of the cord lies in the thoracolumbar region of the spinal canal and it tapers to a point (the conus), which generally terminates at the level of the L1–2 disc. Very occasionally, it ends higher or lower in the range between T12 and L3; in spina bifida, an abnormal cord may terminate lower than normally if it is tethered to the meninges. The cauda equina are the motor and sensory roots of the lumbar and sacral spinal nerves, which supply the lower limbs, bladder and bowel, and other pelvic and perineal structures. The spinal cord and cauda equina are contained within the dural sac, which is lined on its inner aspect by the arachnoid membrane; the cord and cauda equina are bathed

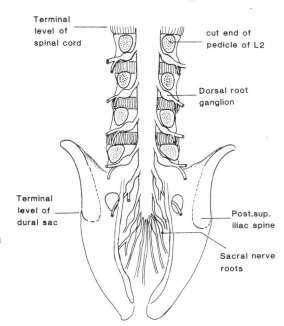

Fig. 1-23 A dorsal view of the lumbosacral spine, from which the vertebral arches have been removed, reveals the dural sac in the spinal canal. The dural sac contains the cauda equina bathed in cerebrospinal fluid. The spinal nerves emerge laterally, where a sheath of dura mater forms the outer fibrous covering of each nerve.

in cerebrospinal fluid within the subarachnoid space. The dural sac and the subarachnoid space terminate at the S2 level, marked by the posterior superior iliac spines (Fig. 1-23). Above this level, there is an angled hollow at the lumbosacral junction, and the lumbar spinous processes above this can be readily palpated.

The nerve rootlets that form the spinal nerves arise in bilateral, parallel, continuous lines along the front and back of the spinal cord. Sets of anterior or posterior rootlets converge to form single anterior and posterior roots, which in turn unite to form a spinal nerve. The thicker, posterior sensory roots contain about three times as many axons as the anterior roots. The anterior roots transmit the somatic motor fibers from the anterior horn cells (lower motor neurons), and sympathetic preganglionic fibers from the lateral horn of grey matter in the spinal cord, to the sympathetic ganglia. The dorsal roots transmit a variety of sensory fibers. Those parts of the nerves within the dural sac do not have strong connective tissue coverings; they receive these fibrous coverings as they pierce the dura to enter the intervertebral foramina. Therefore the central rootlets are not so strong as the peripheral spinal nerves. The cerebrospinal fluid that bathes the roots supplies some nutrition to the nervous tissue of the cord and provides some protection from mechanical forces. Where the nerve roots pierce the arachnoid and the dura they are surrounded by a short, funnel-shaped sleeve of the arachnoid, which extends into the medial end of the foramen. This "root sleeve" contains cerebrospinal fluid and can be outlined in a myelogram. The sleeves of arachnoid end in the intervertebral foramina, at the dorsal root ganglia, but the dura continues as a connective tissue sleeve along each spinal nerve, forming its epineurium. Peripheral nerves are strong and resistant to stretching forces, as a high proportion of each nerve is connective tissue; each axon has a thin, tube-like connective tissue sheath; bundles of axons are enclosed in a fibrous perineurium, and the surface epineurium of the spinal nerve is also fibrous. The nerves contain many small vessels and can become red, swollen, and edematous when "irritated" by noxious mechanical or chemical stimuli. Within the foramen, or in the lateral recess of the spinal canal, each dorsal nerve root forms a fusiform swelling—the dorsal root ganglion. This contains the cell bodies of all sensory neurons, both somatic and visceral, whether they be from skin, muscle, bone, viscera, blood vessels, or the dura itself. The dorsal root ganglia are very vascular structures and they are also sensitive to painful stimuli, as they have their own nerve supply. They are vulnerable to stretch injuries.[78]

The dimensions and shape of the spinal canal vary according to spinal level and age.[79] At L1, the canal is usually oval in transverse section; at this level, the average sagittal diameter of the bony canal is 20 mm and the average coronal (interpedicular) diameter is 25 mm. Below L1 the canal changes to a triangular outline. It becomes trefoil in shape in older people, especially at lower lumbar levels,[80,81] due to facet hypertrophy and osteophytosis. At the same time as these age changes in the facets, there is likely to be some age-related shortening of the osteoligamentous column. These common changes, together with posterior disc protrusions, and anterior buckling of the ligamentum flavum, collectively or individually reduce the space for the nerve roots and may produce clinical spinal stenosis, with nerve root impingement or even compression. In young adults, nucleus pulposus tissue is soft enough to be extruded from a ruptured disc, when it may impinge upon and deform the subarachnoid space. This would be visible on a myelogram as a "filling defect." Escaping disc material is irritant to spinal nerves and can cause a "chemical radiculitis."

Vessels in the Epidural Space

The dural sac, containing the cauda equina, is circular in cross section and occupies the central part of the triangular spinal canal. The lateral and posterior angles of the epidural space contain fat, and the lateral angles of the triangular bony space transmit the spinal nerves as they descend obliquely to their foramina. This space can be accessed by a needle passed through the gaps between the lower lumbar laminae or via the sacral hiatus. The epidural space, particularly its anterior part, contains a rich plexus of valveless veins. This internal vertebral venous plexus has widespread connections. Two wide longitudinal venous sinuses ascend and descend on the posterior surfaces of the vertebral bodies and discs, one on each side of the anterior epidural space; these large longitudinal venous channels receive two or three veins through each intervertebral foramen, and each longitudinal vein has a centrally directed cross-connection to the midline, basivertebral vein of each vertebral body. This arrangement forms a ladder pattern of veins within the anterior epidural space. The veins are thin-walled and they vary enormously in their degree of dilation, according to the pressures in the abdominopelvic cavity and the autonomic reflex activity in the nerves that innervate them. They receive veins from pelvic venous plexuses and connections from segmental sacral and lumbar veins; at the upper end of the spinal canal the longitudinal veins are continuous with intracranial venous sinuses and they anastomose with vertebral and other cervical veins in the suboccipital region. Blood can flow in any direction in the venous plexus, according to the regional differences in pressure, affected by respiration, coughing, and straining and the blood can flow in or out of basivertebral veins at any level. If a vena cava is blocked, the epidural plexus can form a bypass route for the venous return to the heart. Cancer cells may spread by it from a primary tumor, e.g., in the breast or prostate, to the vertebral spongiosa, giving vertebral metastases, with the possibility of pathologic fracture.

Small arteries enter the spinal canal from each intervertebral foramen to supply the vertebrae, meninges, and cauda equina. These segmental arteries are mostly very small, but each divides into three branches[83]: one supplies the vertebral body, one follows the nerve roots (radicular branch) to supply neural structures, and one branch supplies the posterior elements. Like the veins they form a ladder pattern of anastomosis with their neighboring vessels in the anterior epidural space. The radicular branches supply the nerve roots and follow them through the dura and arachnoid into the subarachnoid space. One of the lower thoracic or upper lumbar radicular arteries is very important because it supplies the lower thoracic and lumbosacral parts of the spinal cord. This "great spinal artery" of Adamkiewitz usually arises from about T10 level, most often on the left, and it anastomoses with the anterior and posterior spinal arteries of the spinal cord.[83,84] It may be at risk in operations on aortic aneurysms, as its origin is variable. If it is inadvertently damaged, this may cause paraplegia due to severe cord ischemia.

Intervertebral Foramina. The intervertebral foramina are regularly spaced lateral openings from the spinal canal. Each lies between the pedicles above and below, a vertebral body and intervertebral disc in front, and a zygapophyseal joint, covered by the ligamentum flavum, behind. The average adult foramen is oval and measures 15 mm in height and 8.5 mm in its widest anteroposterior extent, except at L5-S1, which is more rounded and averages 12 mm from front to back and 13 mm in height. The space is widest above where it contains the nerve; the lower part is relatively narrow and is occupied by veins, which may be separated from the upper part of the foramen by a small transforaminal ligament. In addition to a spinal nerve, each lumbar foramen transmits a small branch of a segmental artery, two or more quite large veins, and a small recurrent branch of the spinal nerve called a sinuvertebral nerve. The sinuvertebral nerves supply the anterior and lateral dura and posterior longitudinal ligament and participate in the supply of the outer lamellae of the posterior annulus fibrosus. In the sacrum there are anterior and posterior foramina that separately transmit the ventral and dorsal rami of the sacral nerves. The anterior sacral foramina also transmit small lateral sacral arteries and veins.

The lumbar foramina are short canals that range in length from 9 mm at L1–2 to 2 cm at L5-S1,[79] in proportion to the thickness of the pedicles above and below them. Each nerve root canal receives the spinal nerve roots in their dural sheath, in the lateral recess of the spinal canal, and passes obliquely downward and laterally below the pedicle into the upper part of the intervertebral foramen. In the medial part of the foramen, the anterior root and the posterior root (with its ganglion) unite to form a mixed spinal nerve, and the sleeve of dura becomes continuous with the epineurium of the spinal nerve.[85] This nerve, containing motor, sensory, and sympathetic fibers, passes out through the wide upper part of the foramen, behind the lower part of the vertebral body, and above the level of the intervertebral disc. As it exits from the foramen, it immediately divides into ventral and dorsal rami. The lumbar ventral rami form a plexus in the psoas muscle and participate with sacral ventral rami in the lumbosacral plexus, forming femoral, obturator, gluteal, and sciatic nerves to supply lower limb structures. The ventral rami of Sl-3 groove the anterior aspect of the sacrum as they pass laterally from their anterior foramina to join the lumbosacral trunk (L4–5), which descends over the ala of the sacrum. These nerves are stretched fairly taut over the ala and anterior surface of the sacrum as they form the sciatic nerve, which passes out of the pelvis through the greater sciatic notch, above piriformis, then down behind the hip joint. When L4, L5, or S1 is entrapped, combined hip flexion and knee extension stretches the sciatic nerve and pulls on the entrapped nerve and its dural sheath, eliciting pain and reflex muscle spasm. The slump test is a more general test for dural irritation, depending on the same biomechanical principles.

Each dorsal ramus divides into medial and lateral branches; the lateral branch supplies segmental spinal muscles and becomes cutaneous, supplying the skin of the low back and gluteal region; the medial branch winds around the articular pillar of the superior articular process and supplies two zygapophyseal joints.

The intervertebral foramen may be reduced in size by the same age-related and pathological processes that affect the spinal canal. These include motion segment instability, with retrolisthesis of the upper vertebra,[12] disc thinning or vertebral endplate collapse, lordotic posture, and osteophytosis of the zygapophyseal joint. The combination of Z joint osteophytes and reduction in height of the intervertebral foramen are the changes most likely to put the spinal nerve at risk of entrapment (Fig. 1-24). A prolapsed or her-

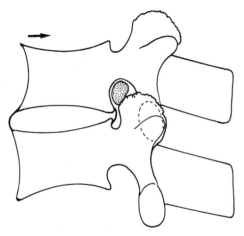

Fig. 1-24 Diagram of a lower lumbar intervertebral foramen, illustrating the narrowing of the foramen that may result from a combination of shortening of the column (from osteoporotic bowing of the endplates or thinning of the disc) and retrolisthesis of the upper vertebra associated with disc degeneration and instability.

niated disc is unlikely to affect the nerve in the foramen unless it migrates upward, as the nerve lies above the level of the disc in the foramen. Disc herniation is more likely to affect the nerve in the lateral recess of the spinal canal as it is descending to the next intervertebral foramen.

Muscles and Fasciae

The lumbar postvertebral muscle masses (erector spinae and multifidus) are larger than the space between the spinous and transverse processes. Thus the tips of the spinous processes are palpated in a longitudinal midline groove between the two muscle masses while the tips of the transverse processes lie deep to the lateral parts of the muscles. The middle layer of the lumbar fascia passes laterally from the tips of the transverse processes, separating quadratus lumborum from erector spinae, and the posterior layer of the lumbar fascia extends laterally from the tips of the spinous processes, the two layers enclosing the erector spinae and multifidus muscles (see Fig. 1-16). This posterior fascia is a strong bilaminar layer with different fiber orientations in the two sheets.[62] The term *erector spinae* is reserved for the superficial, longitudinally running muscle fibers that span many segments. The erector spinae forms a compact mass in the lumbar region and splits as it passes upward into three columns, the spinalis, longissimus, and iliocostalis. Multifidus lies deep and medial to erector spinae. The deeper fascicles of multifidus run in an oblique direction and only span two or three segments. The deeply placed zygapophyseal joints are covered by the deepest fascicles of multifidus (see Fig. 1-19), which may play an important role in stabilizing the zygapophyseal joints.[26,37] The quatratus lumborum is enclosed by the middle and anterior layers of the lumbar fascia and the psoas major has its own fascial sheath. The important roles of the abdominal muscles are discussed in other chapters.

Sacrum and Sacroiliac Joints

The central part of the bony sacrum is formed by the fusion of five centra, but the adult sacrum still contains remnants of intervertebral discs within the bone. The transverse elements fuse to form the alae and lateral masses. The adult sacrum is triangular with its broad base directed upward and forward and its apex directed downward and backward, joined to the coccyx below. Its anterior surface is smooth, with four pairs of anterior sacral foramina lateral to the transverse ridges marking the sites of developmental fusion between the five fused bodies (Fig. 1-25). The posterior surface is roughened by a midline spinous crest, two lateral articular crests, and markings for muscle and ligament attachments. The paired posterior sacral foramina lie between the central and lateral crests. Inferiorly, above the sacrococcygeal joint the posterior wall of the spinal canal is deficient in an inverted **V** shape called the sacral hiatus. This leads into the lower end of the spinal canal, which is filled by fat, plentiful veins and the dural sac, which ends at the S2 level.

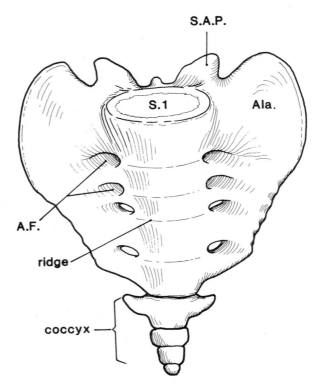

Fig. 1-25 Anterior and superior surfaces of a female sacrum. The superior articular process *(SAP)* of Sl and the anterior sacral foramina *(AF)*, which transmit the ventral rami of sacral spinal nerves, are designated. The ridges mark the positions of fusion between the five centra forming the central part of the sacrum. The ala, or upper end of the sacral lateral mass, is crossed by the lumbosacral trunk (L4,5) as it descends to form the sciatic nerve with Sl, S2, and S3.

On each lateral sacral surface, smooth articular and rough ligamentous areas can be distinguished. The smooth articular area lies in front of the rough ligamentous area. The very strong, posterior and interosseous sacroiliac ligaments suspend the sacrum between the two hip bones (see Fig 1.27). These ligaments join the rough areas on the lateral sacrum to the inner, posterior parts of the iliac crests. The sacroiliac articular surfaces are auricular in shape, each with two "limbs," a short limb directed upward and a longer, lower limb directed backward. The cartilage-covered, articular surfaces are smooth and flat in the child, where rotary movement in the sagittal plane is possible. They become irregular in the mature adult due to the growth of reciprocal ridges and hollows on the opposed surfaces, so that in adults, movements are restricted to a small amount of nutation. The joint is protected behind by its ligaments but it is possible to enter the joint from below, using x-ray control, with a needle directed upward from the upper posterior margin of the greater sciatic notch.

The superior surface of the S1 vertebral body of the sacrum bears the weight of the head, trunk, and upper limbs, transmitted through the lumbar vertebral column. This axial force would tend to rotate the sacrum forward,

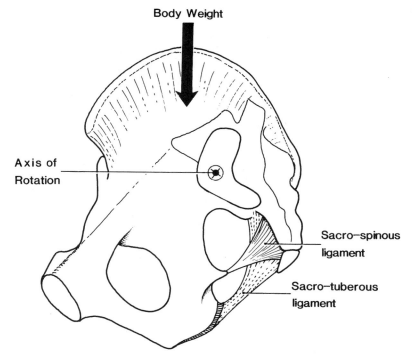

Body Weight

Axis of Rotation

Sacro-spinous ligament

Sacro-tuberous ligament

Fig. 1-26 Diagram illustrating how body weight, acting through the lumbosacral joint, would tend to rotate the sacrum forward if its lower end were not "anchored" by the sacrospinous and sacrotuberous ligaments, which resist the anterior rotational effect of body weight.

but this tendency is resisted by the sacrotuberous and sacrospinous accessory ligaments (Figs. 1-26 and 1-27), which bind the lower parts of the sacrum and coccyx down to the ischial tuberosities and ischial spines. These accessory ligaments assist the posterior sacroiliac ligaments to hold the reciprocal irregularities of the adult articular surfaces close together and resist

Fig. 1-27 The sacrum is "suspended" between the two ilia by very strong posterior sacroiliac ligaments. Body weight tends to compress the ilia against the sacrum at the sacroiliac joints.

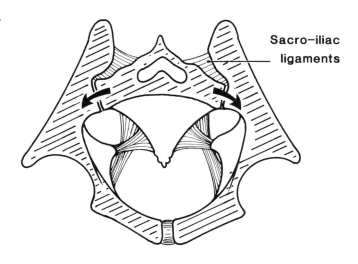

Sacro-iliac ligaments

sacroiliac movements. This makes significant movement almost impossible in most adults.[59,60] In young females, 8 degrees of nutation is said to be possible,[86] and during pregnancy there is a degree of ligamentous laxity, probably due to the effect of hormones on connective tissues.

The sacroiliac joints should not be considered in isolation as they are part of a three-joint complex in the pelvis. A sacroiliac joint cannot rotate without some corresponding movement at the symphysis pubis. Bilateral differences in sacroiliac joint posture are occasionally seen on radiographs of adolescents who have a leg length discrepancy. Pelvic torsion occurs when one sacroiliac joint is rotated more than the other and a "step" is apparent between the right and left pubic bones on the anteroposterior radiograph.[87] The sacroiliac joint is deeply situated, medial and inferior to the posterior iliac spines, and the joint line may be palpated inferior to the posterior superior iliac spine, even though the joint itself is deeply placed.

AGE CHANGES IN THE LUMBAR SPINE

Age Changes in the Anterior Elements

Vertebral Bodies

Measurement studies on a large series of lumbar vertebral columns of all ages[10,11,12,41] demonstrated that the length of the column generally decreased with aging. This was primarily due to loss of vertebral height with gradual, osteoporotic collapse of vertebral end-plates from microfractures in the supporting bony trabeculae. It was not, as a rule, due to loss in disc height. The initial osseous age change is loss of horizontal trabeculae in the vertebral bodies. These horizontal trabeculae form cross ties, stiffening and supporting the vertical trabeculae that are the weightbearing "beams" holding up the vertebral end-plates. The loss of the cross ties allows the unsupported vertical trabeculae, or "beams" of bone, to buckle to the point of fracture (Fig. 1-28).

Measurements in an aging population demonstrated a gradual increase in vertebral end-plate concavity, which appeared earlier in females than in males. In hemisected spines, the increased bowing of the vertebral end-plates was accompanied by "ballooning" of the center of each disc into the adjacent vertebral bodies. The traditional assumption that discs generally get thinner with aging is incorrect. Measurements of average disc thickness and mass in a large series of lumbar spines showed increases in central disc thickness and disc mass in the majority of old lumbar spines.[11]

There were also age changes in the horizontal dimensions of the vertebral bodies, characterized as a "thickening of the waist." These late changes in vertebral shape gradually eliminated the sex differences in vertebral-body shape that were present from adolescence to middle age. The estrogen loss at the female menopause leads to the earlier loss in bone density in aging females. However, osteoporosis with aging is not inevitable. Some loss of bone density is likely but regular exercise, adequate calcium intake, and

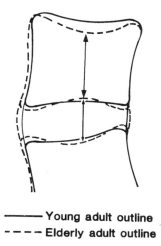

Fig. 1-28 A diagram based on tracings of vertebral bodies and on measurements of vertebral bodies and intervertebral discs shows the changes in their shapes with age. "Ballooning" of the central part of the disc is related to collapse of the vertebral end-plates, and there is some increase in anteroposterior dimension with aging. (From Twomey LT, Taylor JR: Age changes in lumbar intervertebral discs. Acta Orthop Scand 56:496, 1986, with permission.)

————— **Young adult outline**
- - - - **Elderly adult outline**

possibly hormone replacement therapy can reduce or prevent bone loss to the point of symptomatic osteoporosis.[88]

Intervertebral Discs

Contrary to popular belief, aging lumbar discs do not, in the majority of people, become thinner and bulge like underinflated car tires. A minority of the population shows disc thinning and degeneration in one or more lower lumbar discs with aging, but the majority of discs, in a majority of individuals, maintain or even increase their average thickness. Their central expansion in an osteoporotic spine more than counterbalances their tendency to peripheral loss of thickness. When thinning and degeneration are found, they are seen most often in the L4–5 and L5-S1 discs. In subjects over 60 years of age, 30 percent of the L4–5 and L5-S1 discs were classified as degenerate (Rolander grade 3).[10,11] Aging of intervertebral discs is generally associated with a reduction in water content, particularly in the nucleus pulposus, but the greater part of this loss occurs during maturation. The nucleus becomes less well differentiated from the annulus both in its water content and its histologic structure.[8,19] There are increases in the absolute amounts of collagen in the nucleus pulposus and changes in the types of collagen present. There is also an increase in the ratio of keratan sulfate (KS) to chondroitin sulfate (CS) in the disc during childhood growth and maturation, in parallel with some decrease in the water-binding capacity of the disc. The progressive substitution of KS for CS takes place in childhood when growth of the disc is accompanied by a disappearance of its blood vessels. In conditions of oxygen debt, as in a large disc with no blood vessels, KS acts as a functional substitute for CS in maintaining the normal turgor and water content of the disc.[45] The degenerative changes observed in lumbar discs with aging include the appearance of fissures in the annulus, first as circumferential fissures and later as radial fissures. By this stage the nucleus has usually lost some of its fluidity and is firmly bound by collagen, so that it does not prolapse into the fissures. However, if fissures or tears occur in relatively young discs with a high turgor, part of the nucleus may be forced out through the fissure, most often in a posterolateral direction. Disc rupture with extrusion of its nucleus is less frequent than was once supposed. Disc aging is generally accompanied by increased disc stiffness and decreased ranges of movement. Lifetime occupations in heavy manual work and certain sporting activities at an elite level have been shown to increase the likelihood of lumbar disc degeneration, but the increased degeneration is not necessarily associated with increased low back pain. Heavy manual occupations and professional driving are associated with both increased disc degeneration and back disability. On the other hand, while elite weight lifters and soccer players have more disc degeneration than other groups, they suffer less low back pain while they are active in their sports.[89,90,91,92]

Kissing Spines

The shortening of the column associated with osteoporotic collapse of the vertebral end-plates brings the spinous processes closer together and they may come into contact. Histologic studies on four lumbar spines from elderly cadavers showing radiologic evidence of "kissing spines" revealed adventitious joints with a fibrocartilaginous covering on the bone and an interspinous, bursa-like cavity surrounded by fat (Taylor, 1984, unpublished). In the view of Sartoris et al[93] "kissing spines" are attributable to increased lordosis with aging.

Age Changes in Zygapophyseal Joints

Articular Surfaces and Subchondral Bone Plate (SCP)

The geometry of these biplanar joints at different lumbar levels has already been described. Age changes in young and middle-aged adults will be described first.[7,26,37]

Coronal Component (Anteromedial Third of Joint). Compressive loading on the coronal components of the joints, which accompanies forward translation during flexion and loading in the flexed posture, is reflected by changes in the articular cartilage and its supporting SCP. In adolescents and young adults the subchondral bone plate grows thicker in the coronal component of the concave superior articular facet. In middle life, the coronal part of the SCP in the concave facet shows further hypertrophy with intense hematoxylin staining suggestive of sclerosis. In young adults between 30 and 40 years, the articular cartilage lining this thick part of the SCP in the anteromedial third of the joint often shows cell hypertrophy and increased staining of chondrocytes and their pericellular matrix in the articular cartilage of the concave facet. These changes occur in the concave facet first, at the deepest part of its concavity. They occur later in the coronal component of the convex facet. Generally, they do not affect the sagittal component of either facet. In the fourth decade of life the articular cartilage changes often progress to vertical splitting (chondromalacia) of the cartilage[7] (Fig. 1-29, *B*). These bone and cartilage changes are probably reactions to compressive loading, which would occur in flexion, as the convex inferior articular process (IAP) glides upward and presses forward in the concavity of the superior articular process (SAP). The resistance to forward translation of the IAP against the SAP would create compressive loading. Loading of the spine in flexion, due to lifting loads, would also compress the facets together. The changes described are analogous to those of patellofemoral chondromalacia, where the gliding movement is also accompanied by compression of the convex patella against the concave trochlea of the femur.

Sagittal Component (Posterior Two Thirds of Joint). The age changes in the posterior, sagittally oriented two thirds of the zygapophyseal joints are different in character and tend to occur at a later stage than the changes described in the coronal component of the articular facets. The sagittally oriented parts of the SCPs are thin, suggesting less-compressive loading. In middle-aged or elderly adults, a number of joints show partial separation of the articular cartilage from the SCP near the posterior joint margin (Fig. 1-29). This is related to a capsular attachment to the posterior margin of the articular cartilage. We have frequently observed a direct attachment of the posterior fibrous capsule to the posterior margin of the articular cartilage. This was seen most often at the posterior margin of the superior articular facet. The potential for biomechanical derangement is accentuated by the partial insertion of multifidus through the posterior capsule. Frequently repeated tension transmitted to the cartilage from the capsule may shear the articular cartilage from the subchondral bone. Tension in the posterior capsule may be increased in a motion segment that has lost its original mechanical efficiency due to motion segment injury, and parts of the posterior articular cartilage may be detached from their SCP. This has the potential to interfere significantly with normal movements.

Meniscoid Inclusions, Back Pain, and "Locked Back"

In a previous section we described the normal, synovial lined, vascular fat pads, which project up to 3 mm between the articulating surfaces from the polar joint recesses of a normal joint. They are particularly large in the inferior joint recesses of the lowest two lumbar mobile segments.[63,64] Because they are innervated,[66] they are capable of causing back pain if entrapped between articular surfaces. In very sudden movements they may not have time to escape from between the joint surfaces and they may be bruised in traumatic incidents.[9] Much smaller folds from the anterior and posterior capsules fill the small triangular gaps between the rounded joint margins.[82] A survey of 80 adult joints found that there are larger fatty pads in older joints, which show the wear and tear changes of osteoarthrosis, than in young-

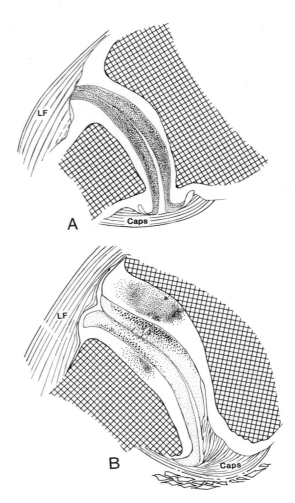

Fig. 1-29 Drawings of midjoint horizontal sections of L3–4 zygapophyseal joints, which were stained by hematoxylin and light green. **(A)** A normal joint from a 20-year-old woman shows smooth articular cartilage with regularly distributed chondrocytes and even staining of the matrix. The subchondral bone plate (white) is slightly thicker anteriorly than posteriorly. The elastic ligamentum flavum *(LF)* forms the anterior capsule, which maintains close apposition of the anterior articular surfaces. In the absence of multifidus, the posterior fibrous capsule *(Caps)* is lax and the posterior part of the joint is open. **(B)** A joint of a 37-year-old man shows chrondrocyte hypertrophy in the articular cartilages of the coronal component. This is most evident in the concave facet of the superior articular process, where two small splits in the articular cartilage are seen. There is further thickening of the SCP in the coronal component. Increased staining of the thickened SCP suggests "sclerosis." The posterior fibrous capsule is covered by fibers of multifidus. Note the continuity of the capsule with the posterior margin of the articular cartilage of the concave facet. Splitting of this cartilage away from the SCP is apparent. *LF* = ligamentum flavum; *Caps* = posterior fibrous capsule.

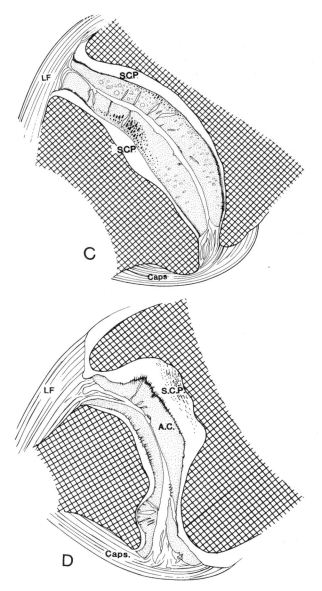

Fig. 1-29 *Continued* **(C)** A joint from a 62 year-old-man showing loss of chondrocytes and loss of staining in the concave facet, with central cell hypertrophy in the convex facet. Fibrillation of both articular cartilages is seen. The SCP has lost thickness compared with the SCP in **(B).** There are developing osteophytes at the posterior joint margin. **(D)** A joint from a 61-year-old-man showing arthritic changes with widespread fibrillation of articular cartilage *(AC)* and infractions with irregularity of the SCP. The coronal component of the SCP appears to have collapsed into the spongy bone of the concave facet.

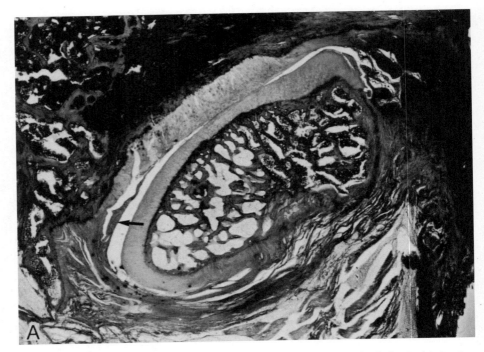

Fig. 1-30 **(A)** The horizontal section from the lower third of a left L3–4 joint in a 37-year-old man shows a joint inclusion, a torn-off portion of the damaged articular cartilage of the concave facet, attached at its base to the posterior fibrous capsule. There is capsule to cartilage continuity around the posterior margin of the facet, with metaplastic articular cartilage formation under the capsule in the form of a "wrap-around bumper" (×4).

adult joints. They appear to act as cushions in the joint recesses, or to extend further between articular surfaces where cartilage loss has occurred (Taylor and Connell, 1983).

In our further study of aging in zygapophyseal joints[7,37] we found instances of fibrocartilaginous inclusions projecting into the posterior aspect of zygapophyseal joints, which appeared to be torn-off portions of articular cartilage that remained attached to the fibrous capsule. Their origin in the articular cartilage is attested by their template-like fit on the underlying damaged cartilage, which is repairing (Fig. 1-30). They may behave like torn menisci in the knee joint, which could be displaced or buckle within the joint. Their entrapment could cause a sharp reduction in the normal range of spinal movement, or "locked back." This may be painful because of traction on the joint capsule and overlying muscle "spasm." The normal action of multifidus in controlling accurate apposition of the joint surfaces may be compromised in some chronic pain states where the muscle atrophies (see chapter 7). If joint congruity is not maintained, there would be an opportunity for the torn portions of cartilage to be displaced, with increased risk of locking. Manipulative techniques would be appropriate in "freeing" such entrapped torn pieces of articular cartilage. On the other hand, forceful lever-

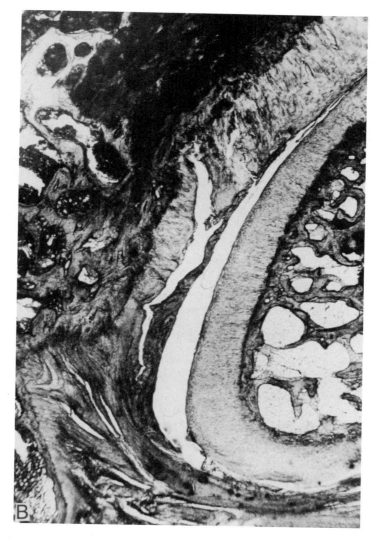

Fig. 1-30 *Continued*   **(B)** A higher power view of the joint inclusion shown in **(A)** shows the template-like fit of the inclusion on the underlying damaged cartilage which shows signs of repair. (**B** from Taylor JR, Twomey LT: Structure, function, and age changes in the lumbar zygaphophyseal joints. Spine 11:739, 1986.)

ing manipulative techniques that "gap" the joints too forcefully might damage joints with capsule-cartilage continuity by "shearing off" articular cartilage.

In comparative anatomic and radiologic studies of "unstable segments," Taylor et al[63,74] showed that loose joints may contain enlarged fat pads that extend from a polar recess down to mid-joint levels. These may represent an attempt to fill the potential space in unstable joints with a loose capsule. Additional changes in the facets of unstable motion segments due to remodeling of subluxed facets were described.

Age Changes in Middle-Aged and Elderly Zygapophyseal Joints

These include changes already described: the chondromalacia and subchondral sclerosis in the coronal components of the facets, and the loosening or "shearing off" of articular cartilage flaps at the posterior joint margins from wear and tear associated with capsule-cartilage continuity. They also include the more general age changes of osteoarthrosis: surface fibrillation and irregularity, thinning or loss of articular cartilage, osteophytic lipping, facet hypertrophy, and sclerotic thickening of the subchondral bone.[37] Subchondral bone cysts are also found. Constant rubbing of enlarged posterior joint margins against a thickened capsule leads to the extension of metaplastic cartilage around the posterior joint margins under the posterior fibrous capsule. These "wrap-around bumpers" are often seen in joint sections and may be recognized on CT scans of the joints.[74]

Measurements of articular cartilage thickness suggest that a slight increase in central thickness may occur in middle age when histologic examination shows chondrocyte hypertrophy with swelling of the matrix. This swelling may disrupt or split the cartilage, perpendicular to the subchondral bone, parallel to the collagen fibers of the mid zone. The underlying subchondral bone plate shows thickening, or infractions, of its anterocentral portion. Measurements of concavity indices of the zygapophyseal joints at L1–2, L3–4 and L4–5, from 70 lumbar spines of all ages, showed increased concavity of the superior articular facets in old age. The concurrent increase in central cartilage thickness may simply represent an attempt to maintain joint congruity. Some osteoporotic joints with very thin SCPs show a marked increase in concavity. Other joints show infractions or local collapse of central parts of the subchondral bone plate. This phenomenon is similar to the osteoporotic collapse of the vertebral body end-plate, which has reduced bony trabecular support.

Spinal Stenosis

This is dealt with in chapter 10, but it is appropriate to comment here on the influence of facet hypertrophy in lateral recess stenosis. Disc and ligamentum flavum bulging and facet hypertrophy may all contribute to narrowing of the lateral recess of the spinal canal (Fig. 1-24) but the change in spinal canal outline from triangle to trefoil is predominantly due to facet and adjacent laminar hypertrophy. Our measurement studies of facet size on over 200 CT scans from patients of all adult ages showed an average 15% increase in superior articular facet size from between the ages of 25 and 60 years.

Relation of Age Changes in Discs and Facet Joints

It is claimed[94] that disc degeneration (as a primary change) leads to secondary zygapophyseal joint degeneration, and clinical observations suggest that facet pain is seen in an older group of patients than those showing disc pain. The coexistence of disc and facet changes in advanced degeneration of the motion segment is often observed but it cannot be assumed that facet changes are always secondary to disc degenerations.[7,95] The facets are vitally important in protecting the discs from damage, and in fulfilling this function they endure repetitive load bearing. In spondylolysis, when the protective influence of the zygapophyseal joint is removed, secondary damage to the intervertebral disc will usually ensue. The anterior, coronally oriented parts of lumbar zygapophyseal joints protect intervertebral discs from translational shearing forces and they bear high loads when they bring flexion to a halt at the end of the physiologic range or when the spine is loaded in a flexed position. The facets also limit the range of extension when the tips of the inferior articular processes abut on the subjacent laminae. The observation of a build-up of sclerotic compact bone in the laminae at the inferior joint recesses in adults of all ages is witness to this effect. The important protective effects of the zygapophyseal joints on the intervertebral discs are largely substantiated by the evidence we have presented.[7,23,37,57] The significantly increased ranges of movement that result from experimental sectioning of pedicles place additional strain on the intervertebral discs. It is apparent from our studies of discs and zygapophyseal joints from the same individuals that in some cases the zygapophyseal joints show more advanced degeneration than is apparent in the intervertebral discs. The mobile segments interact in a mutually dependent way, and it is likely that any defect in one joint of the articular triad would adversely influence the other joints of the triad. Spinal surgeons who perform a laminectomy for spinal stenosis try to preserve as much of the facets as possible to avoid instability.

Common Injuries to the Lumbosacral Spine

Contrasts in Cervical and Lumbar Aging and Injuries

From our experience of sectioning about 300 lumbar spines and over 300 cervical spines from autopsies, a substantial proportion of them from acute injuries, we have observed a wide variety of bone and soft tissue injuries. It is interesting to contrast the injuries in the two regions because their different biomechanical behaviors result in different regional patterns of injury.[4,5,9,69,96]

The 45-degree orientation of cervical facets contrasts with the almost "vertical" orientation of lumbar facets, parallel to the long axis of the spine. Cervical movements, around a center of motion in the vertebral body below, show wider ranges of motion at each segment with a greater degree of translation than in the lumbar spine, where the center of motion is within the disc. Cervical translation exposes the cervical disc to shearing forces, but in the lumbar spine the vertical lumbar facets severely limit translation, protecting the thicker disc from shearing. Lumbar flexion and extension are mainly rocking movements of one vertebral body on another, accompanied by upward and downward gliding between the facets. The thickness of the disc can accommodate the small amount of translatory movement. On the other hand, the forward slide of one cervical vertebra on the next vertebra, which accompanies flexion or extension, produces shearing forces within the disc. This produces transverse fissuring in cervical discs at an early age, first at the uncovertebral clefts before adolescence. From these clefts, fissures gradually extend transversely across the posterior half of the disc in young adults. By contrast with this almost universal cervical disc fissuring at a relatively early age, fissuring of lumbar discs is seldom present in young adults. Lumbar disc fissures appear in later life and are less universal and usually less obvious than in cervical discs.

Contrasting Vulnerability in Flexion and Extension

The nature of injuries to the lumbar or cervical spines is influenced by the different regional biomechanics described. In rapid neck flexion, the cervical spine is protected by a large mass of posterior muscles against the small forward momentum of the 4 kg head, but the erector spinae of the rapidly flexed lumbar spine has to accommodate the much larger mass of the 40 kg torso. Unless the cervical flexion injury is very severe, the posterior muscles prevent dislocations and protect the discs from serious injury. In severe high-speed deceleration injuries, the posterior muscles and the posterior ligamentous complex may not provide adequate protection. They are likely to be strained or torn with risk of facet subluxation with shearing of the disc from the adjacent vertebra and a high risk of spinal cord damage.

The cervical spine is more vulnerable to rapid forceful extension because the small anterior muscles give inadequate protection against extension injury, especially in the typically slender female neck. There are anterior distraction injuries to the discs. First the anterior annulus tears from the vertebral rim. With severe trauma, there is partial avulsion of the disc from the vertebral body, with strain or tear to the anterior longitudinal ligament. The last structures to tear are the compliant longus colli muscles. Posterior compression injuries to the zygapophyseal joints vary from bruising of the vascular synovial folds to articular cartilage fractures or fractures of the facet tips. Vertebral body fractures are relatively rare except for dens fractures.

By contrast, lumbar flexion injuries more frequently result in vertebral body fractures. In flexion-deceleration, the vertical lumbar facets absorb the first force. Small facet fractures, with avulsion of the mamillary process or infraction of the articular surface of the superior articular process, are common. In more severe injuries a facet may fracture across its base, or through the adjacent lamina. If the facets are not severely fractured or dislocated in the flexion-deceleration injury, the motion segment "hinges" forward on the facets and the anterior elements are compressed. This results first in a vertebral end plate fracture with bleeding into the adjacent disc. Higher forces cause a wedge compression fracture of the vertebral body, with or without disc disruption, most frequently at T12 or L1. When the facets are fractured or dislocated, the disc or vertebra may be sheared through, with a whole-segment fracture dislocation. Disc injury is less common as an isolated injury than in the cervical spine. In the lumbar spine it usually accompanies vertebral fracture with intradiscal bleeding or a variable degree of disc disruption, disc contusion, or traumatic herniation, but the disc is protected from shearing disruption so long as the facets remain intact. In acute motor vehicle trauma, lumbar disc tears are less frequent than cervical annular tears. However, annular tears may occur in lower lumbar discs as a result of bending-twisting-lifting trauma, when the Z joints are less congruous than in the extended spine and offer less resistance to axial rotation strains to the spiraling fibers of the annulus. Disc damage of this kind can lead to accelerated disc degeneration.[97,98]

Extension injuries to the lumbar spine are uncommon in motor vehicle accidents, but they may occur as occupational or sporting injuries. If the inferior facets are forcibly driven down against the lamina below, this may fracture the isthmus of the pars interarticularis. This injury may occur either as an acute extension injury, e.g., in a football injury, or as a fatigue fracture after repetitive flexion and extension with rotation, as in fast bowling in cricket, or in repeated hyperextension as in gymnastics.[69,96]

SUMMARY

1.   The strong construction of lumbar vertebrae and motion segments reflects the need for regional stability in weightbearing and movement.

2.   The thick young discs, rich in proteoglycans, are designed to allow useful ranges of movements and bear high compressive loads.

3.   The biplanar facets restrain torsion and translation, protecting the annular fibers of the discs from the stresses to which they are most vulnerable.

4.   In resisting translation in flexion, the coronal components of the facets may develop chondromalacia and thickening of the subchondral bone plate in young adults.

5.   In protecting the discs in deceleration injuries the facets show infractions of their articular surfaces. In flexion compression injuries, the motion segment hinges on the facets and the vertebral bodies are compressed, with end-plate fractures or vertebral wedging.

6.   Spondylolysis in young athletes implies failure of the facet function, with consequent exposure of the disc to shearing forces, which may lead to spondylolisthesis.

7.   Degenerative spondylolisthesis in the elderly implies slow failure of the facets' protective function with segmental instability.

8.   In the "dysfunctional" phase of early loosening of the motion segment, with disc fissuring, tension at the posterior facet margins, where the capsule and articular cartilage are continuous, may "shear off" a flap of articular cartilage forming a loose cartilaginous inclusion in the joint, with the possibility of locking of the joint.

9.   In elderly spines, osteoporosis leads to vertebral endplate collapse with "ballooning" of discs into the concave vertebral end-plates and shortening of the spine; this reduces the vertical dimensions of the nerve root canals.

10.   Loosening of the motion segment may allow vertebral retrolisthesis with reduction in the dimensions of the nerve root canals.

REFERENCES

1. Giles LGF, Taylor JR: Lumbar spine structural changes associated with leg length inequality. Spine 7:159–162, 1982
2. Giles LGF, Taylor JR: The effect of postural scoliosis on lumbar apophyseal joints. Scand J Rheumatol 13:209–220, 1984
3. Walker ML, Rothstein JM, Finucane SD, et al: Relationships between lumbar lordosis, pelvic tilt and abdominal muscle performance. Phys Therapy 67:512–516, 1987
4. Finch PM, Taylor JR: Functional anatomy of the spine. In Waldeman SD, Winnie AP (Eds.): Interventional Pain Management. W.B. Saunders, Philadelphia, 1996, pp. 39–64
5. Kakulas BA, Taylor JR: Pathology of injuries of the vertebral column and spinal cord. In Frankel HL (Ed): Handbook of Clinical Neurology. Elsevier Science Publishers, New York, 1992, pp. 21–51
6. Taylor JR: Growth of lumbar vertebral bodies and intervertebral discs in relation to weightbearing in the erect posture. J Anat 119:413, 1975
7. Taylor JR, Twomey LT: Age changes in lumbar zygapophyseal joints: observations on structure and function. Spine 11:739–745, 1986
8. Taylor JR, Twomey LT: Development of the human intervertebral disc. In Ghosh P (Ed.): Biology of the Intervertebral Disc. CRC Press: Boca Raton, Florida, 1988, pp. 39–82,
9. Taylor JR, Twomey LT, and Corker M: Bone and soft tissue injuries in postmortem lumbar spines. Paraplegia 28:119–129, 1990
10. Twomey LT: Age Changes in the Human Lumbar Vertebral Column. PhD thesis, University of Western Australia, Perth, 1981.
11. Twomey L, Taylor J: Age changes in lumbar vertebrae and intervertebral discs. Clin Orthop 224:97–104, 1987
12. Twomey LT, Taylor JR: Age-related changes in the lumbar spine and spinal rehabilitation. CRC critical review. Phys Rehab Med 2:153–169, 1991
13. Twomey L, Taylor J: Development and growth of the cervical and lumbar spine. In White AH, Schofferman AJ (Eds.): Spine Care. Mosby, St Louis, 1995, pp. 792–808
14. Wolpert L: The cellular basis of skeletal growth during development. Brit Med Bull 37:152–159, 1981
15. O'Rahilly R, Meyer DB: The timing and sequence of events in the development of the human vertebral column during the embryonic period. Proper Anat Embryol 157:167–176, 1979
16. Taylor JR, Twomey L: Factors influencing growth of the vertebral column. In Grieve GP (Ed.): Modern Manual Therapy. Churchill Livingstone, Edinburgh, 1986, pp 30–36
17. Taylor JR, Twomey L: The role of the notochord and blood vessels in development of the vertebral column. In Grieve GP (Ed.): Modern Manual Therapy of the Vertebral Column. Churchill Livingstone, Edinburgh, 1986, pp. 21–29
18. Verbout AJ: The development of the vertebral column. In Beck, Hild, and Ortmann (Eds.): Advances Anatomy, Embryology & Cell Biology. Vol. 90. Springer Verlag, Berlin, 1985, pp. 1–122

19. Taylor JR: Growth and development of the human intervertebral disc. PhD thesis, University of Edinburgh, 1973

20. Taylor JR: Scoliosis and growth: patterns of asymmetry in normal growth. Acta Orthop Scand 54:596–602, 1983

21. Taylor JR: Persistence of the notochordal canal in vertebrae. J Anat 111:211–217, 1972

22. Dale Stewart TD, Kerley ER: Essentials of Forensic Anthropology. Springfield, Illinois, Charles C Thomas, 1976, p. 136

23. Taylor JR, Twomey LT: Vertebral column development and its relation to adult pathology. Aust J Physiother 31:83–88, 1985

24. Tanaka T, Uhthoff HK: The pathogenesis of congenital vertebral malformations. Acta Orthop Scand 52:413–415, 1981

25. Watterson RL, Fowler I, Fowler BJ: The role of the neural tube and notochord in development of the axial skeleton of the chick. Am J Anat 95:337–382, 1954

26. Taylor JR: Age changes in lumbar zygapophyseal joints. In Archives of Biology VIIth Symposium Internationale des sciences morphologiques, Louvain-en-Wolue, 1986, p. 121

27. Taylor JR: Growth of human intervertebral discs and vertebral bodies. J Anat 120:49–68, 1975

28. Taylor JR, Twomey LT: Sexual dimorphism in human vertebral growth. J Anat 138:281–286, 1984

29. Schultz AB: Spine slenderness and flexibility in idiopathic scoliosis. J Biomech 14:491, 1981.

30. McFadden KD, Taylor JR: End-plate lesions of the lumbar spine. Spine 14:867–869, 1989

31. Walmsley R: The human intervertebral disc: development and growth. Edin Med J 60:341–364, 1953

32. Dietz GW, Christensen EE: Normal "Cupid's bow" contour of lower lumbar vertebrae. Radiology 121:577–579, 1976

33. Schmorl G, Junghanns H: Displacement of intervertebral disc tissue. In Besemann EF (Ed.): The Human Spine in Health & Disease (2nd ed.). Grune & Stratton, New York, 1971, pp. 158–165

34. Bradford DS, Moe JH: Scheuermann's juvenile kyphosis: A histological study. Clin Orthop 110:45–53, 1975

35. Taylor JR: Vascular causes of vertebral asymmetry and the laterality of scoliosis. M J A 144:533–535, 1986

36. Dickson R, Lawton JO, Butt WP: Pathogenesis of idiopathic scoliosis. In Dickson R, Bradford D (Eds): Management of Spinal Deformities. Butterworths, London, 1984

37. Taylor JR, Twomey LT: Structure and function of lumbar zygapophyseal (facet) joints. In Boyling JD, Palastanga N (Eds.): Grieve's Modern Manual Therapy of the Vertebral Column. Churchill Livingstone, Edinburgh, 1994, pp. 99–108

38. Van Shaik JPJ, Verbiest H, Van Shaik FDJ: The orientation of laminae and facet joints in the lower lumbar spine. Spine 10:59–63, 1985

39. Taylor JR, Corker M: Age-related responses to stress in the vertebral column: a review. In The Growing Scope of Human Biology: Proceedings of the Australasian Society for Human Biology. Centre for Human Biology, University of Western Australia, Perth, 1989

40. Taylor JR, Slinger BA: Scoliosis screening and growth in Western Australian students. Med J Aust 1:475–478, 1980

41. Twomey LT, Taylor JR, Furniss B: Age changes in the bone density and structure of the lumbar vertebral column. J Anat 136:15–25, 1983

42. Hutton W, Adams MA: The forces acting on the neural arch and their relevance to low back pain. Engineering Aspects of the Spine. London, Mechanical Engineering, 1980, pp. 49–55

43. Davis PR: Human lower lumbar vertebrae: Some mechanical and osteological considerations. J Anat 95:337, 1961

44. Horton WG: Further observations on the elastic mechanism of the intervertebral disc. J Bone Joint Surg 40B:552–557, 1958

45. Taylor JR, Scott JE, Cribb AM, et al: Human intervertebral disc acid glycosaminoglycans. J Anat 180:137–141, 1992

46. Nachemson A, Elfstrom G: Intravital dynamic pressure measurements in lumbar discs. Scand J Rehab Med 1:1–40, 1970

47. Taylor JR, Twomey LT: Innervation of lumbar intervertebral discs. Med J Aust 2:701–702, 1979

48. Taylor JR, Twomey LT: Innervation of lumbar intervertebral discs. NZ J Physio 8:36–37, 1980

49. Freemont A, Peacock T, Goupillie P, et al: Nerve ingrowth into diseased intervertebral discs in chronic low back pain. Lancet 350:178–181, 1997

50. Sachs BL: Dallas discogram description: A new classification of CT discography in low back disorders. Spine 12:287–294, 1987

51. Hirsch C, Schazowicz F: Studies on structural changes in the lumbar annulus fibrosus. Acta Orthop Scand 22:184–231, 1953

52. Bogduk N: The innervation of the lumbar spine. Spine 8:286–293, 1983

53. Maroudas A, Nachemson A, Stockwell RA: Factors involved in the nutrition of the human lumbar intervertebral disc: cellularity and diffusion of glucose in vitro. J Anat 120:113–130, 1975

54. Buckwalter JA: Aging and degeneration of the human intervertebral disc. Spine 20:1307–1314, 1995

55. Holm S, Nachemson A: Nutrition of the IVD: acute effects of cigarette smoking. Upsala J Med Sci 93:91–99, 1988

56. Holm S, Nachemson A: Variation in the nutrition of the canine intervertebral disc induced by motion. Spine 8:866–874, 1983

57. Twomey LT, Taylor JR: Sagittal movements of the human lumbar vertebral column: A quantitative study of the role of the posterior vertebral elements. Arch Phys Med Rehab 64:322–325, 1983

58. Twomey L, Taylor J: Age changes in the lumbar articular triad. Aust J Physiother 31:106–112, 1985

59. Bowen V, Cassidy JD: Macroscopic and microscopic anatomy of the sacro-iliac joint from embryonic life until the 8th decade. Spine 6:620–628, 1981

60. Palfrey AJ: The shape of sacroiliac joint surfaces. J Anat 132:457, 1981

61. Taylor JR, Twomey L: Sagittal & horizontal plane movement of the lumbar vertebral column in cadavers and in the living. Rheum Rehab 19:223–232, 1980

62. Bogduk N, Macintosh JE: The applied anatomy of the thoracolumbar fascia. Spine 9:164–170, 1984

63. Taylor JR, McCormick CC: Lumbar facet joint fat pads. Neuroradiology 33:38–42, 1991

64. Giles LGF, Taylor J: Intra-articular synovial protrusions in the lower lumbar apophyseal joints. Bull Hosp Joint Dis 42:248–254, 1982

65. Wyke B: The neurology of joints: A review of general principles. Clin Rheum Dis 7:223–239, 1981

66. Giles LG, Taylor JR, Cockson A: Hyman zygapophyseal joint synovial folds. Acta Anatomica 126:110–114, 1986

67. Taylor JR, Twomey LT: Lumbar multifidi: Rotator-cuff muscles of zygapophyseal joints. J Anat 149:266–267, 1986
68. McCormick CC, Taylor JR, Twomey LT: Facet joint arthrography in lumbar spondylolysis: Anatomic basis for spread of contrast. Radiology 171:193–196, 1989
69. Twomey LT, Taylor JR, Oliver M: Sustained flexion loading, rapid extension loading of the lumbar spine and the physiotherapy of related injuries. Physiother Pract 4:129–138, 1988
70. Hardcastle P, Annear P, Foster DH, et al: Spinal abnormalities in young fast bowlers. J Bone Joint Surg 74B:421–425, 1992
71. Spangfort EV: The lumbar disc herniation. Acta Orthop Scand 142(suppl):1–80, 1972
72. McRae DL: Radiology of the lumbar spinal canal. In Weinstein PR, Ehni G, and Wilson CB (Eds). Lumbar Spondylosis: Diagnosis, Management & Surgical Treatment. Year Book Medical Publishers, Chicago, 1977, pp. 92–114
73. Crock HV: Internal disc disruption. Spine 11:650–653, 1985
74. Taylor MM, Taylor JR, McCormick CC: Features associated with subluxation in lumbar facet joints: anatomical and radiological comparisons. In Bruce NW (Ed.): Proc Australasian Soc Human Biol. Vol. 5. Centre for Human Biol UWA, 1992, pp. 359–373
75. Ramsey RH: Anatomy of ligamentum flava. Clin Orthop 44:129–140, 1966
76. Yong-Hing MD, Reilly J, and Kirkwaldy-Willis WH: The ligamentum flavum. Spine 1:226–234, 1976
77. Heylings D: Supraspinous and interspinous ligaments of the human lumbar spine. J Anat 125:127, 1978
78. Taylor JR, Twomey LT, Kakulas BA: Dorsal root ganglion injuries in 109 blunt trauma fatalities. Injury 29:335–339, 1998
79. Twomey L, Taylor JR: Age changes in the lumbar spine and intervertebral canals. Paraplegia 26:238–249, 1988
80. Eisenstein S: The morphometry and pathological anatomy of the lumbar spine in South African negroes and caucasoids with specific reference to spinal stenosis. J Bone Joint Surg 59B:173, 1977
81. Parkin IG, Harrison GR: The topographical anatomy of the lumbar epidural space. J Anat 141:211, 1985
82. Engel R, Bogduk N: The menisci of the lumbar zygapophyseal joints. J Anat 135:795, 1982
83. Dommisse GF: Blood supply of spinal cord. J Bone Joint Surg 56B:225–235, 1974
84. Romanes GJR: The arterial blood supply of the spinal cord. Paraplegia 2:199, 1965
85. Sunderland S: Meningeal-neural relationships in the intervertebral space. J Neurosurg 40:756–763, 1974
86. Clayson SJ: Evaluation of mobility of hip and lumbar vertebrae of normal young women. Arch Phys Med 43:1–8, 1962
87. Bourdillon JF: Spinal Manipulation (2nd ed.). Heinemann, London, 1973
88. Twomey LT, Taylor JR: Old age and physical capacity: use it or lose it. Aust J Physiother 30:115–120, 1984
89. Adams MA, Dolan P: Could sudden increases in physical activity cause degeneration of intervertebral discs? Lancet 350:734–735, 1997
90. Battie MC, Videman T, Gibbons L, et al: Determinants of lumbar disc degeneration. Spine 20:2601–2612, 1995

91. Riihimake H, et al: Disc degeneration in house painters and concrete workers. Spine 15:114–119, 1990

92. Videman T, Sarna S, Battie MC, et al: The long term effects of physical loading and exercise lifestyles on back-related symptoms, disability and spinal pathology among men. Spine 20:699–709, 1995

93. Sartoris DJ, Resnick D, Tyson R, Haghighi P: Age-related alterations in the vertebral spinous processes and intervening soft tissues: radiologic-pathologic correlation. Am J Roentgen 145:1025–1030, 1985

94. Vernon-Roberts B: The pathology and interrelation of intervertebral discs lesions, osteoarthrosis of the apophyseal joints, lumbar spondylosis and low back pain. In Jayson MIV (Ed.): The Lumbar Spine and Back Pain (2nd ed.). Pitman, London, 1985, pp. 83–114

95. Swanepoel MW, Adams LM, Smeathers JE: Human lumbar apophyseal joint damage and IVD degeneration. Ann Rheum Dis 54:182–188, 1995

96. Twomey L, Taylor J, Flynn C: Injuries of the lumbar region in sports physiotherapy: Applied science and practice. Churchill Livingstone, Edinburgh, 1995, pp. 485–506

97. Kaapa E, Holm S, Han X, et al: Experimental trauma to the annulus fibrosus can initiate lumbar disc degeneration. J Orthop Res 12:93–102, 1994

98. Osti OL: Annulus tears and intervertebral disc degeneration. An experimental study using an animal model. Spine 15:762–767, 1990

2

Lumbar Posture, Movement, and Mechanics

Lance T. Twomey
James R. Taylor

The adult vertebral column is a segmented, jointed, flexible rod, which supports the loads of weightbearing in the erect posture, protects the spinal cord and emerging spinal nerves, allows a considerable range of movements in all directions, and serves as the axial support for the limbs. The vertebral column's capacity to fully subserve these functions alters through the different phases of the life cycle. The extremely malleable C-shaped column of the neonate remains almost as flexible and mobile in childhood as it grows and develops its finely balanced curves. Further growth and maturation are associated with progressive increases in the strength and "dynamic" stability of the adolescent and young-adult columns, and with a continuing small decline in its mobility. The middle years demonstrate an increasing incidence of minor traumatic and degenerative pathology, with a further decline in range of movement. In old age, with osteoporotic decrease in bone strength, there is progressive increase in joint stiffness with a considerable decline in movement ranges, and a flattening of the lumbar spine. The lumbar spine is markedly lordotic in children, with a small decline in lordosis in adolescents and young adults, and a pronounced flattening of the region in middle life and old age.

Posture is a term that indicates the relative position of the body segments during rest or activity, whereas the term *stature* indicates the height of a subject. In most individuals their resting supine length exceeds their standing height (or stature) by about 2 cm.

POSTURE

Posture refers to a composite of the positions of all of the joints of the body at any given moment.[1] A minimum of muscle work is required for the maintenance of good posture in any human static or dynamic situation. In "good standing" posture, the head is held tall and level, while the spine is nicely balanced so that its sagittal curves allow free movement of the chest and abdomen and prevent the shoulders from sagging forward. The lower limbs

line of gravity

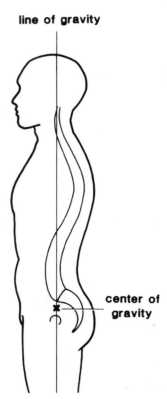

center of
gravity

Fig. 2-1 The relationship between the vertebral column and the line of gravity.

serve as balanced support. In a side view of most individuals, a plumb line would intersect the mastoid process, the acromion process, and the greater trochanter. It would pass just anterior to the center of the knee joint and through the ankle joint.

The usual static posture for the lumbar spine is that of lordosis. Normal spinal posture is expressed as a balanced series of curves when viewed from the side (Fig. 2-1). The adult spine is supported on a symmetric level pelvis by two equal-length lower limbs. In normal sitting posture, the level pelvis is supported with body weight distributed equally through both ischial tuberosities. There is no discernible lateral curvature or rotation of the spine when viewed from the front or behind.

The cervical lordosis begins to appear at birth and develops as a permanent curve at about 3 months of age, while the permanent lumbar lordosis appears with the extension of the legs and weightbearing in the erect posture, usually between 12 and 18 months of age. These curves continue to change until the completion of spinal growth, usually between the ages of 13 and 18 years.[2,3,4]

Sagittal Pelvic Tilt and Muscle Action

Pelvic tilt in the sagittal plane and lumbar lordosis are inextricably linked together, as the lumbar spine and the sacrum are united at the strong, relatively

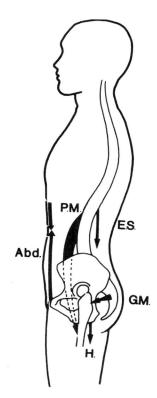

Fig. 2-2 The muscles responsible for the maintenance of pelvic tilt. *Abd,* abdominal muscles; *ES,* erector spine; *GM,* gluteus maximus; *H,* hamstring; *PM,* psoas major.

immobile sacroiliac joints. Thus, when the pelvis is tilted further forward, it brings about an increase in lordosis, and when tilted backward, the lumbar spine flattens. The muscles responsible for pelvic posture include erector spinae (sacrospinalis), abdominals (rectus abdominus and oblique muscles), psoas major and iliacus, gluteus maximus, and hamstrings (Fig. 2-2).

It is the interaction between these muscles that is the major factor determining pelvic tilt and lumbar lordosis at any point in time. Thus, while the back extensor muscles primarily increase lumbar lordosis, the abdominal muscles, gluteals, and hamstrings act together to flatten lumbar lordosis by their action about the lever of the pelvis. The psoas muscles, which attach to the lateral margins of the lumbar vertebrae, can also increase lumbar lordosis when the lower limbs are extended by pulling the lumbar vertebrae forward around the "pulley" of the hip joint (Fig. 2-2). In this way they pull the pelvis and lumbar vertebrae ventrally. In the course of everyday activity we are constantly adjusting our posture to allow for comfort, ergonomic advantage, and in response to our environment. Muscle tightness affecting any of the muscle groups listed can change both habitual resting posture and the total range of dynamic postures available. Tightness of psoas major and hamstring muscles is associated with increased lordosis in some individuals. Shortened hamstrings pull down on the pelvis and flatten the lumbar spine. For this reason, it is possible that tight hamstrings are the result of lordotic posture rather than its cause. There is no evidence that abdominal muscle strength has any influence on pelvic tilt and lumbar lordosis.[5]

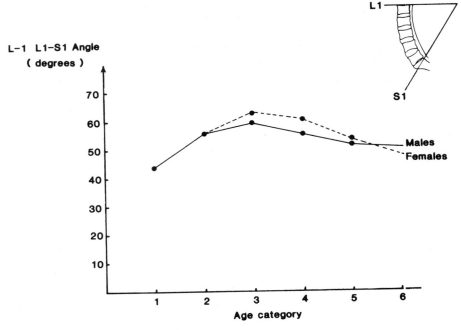

Fig. 2-3   Changes that occur through life to the L5-S1 angle (for age categories see Fig. 2-7).

Analysis of the Lumbar Curve

The lumbosacral lordosis is a compound curve (Fig. 2-3) with the degree of curvature greatest at the L5-S1 level, and least at the Ll-2 level. In general, at all ages the intervertebral discs contribute to a greater proportion of the lordosis in both sexes than do the vertebrae. However, at the lumbosacral junction, the L5 vertebral body makes a significant contribution. The L5-S1 disc is also more wedge-shaped than any of the higher discs.

Sexual Dimorphism

During the childbearing years (i.e., between adolescence and middle age) the Ll-S1 angle of lumbar lordosis is greater in women than in men.[6] This sexual dimorphism is not apparent in childhood and disappears again in old age. Although the reasons for this difference remain obscure, its place in the life cycle suggests that it has a hormonal basis. One of the hormones that may be involved consists of three closely related polypeptides collectively called relaxin. Relaxin is secreted by the ovary and has been shown to relax the symphysis pubis, sacroiliac joints, and spinal ligaments.[7] These hormones, which are secreted in relatively large amounts by the corpus luteum of pregnancy, are also found in small amounts in the circulating blood of nonpregnant women of childbearing age. It is suggested that the effects of relaxin in "loosening" pelvic and lumbar ligaments may coincidentally allow an increase in the lumbar curve during that period in the female life cycle (adolescence and early-adult life) when the hormones are present in relatively large amounts.

Another suggestion advanced to explain the gender differences in lordosis relates to Treanor's demonstration[8] that the wearing of high-heel shoes tips the body's center of gravity forward and brings about an associated increase in pelvic tilt and an increase in lumbar lordosis as lumbar lordosis is dependent on pelvic posture (Fig. 2-4). The habitual wearing of high heels in the "developed" countries may eventually provide a contribution to a difference in lordosis between men and women in Western societies.[9] Other studies[9, 10] show that an increase in pelvic tilt due to high heels does not always bring about an increase in lumbar lordosis in nonpregnant young women. An equal number of women demonstrated a flattening of their lumbar curve as showed an increase. However, pregnant women showed a significant increase in lordosis when wearing 2-inch-high heels. The response of the lumbar spine to changes in pelvic posture would appear to relate to

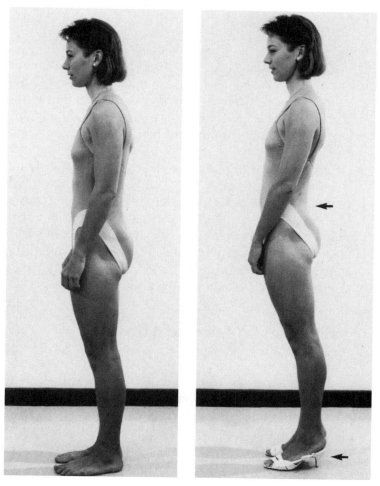

Fig. 2-4 The increase in lumbar lordosis due to wearing high-heel shoes.

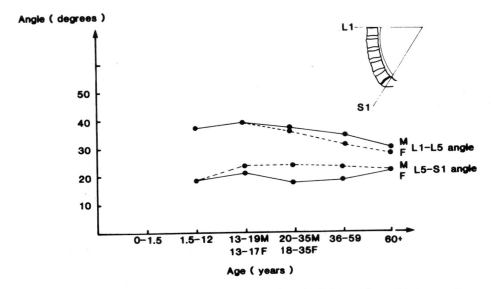

Fig. 2-5   An analysis of the change in L1 to L5 and L5-S1 angles with increasing age.

the location of the center of gravity. In pregnancy, the center of gravity is displaced ventrally and is balanced by an increase in lumbar lordosis.

An analysis of the components of the Ll-S1 angle in a major cadaveric study[6] showed that the principal difference between the lumbar posture of females and males occurs at the lumbosacral junction, as the composite Ll-5 angles are similar throughout life in both sexes (Fig. 2-5). Thus it is the increased sacral and pelvic tilt of females that is primarily responsible for the difference in lordosis during adolescence and early-adult life. In this regard, it is interesting to note that anatomists such as Romanes[11] consider that in normal erect posture, the anterosuperior iliac spines and the symphysis pubis lie in the same plane. This was confirmed in a measurement study of 39 nonpregnant females by Taylor and Alexander.[12] Obstetric experience suggests that the symphysis pubis lies in a more anterior plane than do the iliac spines.[13] The greater L5-SI angle in females may well be related to a greater degree of pelvic tilt during the childbearing years.

Variations in Lumbar Lordosis

Lumbar lordosis is maintained by intrinsic features such as the shape of the vertebrae, discs, and the sacrum, and by extrinsic factors such as position of center of gravity, body weight and its distribution, muscle strength, and sociocultural preferences. In regard to sociocultural preferences, it is commonly observed that an individual's lumbar lordosis and thus habitual posture is based on factors such as fashion (e.g., wearing high heels), repetitive daily activity (e.g., a schoolchild carrying a heavy schoolbag), life-style (e.g., the "typical" military posture), affect and attitude (e.g., depression or elation), and aesthetics or training (e.g., swayback model's posture).[14]

Prolonged Maintenance of the Static Erect Posture

Standing in the upright position for long periods of time tends to produce an increase in lumbar lordosis as muscles begin to fatigue and as the slow "creep" of the soft tissues often emphasizes the natural tendency toward extension of the region. This occurs because the center of gravity is usually ventral to the sacral promontory in most adults.[5] The effect of gravity acting through this center pulls the lumbar spine into a more lordotic posture in those individuals. This postural change accompanies the diurnal decline in height (see Diurnal Variation in Stature). Vertebral column posture is ideally dynamic rather than static, as the tissues adapt to prolonged static loading by further "creep" of the column.[14]

The Effects of Age on Lumbar Lordosis

The lumbar spinal lordosis flattens considerably in old age in both sexes (Fig. 2-5)[2,6] although a few individuals do show small increases in lordosis. Increases are usually associated with increased abdominal girth and weight and declines in abdominal-muscle strength, so that their physique approximates that of a pregnant female. Thus the explanation for an increase in lordosis is the same as that for pregnant women (see above). However, Twomey's[6] large study of a typical Australian society clearly shows a significant decrease in lumbar lordosis with increasing age after adolescence of 32 percent in females and 20 percent in males.

Lumbar Lordosis in Association with Back Pain

Clinicians often report a flattening of the lumbar lordosis during episodes of back pain. However, a study of 600 men between the ages of 23 and 60 years has shown that the distribution and range of lordosis (as viewed on radiographs) does not vary in acute or chronic low-back pain more than it does in men without back pain.[15] However, a more recent study shows impaired postural stability (i.e., the ability to maintain a postural position) to be part of the symptomatology of patients with low back problems.[5,8]

Leg-Length Inequality and Pelvic Obliquity

While pelvic tilt in the sagittal plane is inextricably linked with lumbar lordosis, coronal-plane obliquity of the pelvis is associated with lumbar scoliosis. The most common cause of this functional situation is leg-length inequality.[16] Functional scoliosis must be distinguished from idiopathic structural scoliosis. Structural scoliosis progresses during the growth period, is seen most frequently in girls,[17] and is usually convex to the left in the lumbar spine. Leg length inequality and postural scoliosis have been associated with low back pain, degenerative changes in the intervertebral discs and zygapophyseal joints, and with a higher incidence of osteoarthritic changes in hip and knee joints. Interestingly, it is most often the left leg that tends to be longest, particularly in men,[18] since most right-handed people put more weight on their left foot.[19]

Unequal leg length may be associated with pathologic conditions (e.g., Perthes' disease, previous fracture), but it usually accompanies normal growth. In growing individuals, a degree of asymmetric growth of the lower limbs is very common. It may be associated with asynchronous maturation of paired bones where one of the pair is longer than the other because it is more advanced in its maturity.[18] A leg-length difference of 1 cm or greater is twice as common at the peak of the adolescent growth spurt (13 percent) than at skeletal maturity (7 percent).[20] Indeed, when accurate measurement methods are available, it is rare to find exactly equal leg lengths in normal communities.

Giles and Taylor[21, 22] showed that unequal leg length and the associated "postural" scoliosis are linked with minor structural changes in lumbar discs and vertebral end-plates, and with asymmetric changes to the articular cartilage and subchondral bone of the lumbar zygapophyseal joints. The joints on the convex side of the scoliotic curve show thicker subchondral bone plates and thinner articular cartilage than those from the concave side. This may be related to asymmetric loading, e.g., a response to the greater postural muscle forces necessary on the convex side to prevent buckling of the scoliotic column under axial loading. A number of surveys have shown a statistical association between leg-length inequality and low back pain.[16, 23] Leg-length inequality is twice as common in low back pain patients (13 to 22 percent) than in control populations (4 to 8 percent). Giles and Taylor[16] also suggested that the response to manipulative therapy in chronic or recurrent low back pain associated with leg-length inequality is more long lasting when a foot-raise shoe insert is provided as part of the treatment.

STATURE

Effects of Variations in Stature

The topics of stature and posture are closely related. Stature is affected by posture in a number of ways.

Postural Fatigue

Laxity in posture causes "creep" of soft tissues (see Prolonged Maintenance of the Static Erect Posture).

Diurnal Variation in Stature

In 1777, Buffon noted that a young man was considerably shorter after spending the night at a ball but he regained his previous height after a rest in bed. Merkel (1881) measured his own daily loss in height (2 cm standing, 1.6 cm sitting) by measuring the height of his "visual plane" from the floor.

He found that half his loss in stature occurred in the first hour after rising, and that a greater loss occurred after vigorous exercise.

De Puky[24] measured diurnal variation in stature and found the daily loss in height to average 15.7 mm. Blackman[25] showed a decrease in stature of 0.76 cm 1 hour after rising and 1.77 cm 4 hours after rising. This order of decrease was confirmed by Stone and Taylor,[26] who showed that most of this loss in stature loss was accounted for by loss in sitting height, which was equivalent to 80 percent of the total loss in standing height.

In an interesting study, Tyrrell, Reilly, and Troup[27] showed that average daily variation in stature was about 1 percent of normal stature, and that the greatest loss occurred in the first hour after rising in the morning. Approximately 70 percent of this lost stature was regained during the first half of the night. The carrying of heavy loads increased the rate of shrinkage loss (i.e., by "creep"). Interestingly, rest with the lumbar spine in full flexion produced more rapid gains in stature than in other positions. This also suggests that the diurnal loss involves "creep" into extension (see Prolonged Maintenance of the Static Erect Posture). Adams and Hutton[28] have recently demonstrated that the flexed position induces the transport of metabolites and fluids into the intervertebral discs. If most of the diurnal loss in stature is a loss of trunk length due to small diurnal reductions in disc height,[26] then the use of flexion as a tool to maintain disc height and to preserve normal erect posture without excessive lordosis becomes of clinical interest for physical therapists.

The mechanism involved in diurnal variation in stature is discussed further under later sections on "creep" of vertebral structures.

The Influence of Changes in Posture on Stature

When parents measure their child's stature as a record of their growth rate the usual instructions given are to "stand tall, like a soldier." This implies a general understanding that stature is dependent in part on a person's posture. When "standing tall," the child flattens the spine as much as possible, tucks the chin in, and attempts to push the top of the head as far upward as possible. Similarly, after surgical correction of moderate to severe scoliosis, when the spine is surgically "straightened," children can gain up to 8 cm in height.

The thoracic spine makes the largest contribution to spine length. The lumbar spine constitutes one-third, the cervical spine one-fifth, and the thoracic spine the remainder of the total length of the presacral spine in the adult.[29]

The Effect of Growth and Aging on Stature

The rates of growth and decline in stature are described in Chapter 1. The spinal component in the decline in stature that occurs in old age is much more a result of a decrease in vertebral height than it is a decrease in intervertebral disc height.[30,31] An increasing thoracic kyphosis (particularly in women) also contributes significantly to the loss of stature in old age.

MOVEMENTS OF THE LUMBAR VERTEBRAL COLUMN

At each level in the vertebral column there are three interacting joints allowing and controlling movement. This unique combination is known as the articular triad or as the mobile segment (Chapter 1). Each articular triad allows only a few degrees of movement. However, lumbar movement usually involves a complex interaction of mobile segments at multiple levels. The thickness of each intervertebral disc, the compliance of its fibrocartilage, and the dimensions and shape of its adjacent vertebral end plates are of primary importance in governing the extent of movement possible. The shape and orientation of the vertebral-arch articular facets, with the ligaments and muscles of the arch and its processes, guide the types of movement possible and provide restraints against excessive movement.

Ranges of Disc Movement

The anterior elements (vertebrae and discs) of the articular triads are capable of certain ranges in movement, depending on disc dimensions (thickness and horizontal dimensions) and disc stiffness.

Disc Dimensions

A large range of movement would occur when disc height was relatively great and vertebral end-plate horizontal dimensions relatively short (Fig. 2-6). Adolescent and young-adult females have shorter vertebral end plates (Fig 2-6, *A*) than males, while disc height (Fig. 2-6, *B1, B2, B3*) and disc stiff-

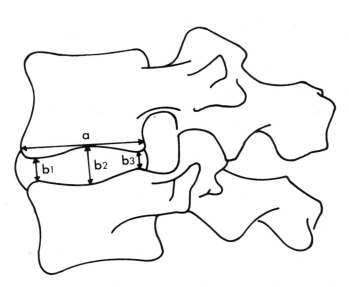

Fig. 2-6 The anterior vertebral elements (mobile segment): *a,* vertebral end-plate; *b,* disc thickness.

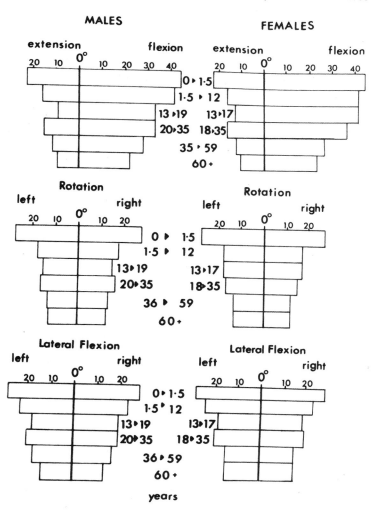

Fig. 2-7 Age changes in the range of lumbar movements in both sexes. (From Taylor and Twomey,[32] with permission.)

ness are substantially the same. Thus females possess the necessary combination of dimensions for a larger range of movements than is possible in males.[6,32] In old age, when male and female vertebrae and disc shapes become very similar and hormonal differences are reduced, the range of movement of men and women become almost identical (Fig. 2-7).

Disc Stiffness

The general reduction in movement ranges in both sexes is attributable to increased disc stiffness. This has been demonstrated by the posterior release experiment of Twomey and Taylor,[33] which demonstrated a 40 percent increase in disc stiffness in the elderly.

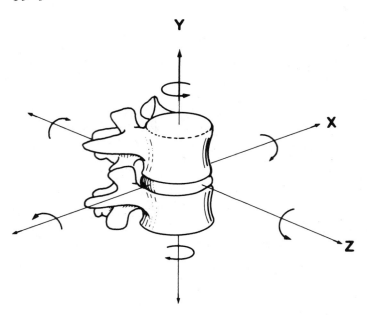

Fig. 2-8   Planes and axes movement. Sagittal plane movements occur along the *x* axis; rotational plane movements occur along the *y* axis; and coronal plane movement occurs along the *z* axis.

Planes of Movement

The movements possible at each lumbar-motion segment are traditionally described as being in the sagittal (flexion-extension), coronal (lateral flexion), and horizontal (axial rotation) planes. Each movement occurs along one of three coordinate axes, x, y, and z (Fig. 2-8). Thus, all mobile segments of the lumbar spine possess 6 degrees of freedom, and each movement consists of an angular or rotary displacement together with translation of a vertebra on its subjacent vertebra. It is rare for movement to occur exclusively in a single plane. Movements are generally "coupled" in habitual movement,[34,35] and occur across the standard descriptive planes of motion.

Ranges of Lumbar Movement

Despite the availability of simple, reliable methods for measuring spinal mobility, these have not been applied to studies of normal lumbar spine movement until recently. The literature records considerable variation in the values given for the ranges of movements of the lumbar spine. This variation stems largely from the different measurement methods used and the differences in age, sex, race, and numbers of subjects studied. The clinical measurements most frequently used include indirect estimates of spinal mobility from measurement of (1) the distance from the fingertips to the floor when the patient bends forward and (2) the use of a tape measure to measure the increase in distance between two skin landmarks, often the Sl and Ll spinous processes. These methods are most inaccurate, and give no direct measure of the range (angular deflection) of spinal movement. The former is influenced by hamstring muscle length and the latter fails to show a reasonable level of consistency between repeated measures. Published studies of lumbar spinal movement have mostly concentrated on sagittal and coronal plane movements and include:

1.   Direct measurement in living subjects, utilizing a wide variety of equipment[32, 36–44]
2.   Radiographic studies[35, 46–51]
3.   Cadaveric studies that have mostly involved a single mobile segment in a small number of specimens[3, 49, 52–64]
4.   Photographic techniques[65, 66]
5.   Theoretic studies based on mathematical models.[67,68,69,70,71]

Estimates of the range of sagittal motion of the lumbar region vary widely from 121 degrees in a young male acrobat,[45] to 21.8 degrees in elderly women.[48] However, Begg and Falconer[72] considered 70 degrees to be the "normal" average total range of lumbar flexion-extension. Few studies have attempted to measure axial rotation in the lumbar spine, largely because of methodologic problems. It has proved difficult to measure lumbar axial rotation in the living either directly or radiographically with any degree of accuracy, and cadaveric studies have mostly been confined to single motion segments where facet orientation blocks true axial rotation, rather than to the whole unrestrained lumbar column. Some authorities maintain that rotary movement does not exist as a separate entity in the lumbar region,[73,74,75] or that if rotation does occur, it is in spite of the fact that the facets are designed to prevent it.[76] Other sources have assessed the total range of rotation as between 5 to 36 degrees of movement.[3, 39, 41, 77–79]

Clinical Measurement

In an effort to provide instrumentation that would be relatively easily applied in the clinical situation and provide reasonably accurate objective data, two instruments were devised to measure lumbar sagittal and horizontal plane movement, and were tested in clinical trials.[32,64,80] The lumbar spondylometer is noninvasive, has good interperson and intertest reliability, and measures lumbar sagittal motion (Fig. 2-9). Because its base rests on the sacrum, the measurement is not confounded and invalidated by the inclusion of hip motion. Tests of its accuracy made by comparing living subjects with fresh, cadaveric specimens suggest that it underestimates the range of movement by an average of 1 degree.[32] Inter- and intraoperator repeatability trials show high correlations.[81] The lumbar spondylometer is comparable in accuracy and in some respects in principle with an inclinometer, but with a more complex geometry.[36] It is also easier to use in a clinical situation where separate readings from two inclinometers would be required. Its use requires a thorough knowledge of the surface anatomy of the lumbar re-

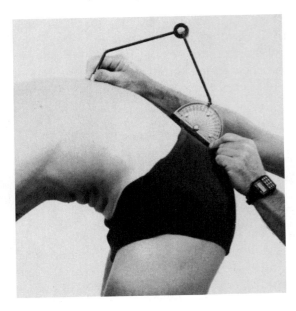

Fig. 2-9   The lumbar spondylometer.

gion, with consistently accurate placement of the cushions, and the precise location of the Ll spinous process.

The cushions of the lumbar spondylometer rest on the dorsal surface of the sacrum, with the top cushion at the level of Sl. The distal end of the instrument rests on the spinous process of Ll (see Fig. 2-9). The physical therapist reads off the initial starting position in degrees, asks the subject to fully extend, and reads off the new position in degrees. The subject returns to the starting position (checked by the operator), and then moves into full-range flexion, with the operator recording the result. Thus flexion, extension, and full-range sagittal motion are recorded. This entire process takes an experienced physical therapist less than 2 minutes to administer and record, and is a useful objective clinical measurement in the assessment of the progress of treatment for back conditions.[80]

The external measurement of rotation in the clinical situation has been made possible by the development of a lumbar rotameter.[32,64] The apparatus consists of a large protractor strapped at right angles to the subject's sacrum, and a belt with a pointer strapped around the trunk at Ll. The tip of the pointer rests just above the protractor (Fig. 2-10). The subject is asked to rotate fully to the right and the left, angular deflections of the pointer being read off on the protractor. Intertrial and interoperator reliability tests show a maximum variation of 5 degrees in a range of 56 degrees, and these measurements correlate well with cadaveric motion.[32] The rotameter is relatively cumbersome, and it takes about 3 minutes for an experienced physical therapist to use it in a clinical setting. For these reasons, it has proved less useful as a clinical tool. It has the additional disadvantage that its reading may be influenced to a minor degree by lower rib cage movements.

Ranges of lumbar movements for both sexes in six age-group categories using the spondylometer and the rotameter, and the gravity inclinometer[38] for side flexion, are listed in Table 2-1.

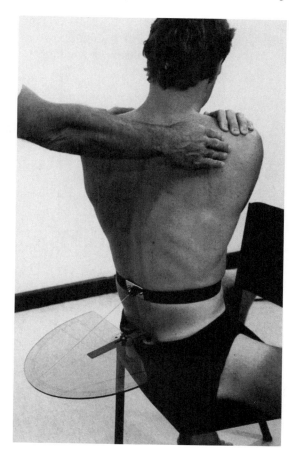

Fig. 2-10   The lumbar rotameter.

Age Changes in Ranges of Movements

Table 2-1 clearly demonstrates a decline in the ranges of all lumbar movements in the living with increasing age. This decline parallels the reductions observed in cadaveric studies by other authors.[6,33,35,82]

In old age the ranges of lumbar movement in men and women become almost identical. It would appear that when hormonal differences are reduced, sexual differentiations in vertebral shape, posture, and spinal movement ranges disappear. The general reduction in ranges in both sexes occurs as a result of increased "stiffening" of the intervertebral disc in association with disc-shape changes involving increases in the anteroposterior length and concavity of the vertebral end-plate.[33] A reason often provided for the decline in average ranges of movements in aging populations (i.e., a general tendency to thinning of intervertebral discs in old age) has recently been shown to be false.[30,31] In old age most discs increase in volume and become thicker and more convex at the disc-vertebral interface. Only about 30 percent of discs become thinner. The principal reason for decreased range of movement is increased disc stiffness.[33]

The 40 percent increase in disc stiffness with age is associated with well-documented histologic and biochemical changes. These include an increase

Table 2-1 The Mean and Standard Deviation for the Total Ranges of Sagittal, Horizontal, and Coronal Plane Movements in Living Subjects (Population 960 Persons)

	Ranges of Movements					
	Sagittal Range (Flexion-Extension)		Horizontal Range (Rotation to Both Sides)		Coronal Range (Side Flexion)	
Age (Yr)	Male	Female	Male	Female	Male	Female
5–12	58° ± 9°	58° ± 9°	34° ± 6°	34° ± 6°	47° ± 6°	47° ± 6°
13–19	45° ± 10°	57° ± 8°	30° ± 4°	34° ± 4°	38° ± 5°	37° ± 4°
19–35	42° ± 6°	42° ± 7°	33° ± 6°	33° ± 6°	40° ± 5°	40° ± 5°
35–59	38° ± 7°	38° ± 7°	26° ± 6°	27° ± 6°	32° ± 4°	30° ± 3°
60+	30° ± 7°	28° ± 6°	22° ± 5°	20° ± 4°	28° ± 4°	30° ± 5°

in the total number of collagen fibers and in the ratio of type I to type II collagen; a decrease in water content; and changes in the proteoglycan content of the discs.[83] There is also an associated increase in "fatigue failure" of collagen in older cartilage. It is uncertain whether it is collagen fibers that undergo "fatigue" or splitting or whether it is the bonds between adjacent collagen fibers that separate. Collectively, these changes and the associated decrease in compliance render the disc fibrocartilage less capable of acting efficiently as a shock absorber or joint, and of transmitting loads along the vertebral column.[33,84,85]

Lumbar Intersegmental Motion

It is an essential part of a physical therapist's examination to determine ranges of movement of the whole lumbar spine. In addition to measurement of these physiologic ranges of movements, the manipulative physical therapist always conducts a manual assessment of lumbar intersegmental motion. This involves the passive displacement of a lumbar motion segment by the application of an external, manual force applied directly through the spinous processes, or indirectly via the ligaments and joints of the adjacent vertebrae. Small rotations and translations about and along the axes of movement can be achieved in this way (Fig. 2-8). No techniques are currently available to allow clinical estimates of increases or decreases in segmental motion to be objectively confirmed. However, although these techniques involve subjective evaluation of vertebral motion, it is interesting to note their excellent correlation with other current diagnostic studies.[39]

Many clinical reports have associated either hypo- or hypermobility with a variety of lumbar disorders and low back pain.[34] At this point in time, there is very little real evidence linking ranges of motion and back pain,[86] although anecdotal and clinical stories abound. Farrell and Twomey[80,81] in a study of acute low-back pain and manipulative therapy demonstrated an improvement in lumbar sagittal motion (measured manually) associated with improvement in back pain symptoms. Giles and Taylor[16] also showed increased lumbar range of movement following recovery from episodes of low back pain, but this increase was only observed in patients under the age of 50 years. Similarly, Jull[87] has shown an increase in intersegmental motion associated with remission of symptoms in patients with low back pain. This is in line with the study by Solomonov et al,[88] which shows a strong relationship between deep lumbar ligaments and muscles, wherein ligamentous damage brought about the recruitment of multifidus muscle to stiffen local motion segments and prevent instability.

BIOMECHANICS

The orientation of the lumbar articular processes facilitates sagittal movement and allows for a considerable range of motion in this plane. From the "normal" erect standing posture, flexion usually comprises about 80 percent and extension 20 percent of the total range of sagittal movement. Flexion ceases due to apposition of lumbar zygapophyseal joint surfaces and tightening of posterior ligaments and muscles, while extension is blocked by bone contact when the inferior joint facets come into contact with the laminae of the vertebra below or the spinous processes meet.[33]

Control of Flexion

Muscular Control of Flexion

The lumbar back muscles exert considerable control over active ranges of lumbar movement (Chapter 4). Erector spinae and multifidis are principally responsible for all movements[89] by exerting an eccentric control (i.e., by paying out) on movements that are gravity assisted. Thus trunk flexion in standing or sitting is controlled by an eccentric contraction of these muscle groups. In exerting this control, the muscles tend to restrict the total range of movements possible, particularly in the sagittal plane.[32,64,78] This helps explain why cadaveric studies show a slightly greater range of lumbar sagittal movement than is usually recorded in the living.[6]

It has been shown that after suitable warm-up exercises, ranges of lumbar flexion increase by a few degrees,[32] and that a change in posture from the upright to the side-lying position brings about an additional increase, which equates with the ranges observed in the cadaveric studies. It would appear that warm-up exercises achieve their effect by relaxation or stretching of the sacrospinalis muscle group, and it is not unreasonable to assume that the slightly larger increase obtained in side lying is due to the elimination of antigravity activity in the long back muscles. Kippers and Parker[6] have shown an "electrically silent" phase in the back muscles at the limit of lumbar flexion. While they conclude that the spine is supported passively by tension in postvertebral connective tissue structures at this point, it may also be due in part to passive elastic tension of the posterior muscles themselves. Indeed, the apposed zygapophyseal facets play the greater restraining role.[33] It also appears that the speed of trunk movements does not affect the trunk flexion relaxation phenomenon.[90]

Each lumbar multifidus muscle attaches strongly to a mamillary process on a superior articular process and also into the capsule of a zygapophyseal joint. Its deep fascicles act like rotator cuff muscles and maintain the close approximation and congruity of the zygapophyseal facets on the posterolateral aspect of the joint. The elasticity of the ligamentum flavum maintains the close apposition of the articular surfaces on the anteromedial side of the joint. The close relation of the multifidus muscle to the posterior joint capsule and its similar innervation would readily explain how with other postvertebral muscles it could limit flexion and rotation in any painful condition of the joints.[88,91]

Other Factors Controlling Lumbar Flexion

In addition to the postvertebral muscles, the posterior elements of the lumbar spine consist of a complex ligamentous system and the articulating bony arches. Over the years there have been a number of conflicting views on the relative roles played by these posterior elements in limiting and controlling the range of lumbar flexion. In general, it has been considered that the interspinous and supraspinous ligaments and the strong elastic ligamentum flavum served principally to act as a "brake" to flexion.[92] In this regard, the elasticity of the ligamentum flavum was seen as important because tension increased as the movement continued, while the dense, strong, and inelastic inter- and supraspinous ligaments acted as a physical barrier to the movement.

Adams, Hutton, and Stott[93] in a sequential posterior release experiment quantitated the relative parts played by the supraspinous-infraspinous ligaments, the ligamentum flavum, the zygapophyseal joint fibrous capsule, and the intervertebral disc in resisting flexion of individual motion segments. They showed that the joint fibrous capsule and intervertebral disc play the more important roles, with the ligamentum flavum and spinous ligaments making lesser contributions. They found it most surprising that the relatively unimpressive fibrous capsule should exert such large restraining forces, and noted that technical problems in sectioning all capsular fibers made it difficult to distinguish the role of capsular forces from articular facet forces exerted through the articular processes.

In the authors' study[33] of the role of the posterior elements, each of the posterior ligaments was sectioned in turn (supraspinous and interspinous ligaments, ligamentum flavum, and capsule), as were the pedicles, to assess the influence of each on the range of lumbar flexion. The range of flexion was measured before and after sectioning each of the elements and the results are listed in Table 2-2. Analysis demonstrated small regular increases in sagittal range on each successive ligamentous release and a large abrupt in-

Table 2-2 Average Increases (Degrees) in Sagittal Range Following Section

Section	Flexion Increase	Extension Increase	Sagittal Range Increase
Supraspinous and interspinous ligaments	2.0	1.5	3.5
Ligamenta flava	2.5	1.0	3.5
Joint capsules	3.0	2.0	5.0
Pedicles	14.0	3.0	17.0

crease in range following section of the vertebral arches (pedicles). Young and middle-age subjects showed almost a 100 percent increase in lumbar sagittal range after removal of all posterior elements, while elderly subjects showed a 60 percent increase (Fig. 2-11).

This study confirms that all the ligamentous elements offer some resistance to lumbar flexion, with the joint capsules having the greatest ligamentous influence, as suggested by Adams, Hutton, and Stott.[93] However, by far the greatest restraining influence on flexion is the increasing pressure between the apposed articular facets during flexion of the zygapophyseal joints. Radiographic analysis of flexion in a young cadaveric lumbar spine showed that the movement includes both forward rotation of a vertebra on the vertebra beneath and along an axis in the posterior part of the intervertebral disc, and an associated forward translation or slide of the superior vertebrae on the inferior vertebra (Fig. 2-12). The zygapophyseal joints guide

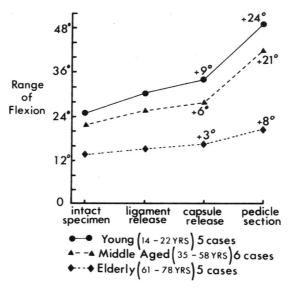

Fig. 2-11 The effects of the release of the posterior vertebral elements on the range of lumbar flexion. (From Twomey and Taylor[33] with permission.)

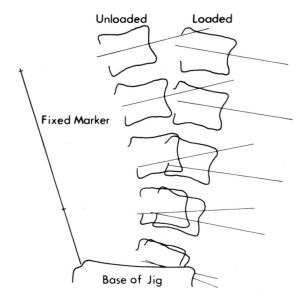

Unloaded   Loaded

Fixed Marker

Base of Jig

Fig. 2-12 Tracings of superimposed radiographic plates showing the range of flexion produced and indicating the types of movement involved. (From Twomey and Taylor[33] with permission.)

the plane of rotation and resist the forward slide. The coronally oriented anterior component of each articular facet bears the resultant load. When the pedicles are cut, a greater degree of forward slide permits further rotation into flexion.

Joint loading in axial weightbearing has been described by Nachemson[94] and by Shah, Hampson, and Jayson.[95] It seems clear from our studies that flexion involves progressive joint loading to the point where the horizontal moment prevents further rotation from occurring. The lumbar vertebral arches through the zygapophyseal joints thus provide an essential restraint limiting the transmission of shearing forces to the intervertebral discs. Excessive shearing could damage the annular fibers of the disc and lead to instability (as in spondylolisthesis).

Age differences in response to the posterior sectioning procedure cited above throw light on the effect of increased stiffness with aging in the intervertebral discs. Following ligamentous release and also more dramatically following pedicle section, the available increase in movement range is much reduced in elderly subjects compared with young subjects. This demonstrates that the increased stiffness or the reduction in disc compliance with aging is the principal reason for the observed age-related decrease in lumbar ranges of movement. The important conclusions drawn from the studies described above are summarized below:

1.   Lumbar flexion involves both forward rotation and slide of one vertebra on the vertebra beneath around a coronal axis located in the posterior anulus of the intervertebral disc.

2.   Flexion of the lumbar vertebral column is restricted more by progressive increase in loading of apposed facetal joint surfaces than by tension in posterior ligaments.

3.   The decline in sagittal range of movement in old age is principally due to increasing stiffness in the intervertebral disc.

"Creep" in the Lumbar Spine

We have argued above that the stiffness in intervertebral discs and the progressive loading of the zygapophyseal joints are the principal factors bringing the normal range of flexion to a halt. However, prolonged loading in flexion (10 minutes or more) does produce further flexion of the spine. This movement is due to "creep," which is the progressive deformation of a structure under constant load when the forces are not large enough to cause permanent damage to the vertebral structures.

Axial "Creep"

In the normal erect posture, approximately 16 to 20 percent of axial compressive load on the lumbar spine is borne by the zygapophyseal joints, while the rest is carried by the intervertebral discs,[94,96] which are well suited to this purpose. When axial loads to intervertebral discs are maintained, the discs progressively lose height until the chemical forces developed within them equal those mechanical forces applied externally.[97] Provided that the forces used are below the levels that would cause permanent damage, the greater the external force, the greater the loss of height that occurs.[97,98]

During the day, a person's body weight acts as an axial compression force through the vertebral column, and the subsequent "creep" brings about a reduction in stature. When body weight is relieved in recumbent posture and axial loading is reduced, the intervertebral discs and other soft tissues are able to rehydrate and stature increases.[99] It has recently been demonstrated that a period of recumbent rest in full flexion brings about a more rapid increase in stature than does rest in the fully extended position.[27] This presumably occurs because flexion acts as a distracting force on the lumbar region, causing the discs to "suck in" water at a greater rate.

"Creep" in Flexion

When full-range lumbar flexion is maintained under load for a period of time, the articular triad is distorted so that the anterior disc region is "squeezed" while its posterior region is stretched; the zygapophyseal joint surfaces are compressed tightly together as the coronal part of the articular surfaces bear most of the load; and the soft tissues adjust by "creep."[94,97,98,100]

"Creep" in flexion is observed as progressive ventral movement into further flexion, so that the end point of flexion is increased (i.e., range increases). The amount of "creep" in the elderly is greater than in the young and both the "creep" and the recovery from "creep" take place over a longer period of time. This age-related increase in creep is associated with a reduced water-binding capacity in the disc proteoglycans with aging. During the creep process, fluid is extruded from the soft tissues and they become relatively deprived of their nutrition.[101] Repetitive loading causes cartilage degeneration and bone hypertrophy in the various elements of the articular triad.[102]

If the amount of "creep" involved after prolonged loadbearing in flexion is considerable, then recovery back to the original starting posture (hysteresis) is extremely slow. It takes a considerable time for the soft tissues to imbibe fluid after it has been expressed during prolonged flexion loading. Many occupational groups (e.g., stonemasons, bricklayers, roofing carpenters, and so on) regularly submit their lumbar spines to this category of insult. They work with their lumbar column fully flexed and under load for considerable periods of time. There is often little movement away from the fully flexed position once it has been reached and little opportunity for recovery between episodes of work in this position. It is therefore not at all surprising to find so many bricklayers, for instance, with chronic back pain and with recurrent episodes of acute pain. These occupational groups need considerable ergonomic advice and require alterations to their working conditions if this situation is to be rectified.[98]

Control of Extension

The Role of Muscles

The control of lumbar extension has not been investigated and analyzed to the same extent as flexion. In the erect standing or sitting postures, the movement is initiated by contraction of the long back-extensor muscles, and then controlled by the eccentric contraction of the abdominal muscle group once the movement has begun. The range of extension from the neutral erect standing position is much less than the range of flexion, but the muscular control mechanisms are very similar.

Other Contributing Factors

It seems probable that the range of extension is not controlled by ligamentous tension, but that it ceases when the two inferior articular processes at any level are forced against the laminae of the vertebrae below or perhaps when the spinous processes "kiss." This is witnessed by the build-up in compact bone, which is evident in the lamina of the inferior joint recess, beneath the inferior process. Extension occurs along an axis in the posterior part of the intervertebral disc at that level. This position probably does not place the soft tissues under the same constant strain as flexion does except at the limits of lordosis after prolonged standing, when zygapophyseal joints probably take a larger amount of the load of body weight. When hyperextension occurs, it is likely that the axis of movement shifts even further posteriorly and is located where the tips of the inferior facets articulate with the laminae. This would cause stretching of the anterior soft tissues, notably the anterior longitudinal ligament and the anterior annulus fibrosus, which are extremely strong and capable of withstanding such forces. It is apparent from our investigations that considerable osteoarthritic change takes place in the articular cartilage and subchondral bone. This change occurs at the polar region of the inferior recesses of the zygapophyseal joints corresponding to the areas of extension impact and compression.[102]

Loading in Extension

Prolonged maintenance of an extended posture or of constant loading in extension is rare, and few if any occupational groups have such a working situation. However, there has been at least one in-vitro study which examined extension creep in the lumbar spine.[103] This investigation recorded a characteristic creep response and also the important role of the zygapophyseal joints in limiting extension. The position of the line of gravity is described as passing anterior to the thoracic vertebrae and through the lumbar vertebrae.[104] Theoretically, prolonged standing, (i.e., axial loading with body weight) would tend to increase thoracic kyphosis (by "creep") but not alter lumbar lordosis. However, present evidence indicates that in prolonged standing there is a tendency for the axial load of body weight to increase lumbar lordosis. In this way, the zygapophyseal joints will take an increasing proportion of the load of body weight. Although long, continued lordotic posture and loading are rare, a number of sports activities involve full extension movements of an explosive nature. These may be repetitive movements and may involve high peaks of loading in full extension. Thus, fast bowlers in cricket, gymnasts, and high jumpers are three groups who place tremendous impact forces through this posterior arch complex. At heel strike during these sports, the chisel-like inferior articular processes are forced down suddenly into the laminae of the vertebrae below. The forces involved are very considerable, as the load borne by the facets increases dramatically with the amount of extension of the region.[105] Repetition over long periods of time results in soft-tissue inflammation and bone sclerosis that may become obvious on radiographic examination, but which may later result in fracture and perhaps displacement. The bone area that absorbs this force is the isthmus between the upper and lower zygapophyseal facets of each vertebra, i.e., the pars interarticularis. As is well known, this is the site at which spondylolysis occurs. It is even more likely that the repetitive combination of alternative explosive full extension followed suddenly by full flexion places enormous strain on the pars interarticularis region. This extension/flexion repetition moment at the pars may cause fatigue fracture in a similar way to that of fatigue in metal caused by successive bending in opposite directions.[96]

VULNERABILITY OF THE DISC TO LOADING: INTRADISCAL PRESSURE

The nucleus of the intervertebral disc is contained under pressure within its protective fibrous and cartilaginous envelope. Intradiscal pressure is a useful index of disc function and has been shown to vary according to posture, movement, external loading, and age. Nachemson's[94] comprehensive study on lumbar intradiscal pressure in 128 discs from 38 cadavers of both sexes from 6 to 82 years concluded the following:

1.   The loaded disc behaves hydrostatically in that the nucleus acts as a fluid, distributing external pressures equally in all outward directions to the annulus.

2.   Axial loading produces lower pressure readings in children below the age of 16 years than in adults.

3.   The level of the lumbar spine does not influence the pressures recorded in "loaded" or resting discs (the L5-S1 disc was not included in the study).

4.   The posterior vertebral structures (pedicles and articular processes) absorb 16 to 20 percent of the axial loading forces.

5.   "Moderately degenerated" discs (as suggested by disc "thinning") show similar pressure behavior to "intact" discs, and the mechanical behavior of a lumbar disc does not change appreciably provided "degeneration" is not advanced.

Since Nachemson's[94] original study, it has been shown in living subjects that intradiscal pressures are higher in the sitting than the standing posture[106,107]; they are less in the physiologic lordotic posture than in the straight or kyphotic posture[107]; pressures are increased with passive lumbar flexion of 20°[108]; they are further increased during active trunk flexion exercises[109]; and the largest increases accompany heavy lifting, particularly when the Valsalva maneuver is performed.[110] Nachemson, Schultz, and Berkson[30] and Merriam et al[111] showed that abnormal degenerated discs did not behave in a consistent way, as they showed patterns of pressure changes in different postures that were often dissimilar from those shown by normal discs. Similarly, other studies have shown that the ability of the disc to withstand compressive forces depends on both the integrity of the disc envelope and the turgor of the contained nucleus pulposus.[55,112,113] This contrasts with the claim of Belytschko et al[114] that in a theoretic model annular tears would reduce intradiscal pressures more than degenerative nuclear lesions.

Clinical Considerations

The effects of different postures, exercises, and loading conditions on intradiscal pressure are of interest to the physical therapist as an indicator of how the disc responds to these variables and of the possible abnormal response in disc degeneration. However, intradiscal pressure alone does not appear to be able to indicate which activities are likely to be either safe or dangerous for a patient's back. Although it is probably important to take the environmental condition of the disc into account when prescribing exercise, as yet there are no clear indications that any particular exercises are contraindicated on the grounds that a rise in intradiscal pressure would be prejudicial to the disc or risk injury to the vertebral end-plates.

It is quite clear that movements such as lumbar flexion and lateral bending and tasks such as the lifting of heavy weights increase intradiscal pressure. For this reason, many clinicians approach these activities with considerable care and watch their patients very carefully when they begin such activities. Similarly, patients need to be aware of the effect of these activities on their lumbar spine and approach tasks that involve rises in intradiscal pressure with reasonable care. In the same way, since it is known that intradiscal pressure is lowest in supine and prone lying, is lower in standing than in sitting, and remains quite low in activities involving lumbar extension and rotation, then some clinicians may wish to utilize this information in the exercise programs they prescribe. While this may be useful, no direct link has yet been established between a rise in intradiscal pressure and the production of a disc lesion. Similarly, ergonomic advice as to lifting technique, seat design (including car seat design), working posture, and activities of daily living that emphasizes the maintenance of a lordosis is often given on the basis of the effects of these tasks on intradiscal pressure. It still remains uncertain just what role raised intradiscal pressure may play in the production of disc lesions and low back pain or whether reduced pressure may prevent disc lesions. Therefore it remains an interesting observation that may ultimately prove to be of practical use, but at present its relevance is uncertain.

THE INFLUENCE OF INTRATRUNCAL PRESSURE

Intrathoracic and intra-abdominal pressure have been considered to be important in relieving the spine of a large part of the axial compression and shear loads by converting the trunk into a more solid cylinder and transmitting part of the load over the wider area. It was considered highly likely that intra-abdominal pressure exerted a major force in this regard by the simultaneous contraction of abdominal muscles, the diaphragm, and the muscles of the pelvic diaphragm. These are mostly transverse and obliquely oriented muscles, all capable of exerting considerable torque and compressive force on the cavity they enclose.

The thoracic spine bears less weight than the lumbar spine and is supported ventrally and laterally by the physical presence of the ribs and to a lesser extent, when the glottis is closed, by a rise in intrathoracic pressure. The role of intra-abdominal pressure in reducing forces acting on the spine and protecting vulnerable vertebral bodies and intervertebral discs from excessive loading was initially investigated by Bartelink[115] and since then has excited the imagination of other researchers.[110–126]

Contraction of the muscles of the trunk cavity to raise intra-abdominal pressure probably functions as a protective reflex mechanism, both to protect abdominal viscera from damage by a blow and to assist in protecting the vertebral column from excessive loading. Thus, when loads are placed on the vertebral column, the muscles are involuntarily called into action to fix the rib cage and to restrain and compress the contents of the abdominal cavity so that it becomes like a "balloon".[119] The positions of the trunk and the load influence the extent of any rise in intra-abdominal pressure. The more the spine is flexed and the further the load is away from the body the greater is the increase in intra-abdominal pressure required to balance the load and help distribute the compression forces.

The mechanism may be compared to an inflated balloon, which acts on an anterior moment arm two or three times the length of the posterior moment arm of the back extensor muscles. Pressures generated in the abdominal cavity will produce a net positive moment, and tend to restore the lordotic curvature of the lumbar spine. This will counteract the flexion moments produced by the upper body and the anterior load carried. Eie[118] described the relieving force of intra-abdominal pressure as reducing by about 40 percent the required compressive effect of the contraction force of the erector spinae muscles.

However, other studies have clearly shown that the effect is nowhere near as substantial as had been claimed.[30] They have shown a much smaller relieving net effect due to intratruncal pressure and have also demonstrated that there is not a linear relationship between the increase in intratruncal pressure and the strength of contraction of the abdominal musculature.[30,121]

Intra-abdominal pressure thus plays a small role in stabilizing the spine and pelvis at the onset of the lift by resisting trunk flexion, although it may do little to reduce intervertebral compression forces. This helps allow the pelvis to be rotated backward and the lumbar curve to be flattened by the powerful gluteal and hamstring muscles, which have a longer moment arm and a greater cross sectional area (and thus power) than do the spinal extensors. Thus they are the most suitable and capable muscles to be recruited in initiating the task of heavy lifting,[122] help to reduce the moment of the load, bring about abdominal hollowing[120] and allow the erector spinae muscles to take over and extend the spine on a stable pelvis.[123]

While the suggested ability of intratruncal pressure to relieve loads acting on the lumbar spine received significant support in the 30 years since Bartelink,[115] there are currently many questions raised about its validity. These have arisen because studies of lifting have not demonstrated sufficiently large rises in intra-abdominal pressure that correlate with either the size of the load being lifted or the stresses measured on the vertebral column.[30,110,121,124] Similarly, increasing intra-abdominal pressure by using the Valsalva maneuver may actually increase the load on the lumbar spine, while strengthening abdominal muscles in normal people or in those with back pain does not appear to increase the capacity to raise intra-abdominal pressure as measured during lifting.[30,110,121,124] It should also be taken into account that it has been clearly shown that to raise intra-abdominal pressure high enough to generate a sufficient antiflexor moment, the pressure would be so high as to obstruct blood flow in the vena cava and abdominal aorta,[125] a point which Bartelink[111] noted in his early study.

The lowest intra-abdominal pressures have been recorded in the smallest people while largest pressures are evident in taller, heavier subjects.[123] Strong athletes are able to produce enormous rises in intra-abdominal pressure.[124] Gait shows phasic changes in this pressure, with increases as the speed of the activity increases. Jumping in place or from a height raises the pressure, as do pushing and pulling activities. It is uncertain whether or not the Valsalva maneuver or the use of a lumbosacral corset does any more than produce marginal increases in intra-abdominal pressure.

More recently, Mueller et al[126] have shown a relationship between intramuscular pressure movements in the erector spinae and body posture, with little change in intra-abdominal pressure. This is presumed to help explain the protective trunk "stiffening" which occurs during lifting without an associated rise in intra-abdominal pressure.

Clinical Considerations

In the past, intra-abdominal pressure was considered to be a potent influence for reducing the loads applied to the spine. This rationale was used to explain the need for the development of strong abdominal musculature surrounding the abdomino-pelvic cavity. However, other research has demonstrated that intra-abdominal pressure does not dramatically reduce loads on the spine. The previous estimate of the loads generated at the L5-S1 junction during maximal lifting were an overestimate, and the back musculature has been shown to be stronger and able to generate a considerably greater power than was first estimated.[121] These observations, together with a greater understanding of the role of the thoracolumbar fascia in assisting in distributing a small percentage of the load and in "tying" the long back muscles down (Chapter 4) has meant that the inherent strength of the back mechanism as a whole is better recognized. Similarly, Waddell[127] has demonstrated that those with back pain respond very favorably to programs of intensive exercise, including a strong trunk strengthening program. This adds weight to the argument that musculoskeletal fitness is a major factor in the management of back pain and lifting disorders. The role of intra-abdominal pressure in this equation is now under serious debate and would benefit from further research. It may well be that improvements in abdominal muscle strength achieve their effect through the better control of pelvic and spinal posture rather than by a greater capacity to raise intra-abdominal pressure.

ZYGAPOPHYSEAL JOINT INTRACAPSULAR PRESSURE

In 1983, physical therapists Giovanelli, Thompson, and Elvey[128] conducted a pilot trial investigating lumbar zygapophyseal intracapsular joint pressures in living subjects. They placed two needles within the joint under radiographic control, one needle to inject saline and the other to record pressure changes. They showed that there is no intracapsular pressure at rest. Once fluid was injected into the joint, most active and passive movements caused a drop in the pressure produced by the injection, the pressure rising again on return to the starting position. The greatest drops in pressure occurred when passive techniques were directed specifically to the joint concerned. This highlighted a possible mechanism of pain relief by the use of localized manipulative and mobilizing techniques because raised intracapsular pressure with outpouring of fluid may result from some forms of joint pathology. This pilot trial has never been extended and thus too much regard should not be placed on its conclusions, but it does provide interesting information useful to the manipulative physical therapist on the ways in which manipulative techniques directly influence the joints moved. The anatomic studies of the fat pads of the lumbar facet polar recesses show that in movement, the fat moves in and out of the joint in response to any changes in pressure.

SKELETAL HEALTH AND EXERCISE

As described in Chapter 1, the internal architecture of lumbar vertebrae consists of vertical bony trabeculae (beams or struts of bone) supported by horizontal trabeculae, which are aligned parallel to the lines of stress. Thus the vertical trabeculae absorb the axial loads of weightbearing and transmit the load downward and outward to the vertebral shell via the transverse trabeculae, which resist buckling of the vertical weight-bearing beams. It is likely that the horizontal trabeculae are also important in absorbing and transmitting the lateral forces applied through the body as a consequence of muscular activity. Old age is associated with a significant selective decline in the numbers of horizontal trabeculae. The compressive load of body weight, which is usually maintained in old age, brings about fractures of the now less-well-supported vertical trabeculae, with collapse of the vertebral endplate. Lumbar vertebrae become shorter and wider in old age, and more concave at the disc-vertebral junction.[129] This pattern of selective bone loss and associated changes in vertebral body shape is part of the general picture of osteopenia and osteoporosis seen in the elderly. In western society at age 65, radiographic comparison with a "standard" suggests that 66 percent of women and 22 percent of men have osteoporosis. In women the incidence increases by about 8 percent for each additional decade, whereas a large increase does not occur until after the age of 76 in men.[130] The principal sites of fracture and pain due to osteoporosis are the vertebral column, the distal radius, and the neck of the femur. It causes over 200,000 hip fractures annually in the United States, while pain and shortened stature accompanied by "dowager's hump" or hunchback in elderly women are major symptoms of advanced osteoporosis, which often lead to vertebral collapse and functional disability.[131]

The prevention of osteoporosis at present focuses on the need for relatively high levels of dietary calcium (1000 to 1200 mg per day), particularly in women, and for estrogen replacement therapy in some women.[132,133] Considerable attention has also been paid to the important role of exercise in prevention. Important studies by Aloia et al[134] and Smith et al[135] have shown bone gain to follow exercise even in the very elderly. Physical therapists concerned in the prevention and treatment of back pain and disability need to stress these factors with their middle-aged and elderly patients. There is no doubt that bone loss occurs in the absence of physical activity, and that bone hypertrophy follows increased exercise activity.[136] It is likely that the incidence of osteoporotic bone fractures in the elderly could be reduced if regular exercise was generally maintained into old age. This reduced risk of fracture may relate as much to the maintenance of muscle strength and neuromuscular coordination as to the associated maintenance of bone mass.

REFERENCES

1. Kendall FP, McCreary EK: Muscles, Testing & Function (3rd ed.). Williams & Wilkins, Baltimore, 1983
2. Schmorl G, Junghanns H: The Human Spine in Health and Disease (2nd ed.). Grune & Stratton, New York, 1971
3. Horak FB: Clinical measurement of postural control in adults. Phys Ther 67(12):1881,1987
4. Taylor JR: Growth of human I/V discs and vertebral bodies. J Anat 120:1, 49, 1975
5. Day JW, Smidt GL, Lehmann T: Effect of pelvic tilt on standing posture. Phys Therapy 64(4):510, 1984
6. Twomey LT: Age changes in the human lumbar spine. PhD thesis, University of Western Australia, Perth, 1981
7. Landau BR: Essential Human Anatomy and Physiology (2nd ed.). Scott, Foresman, Glenview, Illinois, 1980
8. Treanor WJ: Motions of the Hand & Foot. In Licht SH (Ed.): Therapeutic Exercise. Waverly Press, Baltimore, 1965
9. Opila KA, Wagner SS, Schiowit Z, Chen J: Postural alignment in barefoot and high heel stance. Spine 13(5):542, 1988
10. Youngman A, Elliott M: The effect of high heel shoes on lumbar lordosis. BAppSc project, Western Australian Institute of Technology, Perth, 1985
11. Romanes CJ: Cunningham's Textbook of Anatomy (11th ed.). Oxford University Press, Oxford, 1972
12. Taylor JR, Alexander R: BSc project, University of Western Australia, Perth (unpublished), 1983
13. Ostgaard HC, Andersson GBJ, Karlsson K: Prevalence of back pain in pregnancy. Spine 16(5):549,1991
14. Raine S, Twomey LT: Attributes and qualities of human posture and their relationship to musculoskeletal pain. Clin Rev Physical Rehabil Med 64:409, 1994
15. Hansson T, Sandstrom J, Roos B, et al: The bone mineral content of the lumbar spine in patients with chronic low back pain. Spine 10:158, 1985
16. Giles LGF, Taylor JR: Low back pain associated with leg length inequality. Spine 6(5):510, 1981
17. Willner S: A study of height, weight and menarche in girls with idiopathic structural scoliosis. Acta Orthop Scand 46:71, 1975
18. Taylor JR, Halliday M: Limb length asymmetry and growth. J Anat 126:634, 1978
19. Ingelmark BE, Lindstrom J: Asymmetries of the lower extremities and pelvis and their relationship to lumbar scoliosis. Acute Morphol Neerl Scand 5/6:227, 1963
20. Taylor JR, Slinger BS: Scoliosis screening and growth in Western Australian students. Med J Aust 1:475, 1980
21. Giles LGF, Taylor JR: Intra-articular synovial protrusions. Bull Hosp J Dis Orthop Inst 42(2):248, 1982
22. Giles LGF, Taylor JR: The effect of postural scoliosis on lumbar apophyseal joints. Scand J Rheumatol 13:209, 1984
23. Terjesen T, Benum P, Rossvoll I, et al: Leg length discrepancy measured by ultrasonography. Acta Orthop Scand 62(2):121, 1991
24. De Puky MD: Diurnal variation in stature. Acta Orthop Scand 6:338, 1935

25. Blackman J: Experimental error inherent in measuring the growing human being. In Boyd E (Ed.): Am J Phys Anthropol 13:389, 1924
26. Stone M, Taylor JR: Factors influencing stature. BSc anatomy dissertation, University of Western Australia, Perth, 1977
27. Tyrrell AR, Reilly T, Troup JDG: Circadian variation in stature and the effects of spinal loading. Spine 10(2):161, 1985
28. Adams MA, Hutton WC: The effect of posture on the lumbar spine. Bone Joint Surg 67B(4):625, 1985
29. Sullivan WE, Miles M: The lumbar segment of the vertebral column. Anat Rec 133:619, 1959
30. Nachemson AL, Schultz AB, Berkson MH: Mechanical properties of human lumbar spine motion segments. Spine 4(1):1, 1979
31. Twomey LT, Taylor JR: Age changes in the lumbar intervertebral discs. Acta Orthop Scand 56:496, 1985
32. Taylor JR, Twomey LT: Sagittal and horizontal plane movement of the human lumbar vertebral column in cadavers and in the living. Rheumatol Rehabil 19:223, 1980
33. Twomey LT, Taylor JR: Sagittal movements of the human lumbar vertebral column: A quantitative study of the role of the posterior vertebral elements. Arch Phys Med Rehabil 64:322, 1983
34. White AA, Panjabi MM: The Clinical Biomechanics of the Spine. JB Lippincott, Philadelphia, 1978
35. Vachalathiti R, Crosbie J, Smith R: Effects of age, gender and speed on three-dimensional lumbar spine kinematics. Aust J Physiol 41:245, 1995
36. Dunham WF: Ankylosing spondylitis: measurement of hip and spine movements. Br J Phys Med 12:126, 1949
37. Lindahl O: Determination of the sagittal mobility of the lumbar spine: A clinical method. Acta Orthop Scand 37:241,1966
38. Leighton JR: The Leighton flexometer and flexibility test. J Assoc Phys Ment Rehabil 20(3):86, 1966
39. Gregersen G, Lucas DB: An in vivo study of the axial rotation of the human thoraco-lumbar spine. J Bone Joint Surg 49A(2):247, 1967
40. Loebl WY: Measurement of spinal posture and range of spinal movement. Ann Phys Med 9:103, 1967
41. Loebl WY: Regional rotation of the spine. Rheumatol Rehabil 12:223, 1973
42. Macrae IF, Wright V: Measurement of back movement. Ann Rheum Dis 28:584, 1969
43. Moll JMH, Liyanage SP, Wright V: An objective clinical method to measure spinal extension. Rheum Phys Med 11:293, 1972
44. Moll J, Wright V: Measurement of Spinal Movement. In Jayson M (Ed.): The Lumbar Spine and Back Pain, Pitman Medical, Kent, 1976, p. 93
45. Wiles P: Movements of the lumbar vertebra during flexion and extension. Proc R Soc Med 28:647,1935
46. Gianturco C: A roentgen analysis of the motion of the lower lumbar vertebrae. Am J Roentogenol 52(3):261, 1944
47. Hasner E, Schalintzek M, Snorrason E: Roentgenological examination of the function of the lumbar spine. Acta Radiol 37:141, 1952
48. Tanz SS: Motion of the lumbar spine. A roentgenologic study. Am J Roentgenol 69(3):399, 1953
49. Rolander SD: Motion of the lumbar spine with special reference to the stabilizing effect of posterior fusion. Acta Orthop Scand (suppl) 90, 1966

50. Troup JDG, Hood CA, Chapman AE: Measurements of the sagittal mobility of the lumbar spine and hips. Ann Phys Med 9:308, 1967

51. Froning EC, Frohman B: Motion of the lumbosacral spine after laminectomy and spine fusion. J Bone Joint Surg 50A:5, 897, 1968

52. Virgin WJ: Experimental investigations into the physical properties of the intervertebral disc. J Bone Joint Surg 33B(4):607, 1951

53. Hirsch K: The reaction of the intervertebral discs to compression forces. J Bone Joint Surg 37A:1188, 1955

54. Hirsch K, Nachemson A: A new observation on the mechanical behaviour of lumbar discs. Acta Orthop Scand 23:254, 1954

55. Brown T, Hansen RJ, Yorra AJ: Some mechanical tests on the lumbosacral spine with particular reference to the intervertebral discs. J Bone Joint Surg 39A:5, 1135, 1957

56. Evans FG, Lissner HR: Biomechanical studies on the lumbar spine and pelvis. J Bone Joint Surg 41A:278, 1959

57. Roaf, R: Vertebral growth and its mechanical control. J Bone Joint Surg 42B:40, 1960

58. Galante JO: Tensile properties of the human lumbar annulus fibrosis. Acta Orthop Scand (suppl) 100:1, 1967

59. White AA: Analysis of the mechanics of the thoracic spine in man. Acta Orthop Scand (suppl) 127, 1969

60. Farfan HF, Cossette JW, Robertson GH, et al: The effects of torsion on the lumbar intervertebral joints: The role of torsion in the production of disc degeneration. J Bone Joint Surg 52A:468, 1970

61. King AI, Vulcan AP: Elastic deformation characteristics of the spine. J Biomech 4:413, 1971

62. Kazarian L: Dynamic response characteristics of the human lumbar vertebral column. Acta Orthop Scand suppl 146:1, 1972

63. Panjabi MM: Experimental determination of spinal motion segment behaviour. Orthop Clin North Am 8(1):169, 1977

64. Twomey LT, Taylor JR: Physical Therapy of the Low Back (2nd Ed.). Churchill Livingstone, New York, 1994

65. Keegan JJ: Alterations of the lumbar curve related to posture and seating. J Bone Joint Surg 35A:589, 1953

66. Davis PR, Troup JDG, Burnard JH: Movements of the thoracic and lumbar spine when lifting: A chrono-cyclophotographic study. J Anat 99(1):13, 1965

67. Schultz AB, Belytschko TP, Andriacchi TP, et al: Analog studies of forces in the human spine: Mechanical properties and motion segment behaviour. J Biomech 6:373, 1973

68. Panjabi MM: Three-dimensional mathematical model of the human spine structure. J Biomech 6:671, 1973

69. Belytschko TB, Andriacchi TP, Schultz AB, et al: Analog studies of forces in the human spine: Computational techniques. J Biomech 6:361, 1973

70. Panjabi MM, Brand RA, White AA: Mechanical properties of the human thoracic spine. J Bone Joint Surg 58A(5):642, 1976

71. Panjabi MM, Krag MH, White AA: Effects of preload on load displacement curves of the lumbar spine. Orthop Clin North Am 8:1, 181, 1977

72. Begg AG, Falconer MA: Plain radiographs in intraspinal protrusion of lumbar intervertebral discs: A correlation with operative findings. Br J Surg 36:225, 1949

73. Lovett RW: A contribution to the study of the mechanics of the spine. Am J Anat 2:457, 1902
74. Tondury G: Functional anatomy of the small joints of the spine. Ann de Med Phys 15:2, 1971
75. Kapandji IA: The Physiology of the Joints. (2nd Ed.). Vol. 3. Trunk and Vertebral Column. Churchill Livingstone, London, 1974
76. Lewin T, Moffett B, Viidik A: The morphology of lumbar synovial intervertebral joints. Acta Morphol Neerl Scand 4:229, 1961
77. Rissanen PM: The surgical anatomy and pathology of the supraspinous and interspinous ligaments of the lumbar spine with special reference to ligament ruptures. Acta Orthop Scand (suppl) 46, 1960
78. Bogduk N, Twomey LT: Clinical Anatomy of the Lumbar Spine. Churchill Livingstone, Melbourne, 1987
79. Lumsden RM, Morris JM: An in vivo study of axial rotation and immobilisation at the lumbosacral joint. J Bone Joint Surg SOA:1591, 1968
80. Farrell JP, Twomey LT: Acute low back pain: Comparison of two conservative treatment approaches. Med J Aust 1:160, 1982
81. Farrell J: A comparison of two conservative treatment approaches to acute low back pain. MAppSc thesis, Western Australian Institute of Technology, Perth, 1982
82. Nachemson A: Lumbar spine instability: A critical update and symposium summary. Spine 10(3):290, 1985
83. Adams P, Eyre DR, Muir H: Biomechanical aspects of development and ageing of human lumbar intervertebral discs. Rheum Rehabil 16:22, 1977
84. Bushell GR, Ghosh P, Taylor TFK, et al: Proteoglycan chemistry of the intervertebral disc. Clin Orthop 129:115, 1977
85. Nachemson AL: The lumbar spine: An orthopaedic challenge. Spine 1(1):59, 1976
86. Hilton RC, Ball J, Benn RT: In-vitro mobility of the lumbar spine. Ann Rheum Dis 38:378, 1979
87. Jull G: The changes with age in lumbar segmental motion as assessed by manual examination. Master's thesis, University of Queensland, Brisbane, 1985
88. Solomonov M, Zhou B-H, Harris M, et al: The ligaments—muscular stabilizing system of the spine. Spine 23:2552, 1998
89. Bogduk N, Macintosh JE, Pearcy MJ: A universal model of the lumbar back muscles in the upright position. Spine 17(8):897, 1992
90. Steventon C, Ng G: Effect of trunk flexion on flexion relaxation of erector spinae. Aust J Physiol 41:241, 1995
91. Quint U, Wilke HJ, Shirazi-Adl A, et al: Importance of intersegmental trunk muscles for stability of the lumbar spine. Spine 23:1937, 1998
92. Ramsey RH: The anatomy of the ligamenta flava. Clin Orthop 44:129, 1966
93. Adams MA, Hutton WC, Stott MA: The resistance to flexion of the lumbar intervertebral joint. Spine 5(3):245, 1980
94. Nachemson A: Lumbar intradiscal pressure. Acta Orthop Scand (suppl) 43, 1960
95. Shah JS, Hampson WGJ, Jayson MIV: The distribution of surface strain in the cadaveric lumbar spine. J Bone Joint Surg 60B(2):246, 1978
96. Miller JAA, Haderspeck KA, Schultz AB: Posterior element loads in lumbar motion segments. Spine 8(3):331, 1983
97. Kazarian LE: Creep characteristics of the human spinal column. Orthop Clin North Am 6(1):3, 1975

98. Twomey LT, Taylor JR, Oliver MJ: Sustained flexion loading, rapid extension loading of the lumbar spine and the physical therapy of related injuries. Physiother Pract 4:129, 1988

99. Shirazi-Adl A: Finite element simulation of changes in the fluid content of intervertebral discs. Spine 17(2):206, 1992

100. Twomey LT, Taylor JR: Flexion creep deformation and hysteresis in the lumbar vertebral column. Spine 7:2, 116, 1982

101. Adams MA, Hutton WC: The effect of posture on the fluid content of lumbar intervertebral discs. Spine 8(6):665, 1983

102. Twomey LT, Taylor JR: Age changes in the lumbar articular triad. Aust J Physiother 31(3):106, 1985

103. Oliver MJ, Twomey LT: Extension creep in the lumbar spine. Clin Biomech 10:361, 1995

104. Pearsall DJ, Reid JG: Line of gravity relative to upright vertebral posture. Clin Biomech 7:80, 1992

105. Yang KH, King AI: Mechanism of facet load transmission as a hypothesis for low back pain. Spine 9(6):557, 1984

106. Nachemson A, Morris JM: In vivo measurements of intradiscal pressure. J Bone Joint Surg 46A(5):1077, 1964

107. Andersson BJG, Ortengren R, Nachemson A, et al: Lumbar disc pressure and myoelectric back muscle activity during sitting. Scand J Rehabil Med 6:104, 1974

108. Nachemson A: The effect of forward bearing on lumbar intradiscal pressure. Acta Orthop Scand 35:314, 1965

109. Nachemson A, Elfstrom G: Intravital dynamic pressure measurements in lumbar discs. Scand J Rehabil Med (suppl) 1:1, 1970

110. Andersson BJG, Ortengren R, Nachemson A: Quantitative studies of back loads in lifting. Spine 1(3):178, 1976

111. Merriam WF, Quinnell RC, Stockdale HR, et al: The effect of postural changes on the inferred pressures within the nucleus pulposus during lumbar discography. Spine 9(4):406, 1984

112. Virgin WJ: Anatomical and pathological aspects of the intervertebral disc. Indian J Surg 20:113, 1958

113. Panjabi MM, Krag MH, Chung TQ: Effects of disc injury on mechanical behaviour of the human spine. Spine 9(7):707, 1984

114. Belytschko T, Kulak RF, Schultz AB, et al: Finite element stress analysis of an intervertebral disc. J Biomech 4:277, 1974

115. Bartelink DL: The role of abdominal pressure in relieving the pressure on the lumbar intervertebral discs. J Bone Joint Surg 39B(4):718, 1957

116. Morris JM, Lucas DB, Bresler B: Role of the trunk in stability of the spine. J Bone Joint Surg 43A(3):328, 1961

117. Davis PR, Troup JDG: Pressures in the trunk cavities when pulling, pushing, and lifting. Ergonomics 7:465, 1964

118. Eie N: Load capacity of the low back. J Oslo City Hosp 16:73, 1966

119. Kumar S, Davis PR: Lumbar vertebral innervation and intra-abdominal pressure. J Anat 114:47, 1973

120. Allison G, Kendle K, Roll S, et al: The role of the diaphragm during abdominal hollowing exercise. Aust J Physiol 44:95, 1998

121. McGill SM, Norman RW: Portioning of the L4-L5 dynamic movement into disc, ligamentous and muscular components during lifting. Spine 11(7):666, 1986

122. Davis PR, Stubbs DA, Ridd JE: Radio pills: Their use in monitoring back stress. J Med Eng Technol 1(4):209, 1977

123. Ortengren R, Andersson GBJ: Electromyographic studies of trunk muscles, with special reference to the functional anatomy of the lumbar spine. Spine 2(1):44, 1977

124. Ortengren R, Andersson GBJ, Nachemson AL: Studies of relationships between lumbar disc pressure, myoelectric back muscle activity and intra-abdominal pressure. Spine 6:98, 1981

125. Gracovetsky S, Farfan HF: The optimum spine. Spine 11(6):543, 1986

126. Mueller G, Morlock MM, Vollmer M, et al: Intramuscular pressure in the erector spinae and intra-abdominal pressure related to posture and load. Spine 23:2580, 1998

127. Waddell G: A new clinical model for the treatment of low back pain. Spine 12(7):632, 1987

128. Giovanelli B, Thompson E, Elvey R: Measurement of variations in lumbar zygapophyseal joint intracapsular pressure: A pilot study. Aust J Physiother 31(3):115, 1985

129. Twomey LT, Taylor JR, Furniss B: Age changes in the bone density and structure of the lumbar vertebral column. J Anat 136(1):15, 1983

130. Eisman JA: Osteoporosis: prevention, prevention and prevention. Current Therapeutics 33(2):25, 1992

131. Pardini A: Exercise, vitality and aging, Age Ageing 344:19, 1984

132. Dixon AStJ: Non hormonal treatment of osteoporosis. Br Med J 286:999, 1983

133. Spencer H, Kramer L, Lesniak M, et al: Calcium requirements in humans. Clin Orthop 184:270, 1984

134. Aloia JF, Cohn SH, Ostuni JA, et al: Prevention of involutional bone loss by exercise. J Clin Endocrinol Met 43:992, 1978

135. Smith EL, Reddan W, Smith PE: Physical activity and calcium modalities for bone mineral increase in aged women. Med Sci Sports Exerc 13:60, 1981

136. Menard D, Stanish WD: The aging athlete. Am J Sports Med 17(2):187, 1991

3

Innervation and Pain Patterns of the Lumbar Spine

Nikolai Bogduk

Two types of pain can arise from the lumbar spine: somatic pain, which is caused by noxious stimulation of structures or tissues intrinsic to the lumbar spine; and radicular pain, which is caused by irritation of the lumbar or sacral nerve roots that pass through the lumbar vertebral canal or intervertebral foramina. These two types of pain are distinct both in mechanism and clinical features, but confusion of the two is still quite common in contemporary clinical practice.

SOMATIC PAIN

Back pain can be caused by disorders of any of the components of the lumbar spine that receive an innervation. These are the vertebrae, the zygapophysial joints, the intervertebral discs, and the ligaments, muscles, and fasciae of the lumbar spine.

Innervation

Anterior Column

The anterior column of the lumbar spine consists of the vertebral bodies, the intervertebral discs, and the longitudinal ligaments. These structures are surrounded by extensive plexuses of fine nerves.[1] An anterior plexus follows the anterior longitudinal ligament (Fig. 3-1), and a posterior plexus follows the posterior longitudinal ligament (Fig. 3-2). A lesser plexus covers the lateral aspects of the intervertebral discs and vertebral bodies, deep to the psoas major muscle.

The anterior plexus is formed largely by branches of the lumbar sympathetic trunk.[1] The posterior plexus is formed by the lumbar sinuvertebral nerves, which are the recurrent meningeal branches of the lumbar ventral rami.[2] These are mixed nerves that are formed by somatic roots from the lumbar ventral rami and sympathetic roots that arise from the grey rami communicantes near where they join the ventral rami. The lateral plexus is

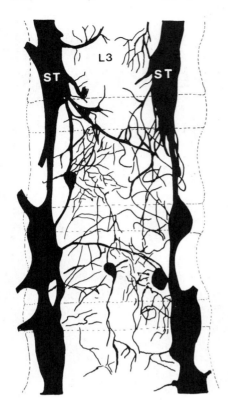

Fig. 3-1   The nerve plexus accompanying the anterior longitudinal ligament at the levels of the L3 and lower vertebrae, as seen in whole mounts of human fetuses. *ST,* lumbar sympathetic trunk. (Adapted from Groen et al,[1] as appeared in Bogduk N: Clinical Anatomy of the Lumbar Spine and Sacrum. (3rd ed.) Churchill-Livingstone, Edinburgh, 1997.)

Fig. 3-2   The nerve plexus accompanying the posterior longitudinal ligament at the levels of the L3 and lower vertebrae, as seen in whole mounts of human fetuses. The large fibers *(arrows)* represent the sinuvertebral nerves. (Adapted from Groen et al,[1] as appeared in Bogduk N: Clinical Anatomy of the Lumbar Spine and Sacrum. (3rd ed.) Churchill-Livingstone, Edinburgh, 1997.)

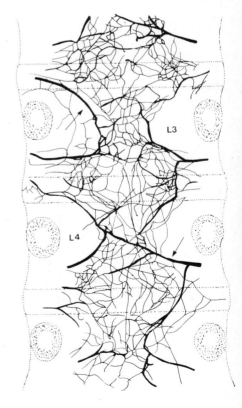

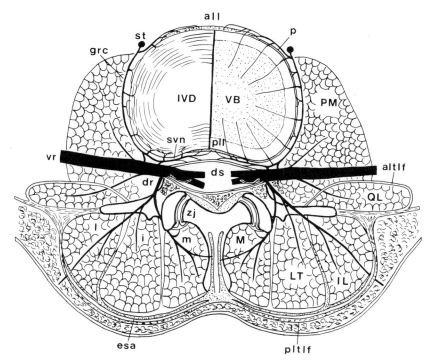

Fig. 3-3 Innervation of the lumbar spine. A cross-sectional view incorporating the level of the vertebral body *(VB)* and its periosteum *(p)* on the right, and the intervertebral disc *(IVD)* on the left. *PM,* psoas major; *QL,* quadratus lumborum; *IL,* iliocostalis lumborum; *LT,* longissimus thoracis; *M,* multifidus; *altlf,* anterior layer of thoracolumbar fascia; *pltlf,* posterior layer of thoracolumbar fascia; *esa,* erector spinae aponeurosis; *ds,* dural sac; *zj,* zygapophysial joint; *pll,* posterior longitudinal ligament; *all,* anterior longitudinal ligament; *vr,* ventral ramus; *dr,* dorsal ramus; *m,* medial branch; *I,* intermediate branch; *l,* lateral branch; *svn,* sinuvertebral nerve; *grc,* grey ramus communicans; *st,* sympathetic trunk. (From Bogduk N: Clinical Anatomy of the Lumbar Spine and Sacrum. (3rd ed.) Churchill-Livingstone, Edinburgh, 1997.)

formed by branches of the grey rami communicantes as they pass from the sympathetic trunks to the ventral rami.[1]

These plexuses innervate their respective longitudinal ligaments and furnish penetrating branches to the lumbar vertebral bodies and to the intervertebral discs (Fig. 3-3). Within the vertebral bodies, long nerves penetrate deeply into the cancellous bone accompanying the vessels that enter the vertebrae.[1,3] A particularly large leash of nerves enters with the basivertebral veins.[3] Within the vertebral body the nerves are widely distributed, most with blood vessels but some in isolation. Some nerve fibers terminate in the subchondral bone of the vertebral end-plate.[4]

Within the intervertebral discs, nerve fibers and nerve endings are abundant in the outermost layers of the annulus fibrosus but can be found regularly throughout the outer third of the annulus.[5,6,7] They are sparse in the middle third and absent in the inner third and in the nucleus pulposus of normal discs. In damaged discs the number of nerve fibers in deeper portions of the annulus, and even in the nucleus, may be increased as invading blood vessels in granulation tissue bring nerve fibers into the deeper portions of the disc.[8]

The disc is endowed with free endings, with complex unencapsulated endings, and with some encapsulated endings.[5,6,7] The latter are found on the outer surface of the disc, particularly in its lateral regions. The former are distributed within the substance of the annulus. Some are associated with blood vessels, but many are isolated. These nerve endings probably subserve a proprioceptive role, by monitoring tension within the annulus fibrosus, but can subserve nociception. They are endowed with the neuropeptides that are also characteristic of nociceptive nerve endings.[9,10]

As the sinuvertebral nerves enter their intervertebral foramina, they furnish posteriorly directed branches to the dura mater (see Fig. 3-3). Nerve endings are abundant in the dural sleeve of the lumbar nerve roots and in the ventral aspects of the dural sac.[1] A sparser innervation is found in the dorsal aspects of the sac.

Posterior Column

The posterior column of the lumbar spine consists of the neural arches of the lumbar vertebrae, their joints and ligaments, and the posterior back muscles. These structures are innervated by the posterior rami of the lumbar spinal nerves.[11] These rami issue from the intervertebral foramina and cross the superior border of the L2 to L5 transverse processes to enter the posterior compartment of the back. The L5 dorsal ramus crosses the superior border of the ala of the sacrum (Fig. 3-4).

Each lumbar dorsal ramus, at levels L1 to L4, divides into three branches (see Fig. 3-4). A lateral branch enters and supplies the iliocostalis lumborum muscle, and those branches from L1 to L3 typically emerge from the lateral border of this muscle to become cutaneous over the buttock. They constitute the superior clunial nerves. In some cases they may be joined by a cutaneous branch from L4. On emerging from the iliocostalis, these nerves pierce the posterior layer of thoracolumbar fascia and are probably the source of nerve endings in this fascia.[12]

The intermediate branches of the L1 to L4 dorsal rami enter the longissimus thoracis muscle and form an intersegmental plexus from which the muscle is supplied.[11] They remain entirely intramuscular.

The medial branches of the L1 to L4 dorsal rami pass around the root of the superior articular process at each level and under the mamillo-accessory ligament[13] to lie dorsal to the lamina. Eventually these nerves enter and supply the multifidus muscle, but each also supplies a branch to the interspinous muscle and ligament of its respective segment. The segmental distribution of the medial branches is such that each nerve supplies only those muscles that arise from the spinous process of the vertebra with the same segmental number as the nerve.[11,14] Each medial branch also supplies artic-

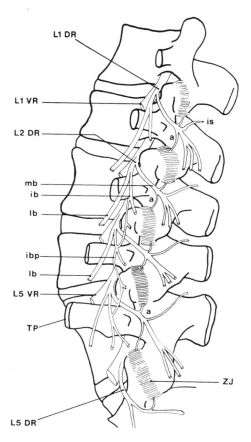

L1 DR

L1 VR

L2 DR

is

a

mb
ib

lb

a

ibp

lb

L5 VR

a

TP

ZJ

L5 DR

Fig. 3-4 Left posterolateral view of the lumbar dorsal rami showing the disposition of their branches. *VR,* ventral ramus; *DR,* dorsal ramus; *mb,* medial branch; *ib,* intermediate branch; *lb,* lateral branch; *ibp,* intermediate branch plexus; *is,* interspinous branch; *a,* articular branch; *ZJ,* zygapophysial joint. (From Bogduk N: Clinical Anatomy of the Lumbar Spine and Sacrum. (3rd ed.) Churchill-Livingstone, Edinburgh, 1997.)

ular branches to the zygapophysial joints above and below its course, so that the L_n medial branch supplies both the $L_n - L_{n+1}$ and the $L_{n-1} - L_n$ zygapophysial joints (see Fig. 3-4). The medial branches are also believed to innervate the thoracolumbar fascia overlying the multifidus[15] and are presumably the source of the few nerve endings found in the ligamentum flavum.

The L5 dorsal ramus differs in that it is a long nerve that crosses the ala of the sacrum, assuming a course that is analogous to that of the medial branch at higher levels, in that it runs along the root of the S1 superior articular process.[11] Opposite the caudal end of this process it divides into two branches: a medial branch that curves medially around the base of the articular process, to innervate the lumbosacral zygapophysial joint and finally to end in multifidus; and a second branch that is analogous to the intermediate branch of higher levels and ends in the longissimus.

The innervation of the iliolumbar ligament is not known. Its relationship to the quadratus lumborum suggests that it most likely derives its nerve supply from nerves in this muscle. However, the longissimus and iliocostalis muscles cover the ligament posteriorly, and an innervation from the lateral or intermediate branches of the L4 dorsal ramus seems possible.

SOMATIC REFERRED PAIN

Somatic referred pain is best defined as pain perceived in regions innervated by nerves other than those that innervate the actual source of pain. In some instances the zone of referral may be remote from the source of pain, or it may be adjacent to it.[16] For example, pain from the lumbar spine may be referred to the thigh or leg, or it may be referred only to the buttock. However, in both instances, the zone of referral is not supplied by the posterior rami or the longitudinal plexuses of the lumbar spine.

Somatic referred pain arises as a result of convergence.[17] Within the spinal cord, afferents from the lumbar spine synapse on second-order neurons that happen also to receive afferents from other regions, particularly those supplied by the ventral rami of the spinal nerves. The second-order neuron has no means to determine exactly which afferent stimulates it. It can only transmit to higher centers the information that it has been activated by nociceptive afferents. Consequently, the brain can interpret the information only as pain arising from somewhere in the tissues innervated by the spinal cord segment that provided the information. Thus the brain thinks not in terms of pain from the back or pain from the thigh, but in terms of pain somewhere in the L5 segment.

This explanation of somatic referred pain should be distinguished from the erroneous concept of sclerotomes. Based on maps of the distribution of referred pain in normal volunteers, some investigators[18] inferred that the maps indicated a segmental pattern of peripheral innervation of deep structures, analogous to myotomes and dermatomes. However, myotomes and dermatomes have an anatomical basis. By dissection, by electrophysiologic means, or by use of tracer substances, motor nerves from a given spinal cord segment can be traced to particular muscles, and sensory nerves from areas of skin can be traced back to the spinal cord segment. The same does not apply to deep, skeletal structures. No one has demonstrated anatomically or otherwise a segmental pattern of innervation of deep structures. Maps of sclerotomes are totally subjective and simply depict where volunteers report that they feel pain. This perception may have more to do with how their central nervous system is wired than with how peripheral nerves are distributed. However, these remarks do not reduce the clinical value of pain maps; they only dispute the traditional, inferred basis of those maps.

Experiments in normal volunteers have shown that somatic referred pain has characteristic features. It is perceived deeply and is dull and aching in quality, or like an expanding pressure. Its boundaries are hard to localize, but the subjects are well aware of where it is centered. Furthermore, somatic referred pain is not phasic or radiating. Once established it remains relatively fixed in its location. However, the area of perceived pain may increase in proportion to the intensity of the primary stimulus that evokes it. Thus pain generated by stimulating a lower lumbar zygapophysial joint may be centered fundamentally over the buttock, but if the stimulus is stronger, the pain extends into the lower limb.[19]

Any of the structures of the lumbar spine can in principle be a source of somatic referred pain. Indeed, explicit evidence is available to indicate that the dura mater, the back muscles, the interspinous ligaments, zygapophysial joints, and sacroiliac joints can be sources of somatic referred pain.

Dura

In volunteer patients the dura mater has been stimulated both chemically and mechanically. Chemical stimulation involved injection of hypertonic saline around the nerve root sleeves.[20] Mechanical stimulation involved pulling on sutures threaded through the dura, or pinching it with forceps, in patients undergoing spinal surgery under local anesthesia.[21,22] In all instances the same sort of pain was produced. It was dull and aching and felt deeply over the buttock. However, this distribution of pain is not diagnostic of dural pain. Rather, the dura is simply one possible source of somatic referred pain in the buttock. No clinical feature distinguishes dural pain.

Muscles

In normal volunteers, noxious stimulation of the lumbar back muscles with injections of hypertonic saline evokes both local pain and referred pain.[23,24] From study to study the distribution of this pain has varied, from the buttock and inguinal region, to the thigh, and even into the leg. In all instances, however, the character of the pain was that of somatic referred pain: deep, dull, and aching.

Ligaments

The interspinous ligaments have been the only ligaments studied for referred pain in normal volunteers. Stimulation of these ligaments with hypertonic saline produces deep, aching pain that extends into the buttock and lower limb.[25,26] Stimulation of ligaments at different segments produces a different distribution pain, suggesting a segmental relationship, but this relationship is not consistent. Different studies have described different patterns of referral from stimuli delivered at essentially the same site.

Zygapophysial Joints

Referred pain patterns from the lumbar zygapophysial joints have been extensively studied. These joints have been stimulated with injections of hypertonic saline,[19,27] and the medial branches that innervate them have been stimulated electrically.[28] The referred pain that is evoked tends to be focused over the ipsilateral buttock and proximal thigh, but more extensive distributions into the lower limb, and even to the foot, have been recorded. As with all other sources of referred pain from the lumbar spine, the pain from the zygapophysial joints is deep and aching.

Stimulation of joints at different segmental levels produces pain in different regions of the lower limb. However, there is no consistent segmental pattern.[27,28] Pain from high lumbar joints tends to be felt higher on the buttock, toward the iliac crest, whereas pain from lower segments tends to be felt lower in the buttock and into the lower limb. However, pain from adjacent segments cannot be reliably distinguished, and the location of referred pain is a poor guide as to the segmental level of its origin. No clinical feature distinguishes zygapophysial joint pain from any other source of somatic referred pain.[29,30,31]

Sacroiliac Joint

Although the sacroiliac joint is not a component of the lumbar spine, it is a nearby relation and a potent source of back pain. In normal volunteers, distending the joint with contrast medium evokes pain that is largely perceived over the buttock.[32] Clinically, however, this pain cannot be distinguished from other sources of somatic referred pain.[33,34,35]

Intervertebral Discs

Intervertebral discs have not been studied in normal volunteers as a source of lumbar spinal pain or referred pain. However, that they can be painful has been established through clinical observations. When affected by discitis, lumbar intervertebral discs are extremely painful,[36] which is evidence that the disc can be rendered painful. Furthermore, unpublished clinical experience in the practice of discography attests to the outer layers of the annulus fibrosus being pain-sensitive to needling.

Discography is not painful if the disc is normal.[37] This is understandable because discography involves stimulating the disc with an injection of contrast medium into the nucleus pulposus, which is not innervated.[38] For discography to be painful the innervated, outer layers of the annulus have to be distended. In a normal disc this is prevented by the intact inner layers of the annulus, which protect the outer layers from distention. Extreme pressures are required to overcome this resistance. However, discography is painful when the internal architecture of the disc is disrupted by radial fissures.[37,38,39] Such fissures occur only in damaged discs, and the presence of fissures correlates strongly with the disc being painful.[40,41] The pain evoked from a damaged disc is felt typically in the back, but may be referred into the buttock and even into the lower limb.

RADICULAR PAIN

Radicular pain is of a totally different character to somatic referred pain. Experiments in volunteer patients have shown that stimulating nerve roots mechanically, by pulling on suture threaded around them,[21] produces lancinating pain that travels along the length of the lower limb in a narrow band not more than a few centimeters wide. This pain differs both in quality and in distribution from somatic referred pain. It is lancinating or electric, as opposed to aching or pressure-like. The pain occurs in a linear distribution, along bands as opposed to wide regions, and it travels or shoots along the length of the lower limb as opposed to nestling in a relatively constant location.

The quality of radicular pain can be understood if its mechanism is understood. Radicular pain does not occur as a result of selective or exclusive stimulation of nociceptive afferent fibers. Traction, compression, or other stimuli of the nerve roots evoke discharges not only in C fibers and Aδ fibers but also in Aβ fibers.[42,43] Thus the patient suffers an afferent barrage in several types of fibers. They have a shocking sensation that they might refer to as pain, but some patients will explain that it is not like "normal" pain, or pain with which they have been familiar elsewhere in the body. The pain is more neuralgic and is related more to the pain of post-herpetic neuralgia than to somatic referred pain.

COMBINED STATES

It had been the convention to attribute any pain referred into the lower limb to disc prolapse compressing a lumbar or sacral nerve root. This inference ignored the experimental and clinical evidence on somatic referred pain. Indeed, somatic referred pain is not only a possible basis for pain in the lower limb but also far more common than radicular pain. Radicular pain occurs in fewer than 12% of patients presenting with a lumbar spine disorder.[44,45]

However, it is possible for both types of pain to occur concurrently. A patient may have a disorder that causes discogenic or zygapophysial joint pain, but the pathology might also secondarily impinge on a nerve root to cause radicular pain. Clinically, the immediate distinction may be difficult and requires analyzing the patient's symptoms carefully. Not all of the pain will be radicular in quality and distribution. Instead, the patient will have radicular pain superimposed on a background of somatic pain. The somatic pain will be deep, aching, and constant in location, whereas the radicular pain will be linear and radiating into the lower limb.

The reason for distinguishing somatic referred pain from radicular pain in combined states is so that misapprehensions about treatment do not arise. Treatment that might benefit radicular pain might not be appropriate for somatic pain, and vice versa. By recognizing that the patient has one or the other type of pain, or both, treatment can be selected specifically for each type of pain. Failure to do so may result in one pain being relieved but not the other. Under these circumstances, a treatment that should and does work for one type of pain may get an undeserved reputation of being ineffective, simply because it did not provide complete relief.

REFERENCES

1. Groen G, Baljet B, Drukker J: The nerves and nerve plexuses of the human vertebral column. Am J Anat 188:282–296, 1990
2. Bogduk N, Tynan W, Wilson AS: The nerve supply to the human lumbar intervertebral discs. J Anat 132:39–56, 1981
3. Antonacci MD, Mody DR, Heggeness MH: Innervation of the human vertebral body: a histologic study. J Spinal Disorders 11:536–531, 1998
4. Brown MF, Hukkanen MVJ, McCarthy ID, et al: Sensory and sympathetic innervation of the vertebral endplate in patients with degenerative disc disease. J Bone Joint Surg 79B: 147–153, 1997
5. Malinsky J: The ontogenetic development of nerve terminations in the intervertebral discs of man. Acta Anat 38:96–113, 1959
6. Rabischong P, Louis R, Vignaud J, Massare C: The intervertebral disc. Anat Clin 1:55–64, 1978
7. Yoshizawa H, O'Brien JP, Thomas-Smith W, Trumper M: The neuropathology of intervertebral discs removed for low-back pain. J Path 132:95–104, 1980
8. Freemont AJ, Peacock TE, Goupille P, et al: Nerve ingrowth into diseased intervertebral disc in chronic back pain. Lancet 350:178–181, 1997
9. Roberts S, Eisenstein SM, Menage J, et al: Mechanoreceptors in intervertebral discs: morphology, distribution, and neuropeptides. Spine 20:2645–2651, 1995
10. Ashton IK, Roberts S, Jaffray DC, et al: Neuropeptides in the human intervertebral disc. J Orthop Res 12:186–192, 1994
11. Bogduk N, Wilson AS, Tynan W: The human lumbar dorsal rami. J Anat 134:383–397, 1982
12. Yahia LH, Rhalmi S, Newman N, Isler M: Sensory innervation of human thoracolumbar fascia: an immunohistochemical study. Acta Orthop Scand 63:195–197, 1992
13. Bogduk N: The lumbar mamillo-accessory ligament. Its anatomical and neurosurgical significance. Spine 6:162–167, 1981
14. Macintosh JE, Valencia F, Bogduk N, Munro RR: The morphology of the lumbar multifidus muscles. Clin Biomech 1:196–204, 1986
15. Stillwell DL: The innervation of tendons and aponeuroses. Am J Anat 100:289–318, 1957
16. Merskey H, Bogduk N (Eds.): Classification of Chronic Pain. Descriptions of Chronic Pain Syndromes and Definitions of Pain Terms. (2nd ed.) IASP Press, Seattle, 1994
17. Gillette RG, Kramis RC, Roberts WJ: Characterization of spinal somatosensory neurons having receptive fields in lumbar tissues of cats. Pain 54:85–98, 1993
18. Inman VT, Saunders JBD: Referred pain from skeletal structure. J Nerv Ment Dis 99:660–667, 1944
19. Mooney V, Robertson J: The facet syndrome. Clin Orthop 115:149–156, 1976
20. El Mahdi MA, Latif FYA, Janko M: The spinal nerve root innervation, and a new concept of the clinicopathological interrelations in back pain and sciatica. Neurochirurgia 24:137–141, 1981
21. Smyth MJ, Wright V: Sciatica and the intervertebral disc. An experimental study. J Bone Joint Surg 40A:1401–1418, 1959
22. Norlen G: On the value of the neurological symptoms in sciatica for the localization of a lumbar disc herniation. Acta Chir Scand 95(Supp):1–96, 1944
23. Kellgren JH: Observations on referred pain arising from muscle. Clin Sci 3:175–190, 1938

24. Bogduk N: Lumbar dorsal ramus syndrome. Med J Aust 2:537–541, 1980
25. Kellgren JH: On the distribution of pain arising from deep somatic structures with charts of segmental pain areas. Clin Sci 4:35–46, 1939
26. Feinstein B, Langton JNK, Jameson RM, Schiller F: Experiments on pain referred from deep somatic tissues. J Bone Joint Surg 35A:981–987, 1954
27. McCall IW, Park WM, O'Brien JP: Induced pain referred from posterior lumbar elements in normal subjects. Spine 4:441–446, 1979
28. Fukui S, Ohseto K, Shiotani M, Ohno K, Karasawa H, Naganuma Y: Distribution of referred pain from the lumbar zygapophyseal joints and dorsal rami. Clin J Pain 13:303–307, 1997
29. Schwarzer AC, Aprill CN, Derby R, et al: Clinical features of patients with pain stemming from the lumbar zygapophysial joints. Is the lumbar facet syndrome a clinical entity? Spine 19:1132–1137, 1994
30. Schwarzer AC, Derby R, Aprill CN, et al: Pain from the lumbar zygapophysial joints: a test of two models. J Spinal Disord 7:331–336, 1994
31. Schwarzer AC, Wang S, Bogduk N, et al: Prevalence and clinical features of lumbar zygapophysial joint pain: a study in an Australian population with chronic low back pain. Ann Rheum Dis 54:100–106, 1995
32. Fortin JD, Dwyer AP, West S, Pier J. Sacroiliac joint: pain referral maps upon applying a new injection/arthrography technique. Part I: asymptomatic volunteers. Spine 19:1475–1482, 1994
33. Dreyfuss P, Michaelsen M, Pauza K, et al: The value of history and physical examination in diagnosing sacroiliac joint pain. Spine 21:2594–2602, 1996
34. Schwarzer AC, Aprill CN, Bogduk N: The sacroiliac joint in chronic low back pain. Spine 20:31–37, 1995
35. Maigne JY, Aivaliklis A, Pfefer F: Results of sacroiliac joint double block and value of sacroiliac pain provocation tests in 54 patients with low-back pain. Spine 21:1889–1892, 1996
36. Bogduk N: The lumbar disc and low back pain. Neurosurg Clin North Am 2:791–806, 1991
37. Walsh TR, Weinstein JN, Spratt KF, et al: Lumbar discography in normal subjects. J Bone Joint Surg 72A:1081–1088, 1990
38. Bogduk N, Aprill C, Derby R: Discography. In White AH (Ed.): Spine Care. Vol. 1. Diagnosis and Conservative Treatment. Mosby, St Louis, 1995
39. Schwarzer AC, Aprill CN, Derby R, et al: The prevalence and clinical features of internal disc disruption in patients with chronic low back pain. Spine 20:1878–1883, 1995
40. Vanharanta H, Sachs BL, Spivey MA, et al: The relationship of pain provocation to lumbar disc deterioration as seen by CT/discography. Spine 12:295–298, 1987
41. Moneta GB, Videman T, Kaivanto K, et al: Reported pain during lumbar discography as a function of anular ruptures and disc degeneration. A re-analysis of 833 discograms. Spine 17:1968–1974, 1994
42. Howe JF: A neurophysiological basis for the radicular pain of nerve root compression. In Bonica JJ, Liebeskind JC, Albe-Fessard DG (Eds.): Advances in Pain Research and Therapy. Vol. 3. Raven Press, New York, 1979
43. Howe JF, Loeser JD, Calvin WH: Mechanosensitivity of dorsal root ganglia and chronically injured axons: a physiological basis for the radicular pain of nerve root compression. Pain 3:25–41, 1977
44. Mooney V: Where is the pain coming from? Spine 12:754–759, 1987
45. Deyo RA, Tsui-Wu YJ: Descriptive epidemiology of low-back pain and its related medical care in the United States. Spine 12:264–268, 1987

4

The Lumbar Muscles and Their Fascia

Nikolai Bogduk

The lumbar spine is surrounded by muscles that, for descriptive purposes and on functional grounds, may be divided into three groups. These are:

1. Psoas major, which covers the anterolateral aspects of the lumbar spine.

2. Intertransversarii laterales and quadratus lumborum, which connect and cover the transverse processes anteriorly.

3. The lumbar back muscles, which lie behind and cover the posterior elements of the lumbar spine.

PSOAS MAJOR

The psoas major is a long muscle that arises from the anterolateral aspect of the lumbar spine and descends over the brim of the pelvis to insert into the lesser trochanter of the femur. It is essentially a muscle of the thigh whose principal action is flexion of the hip.

The psoas major has diverse but systematic attachments to the lumbar spine (Fig. 4-1). At each segmental level, from T12-L1 to L4–5, it is attached to the medial three quarters or so of the anterior surface of the transverse process, to the intervertebral disc, and to the margins of the vertebral bodies adjacent to the disc.[1] An additional fascicle arises from the L5 vertebral body. Classically, the muscle is said to arise also from a tendinous arch that covers the lateral aspect of the vertebral body.[2] However, close dissection[1] reveals that these arches constitute no more than the medial, deep fascia of the muscle, and that the fascia affords no particular additional origin; the most medial fibers of the muscle skirt the fascia and are anchored directly to the upper margin of the vertebral body. Nonetheless, the fascia forms an arcade deep to the psoas, over the lateral surface of the vertebral body, leaving a space between the arch and the bone. This space transmits the lumbar arteries and veins.

The muscle fibers from the L4–5 intervertebral disc, the L5 body, and the L5 transverse process form the deepest and lowest bundle of fibers within the muscle. These fibers are systematically overlapped by fibers from the

105

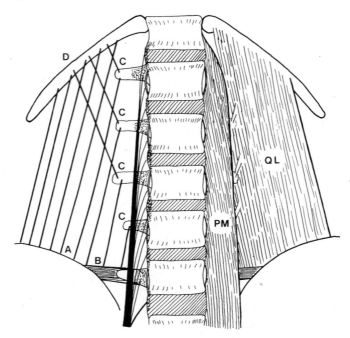

Fig. 4-1   Psoas major *(PM)* and quadratus lumborum *(QL)*. At each segmental level psoas major attaches to the transverse process, the intervertebral disc, and adjacent vertebral margins. The attachments of quadratus lumborum are to the iliac crest (A), the iliolumbar ligament (B), the transverse processes (C), and the 12th rib (D). (Reproduced, with permission, from Bogduk N: Clinical Anatomy of the Lumbar Spine and Sacrum. (3rd ed.) Churchill Livingstone, Edinburgh, 1997.)

disc, vertebral margins, and transverse process at successively higher levels. As a result, the muscle in cross-section is layered circumferentially, with fibers from higher levels forming the outer surface of the muscle and those from lower levels buried sequentially, deeper within its substance. Within the muscle, bundles from individual lumbar segments have the same length, so that those from L1 become tendinous before those from successively lower levels. This isometric morphology indicates that the muscle is designed exclusively to act on the hip.[1]

Biomechanical analysis reveals that the psoas has only a feeble action on the lumbar spine with respect to flexion and extension. Its fibers extend upper lumbar segments and flex lower lumbar segments. However, the fibers act very close to the axes of rotation of the lumbar vertebrae, so they can exert only very small moments, even under maximal contraction.[1] This denies the psoas any substantial action on the lumbar spine. Rather, it uses the lumbar spine as a base from which to act on the hip.

However, the psoas potentially exerts massive compression loads on the lower lumbar discs. The proximity of the lines of action of the muscle to the axes of rotation minimizes its capacity as a flexor but maximizes the axial compression that it exerts. On maximum contraction, in an activity such as sit-ups, the two psoas muscles can exert a compression load on the L5-S1 disc equal to about 100 kg.[1]

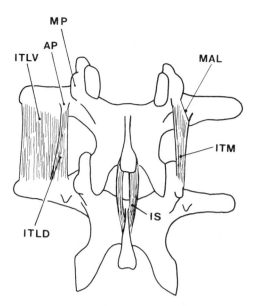

Fig. 4-2 The short, intersegmental muscles. *ITLV*—intertransversarii laterales ventrales. *ITLD*—intertransversarii laterales dorsales. *ITM*—intertransversarii mediales. *IS*—interspinales. *AP*—accessory process. *MP*—mamillary process. *MAL*—mamillo-accessory ligament. (Reproduced, with permission, from Bogduk N: Clinical Anatomy of the Lumbar Spine and Sacrum. 3rd ed. Churchill Livingstone, Edinburgh, 1997.)

INTERTRANSVERSARII LATERALES

The **intertransversarii laterales** consist of two parts: the intertransversarii laterales **ventrales** and the intertransversarii laterales **dorsales.** The ventral intertransversarii connect the margins of consecutive transverse processes, while the dorsal intertransversarii each connect an accessory process to the transverse process below (Fig. 4-2). Both the ventral and dorsal intertransversarii are innervated by the ventral rami of the lumbar spinal nerves,[3] and consequently cannot be classified among the back muscles, which are all innervated by the dorsal rami. On the basis of their attachments and their nerve supply, the ventral and dorsal intertransversarii are considered to be homologous to the intercostal and levator costae muscles of the thoracic region.[3]

The function of the intertransversarii laterales has never been determined experimentally, but it may be like that of the posterior, intersegmental muscles (see below).

QUADRATUS LUMBORUM

The quadratus lumborum is a wide, more or less rectangular muscle that covers the lateral two thirds or so of the anterior surfaces of the L1 to L4 transverse processes and extends laterally a few centimeters beyond the tips of the transverse processes. The muscle is a complex aggregation of various oblique and longitudinally running fibers that connect the lumbar transverse processes, the ilium, and the 12th rib[4] (see Fig. 4-1).

Caudally, the muscle arises from the L5 transverse process, the trough formed by the superior and anterior iliolumbar ligaments, and from the iliac crest lateral to the point of attachment of the iliolumbar ligament. From this series of attachments the most lateral fibers pass directly toward the lower anterior surface of the 12th rib. More medial fibers pass obliquely upward and medially to the anterior surfaces of each of the lumbar transverse processes above L5. These oblique fibers intermingle with other oblique fibers that run upward and laterally from each of the lumbar transverse processes to the 12th rib.

The majority of the fibers of the quadratus lumborum are connected to the 12th rib, and one of the functions of this muscle is said to be to fix the 12th rib during respiration.[2] The remaining fibers of quadratus lumborum connect the ilium to the upper four lumbar transverse processes. These latter fibers are the only components of quadratus lumborum that can execute lateral flexion; but they constitute a variable portion of the mass of the muscle, and their strength as lateral flexors has not been determined. Their anatomy suggests that their contribution to lateral flexion is unlikely to be substantial.

THE LUMBAR BACK MUSCLES

The lumbar back muscles lie behind the plane of the transverse processes and exert an action on the lumbar spine. They include muscles that attach to the lumbar vertebrae and thereby act directly on the lumbar spine, and certain other muscles that, while not attaching to the lumbar vertebrae, nevertheless exert an action on the lumbar spine.

The lumbar back muscles may be divided into three groups:

1. The short intersegmental muscles—the interspinales and the intertransversarii mediales.

2. The polysegmental muscles that attach to the lumbar vertebrae—the multifidus and the lumbar components of longissimus and iliocostalis.

3. The long polysegmental muscles, represented by the thoracic components of longissimus and iliocostalis lumborum, which in general do not attach to the lumbar vertebrae but cross the lumbar region from thoracic levels to find attachments on the ilium and sacrum.

The descriptions of the back muscles offered in this chapter, notably those of the multifidus and erector spinae, differ substantially from those given in standard textbooks. Traditionally, these muscles have been regarded as stemming from a common origin on the sacrum and ilium and passing upward to assume diverse attachments to the lumbar and thoracic vertebrae and ribs. However, in the face of several studies of these muscles[5,6,7,8] it is more appropriate to view these muscles in the reverse direction—from above downward. This is not only more consistent with the pattern of their nerve supply[8,9] but also clarifies the identity of certain muscles and the identity of the erector spinae aponeurosis and reveals the segmental biomechanical disposition of the muscles.

Interspinales

The lumbar interspinales are short, paired muscles that lie on either side of the interspinous ligament and connect the spinous processes of adjacent lumbar vertebrae (see Fig. 4-2). There are four pairs in the lumbar region.

Although disposed to produce posterior sagittal rotation of the vertebra above, the interspinales are quite small and would not contribute appreciably to the force required to move a vertebra. This paradox is similar to that which applies for the intertransversarii mediales and is discussed further in that context.

Intertransversarii Mediales

The intertransversarii mediales can be considered to be true back muscles because, unlike the intertransversarii laterales, they are innervated by the lumbar dorsal rami.[3,9] The intertransversarii mediales arise from an accessory process, the adjoining mamillary process, and the mamillo-accessory ligament that connects these two processes.[10] They insert into the superior aspect of the mamillary process of the vertebra below (see Fig. 4-2).

The intertransversarii mediales lie lateral to the axis of lateral flexion and behind the axis of sagittal rotation. However, they lie very close to these axes and are very small muscles. Therefore, it is questionable whether they could contribute any appreciable force in either lateral flexion or posterior sagittal rotation. It might be argued that perhaps larger muscles provide the bulk of the power to move the vertebrae, and the intertransversarii act to 'fine tune' the movement. However, this suggestion is highly speculative and does not account for their small size and considerable mechanical disadvantage.

A tantalizing alternative suggestion is that the intertransversarii (and perhaps also the interspinales) act as large, proprioceptive transducers; their value lies not in the force they can exert but in the muscle spindles they contain. Placed close to the lumbar vertebral column, the intertransversarii could monitor the movements of the column and provide feedback that influences the action of the surrounding muscles. Such a role has been suggested for the cervical intertransversarii, which have been found to contain a high density of muscle spindles.[11,12,13] Indeed, all unisegmental muscles of the vertebral column have between two and six times the density of muscles spindles found in the longer, polysegmental muscles, and there is growing speculation that this underscores the proprioceptive function of all short, small muscles of the body.[14,15,16]

Multifidus

Multifidus is the largest and most medial of the lumbar back muscles. It consists of a repeating series of fascicles that stem from the laminae and spinous processes of the lumbar vertebrae and exhibit a constant pattern of attachments caudally.[8]

The shortest fascicles of the multifidus are the "laminar fibers," which arise from the caudal end of the dorsal surface of each vertebral lamina and insert into the mamillary process of the vertebra two levels caudad (Fig. 4-3, *A*). The L5 laminar fibers have no mamillary process into which they can insert, and insert instead into an area on the sacrum just above the first dorsal sacral foramen.

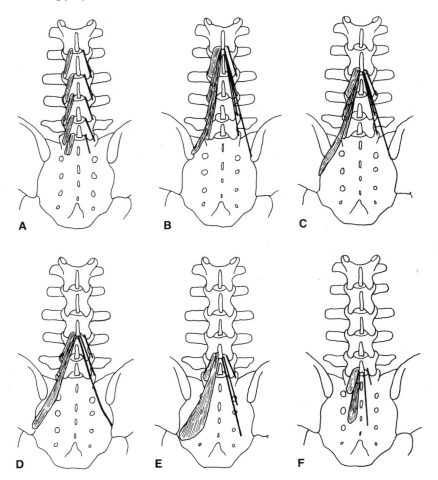

Fig. 4-3   The component fascicles of multifidus. **A:** The laminar fibers of multi-fidus. **B** to **F:** The fascicles from the L1 to L5 spinous processes respectively. (Reproduced, with permission, from Bogduk N: Clinical Anatomy of the Lumbar Spine and Sacrum (3rd ed.) Churchill Livingstone, Edinburgh, 1997.)

The bulk of the lumbar multifidus consists of much larger fascicles that radiate from the lumbar spinous processes. These fascicles are arranged in five overlapping groups, and each lumbar vertebra gives rise to one of these groups. At each segmental level, a fascicle arises from the base and cau-dolateral edge of the spinous process, and several fascicles arise from the caudal tip of the spinous process by way of a tendon referred to as "the common tendon." Although confluent with one another at their origin, the fascicles in each group diverge caudally to assume separate attachments to mamillary processes, the iliac crest, and the sacrum.

The fascicle from the base of the L1 spinous process inserts into the L4 mamillary process, while those from the common tendon insert into the mamillary processes of L5, S1, and the posterior superior iliac spine (see Fig. 4-3, *B*).

The fascicle from the base of the spinous process of L2 inserts into the mamillary process of L5, and those from the common tendon insert into the S1 mamillary process, the posterior superior iliac spine, and an area on the iliac crest just caudoventral to the posterior superior iliac spine (see Fig. 4-3, *C*).

The fascicle from the base of the L3 spinous process inserts into the mamillary process of the sacrum, while those fascicles from the common tendon insert into a narrow area extending caudally from the caudal extent of the posterior superior iliac spine to the lateral edge of the third sacral segment (see Fig. 4-3, *D*). The L4 fascicles insert onto the sacrum in an area medial to the L3 area of insertion but lateral to the dorsal sacral foramina (see Fig. 4-3, *E*), while those from the L5 vertebra insert onto an area medial to the dorsal sacral foramina (see Fig. 4-3, *F*).

It is noteworthy that although many of the fascicles of multifidus attach to mamillary processes, some of the deeper fibers of these fascicles attach to the capsules of the zygapophysial joints next to the mamillary processes.[17] This attachment allows the multifidus to protect the joint capsule from being caught inside the joint during the movements executed by the multifidus.

The key feature of the morphology of the lumbar multifidus is that its fascicles are arranged segmentally. Each lumbar vertebra is endowed with a group of fascicles that radiate from its spinous process, anchoring it below to mamillary processes, the iliac crest, and the sacrum. This disposition suggests that the fibers of multifidus are arranged in such a way that their principal action is focused on individual lumbar spinous processes.[8] They are designed to act in concert on a single spinous process. This contention is supported by the pattern of innervation of the muscle. All the fascicles arising from the spinous processes of a given vertebra are innervated by the medial branch of the dorsal ramus that issues from below that vertebra.[8,9] Thus the muscles that directly act on a particular vertebral segment are innervated by the nerve of that segment.

In a posterior view, the fascicles of multifidus are seen to have an oblique, caudolateral orientation. Their line of action therefore can be resolved into two vectors: a large vertical vector, and a considerably smaller horizontal vector[6] (Fig. 4-4, *A*).

The small horizontal vector suggests that the multifidus could pull the spinous processes sideways and therefore produce horizontal rotation. However, horizontal rotation of lumbar vertebrae is impeded by the impaction of the contralateral zygapophysial joints. Horizontal rotation occurs after impaction of the joints only if an appropriate shear force is applied to the intervertebral discs, but the horizontal vector of multifidus is so small that it is unlikely that multifidus would be capable of exerting such a shear force on the disc by acting on the spinous process. Indeed, electromyographic studies reveal that multifidus is inconsistently active in derotation and that, paradoxically, it is active in both ipsilateral and contralateral rotation.[18] Rotation therefore cannot be inferred to be a primary action of multifidus. In this context, multifidus has been said to act only as a "stabilizer" in rotation,[17,18] but the aberrant movements that it is supposed to stabilize have not been defined (although see below).

The principal action of multifidus is expressed by its vertical vector, and further insight is gained when this vector is viewed in a lateral projection (see Fig. 4-4, *B*). Each fascicle of multifidus, at every level, acts virtually at

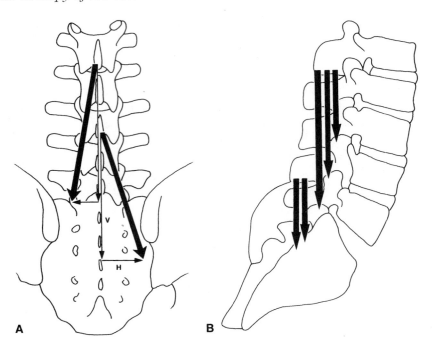

Fig. 4-4 The force vectors of multifidus. **A,** In a posteroanterior view, the oblique line of action of the multifidus at each level *(bold arrow)* can be resolved into a major vertical vector *(V)* and a smaller horizontal vector *(H).* **B,** In a lateral view, the vertical vectors of the multifidus are seen to be aligned at right angles to the spinous processes. (Reproduced, with permission, from Bogduk N: Clinical Anatomy of the Lumbar Spine and Sacrum. (3rd ed.) Churchill Livingstone, Edinburgh, 1997.)

right angles to its spinous process of origin.[6] Thus, using the spinous process as a lever, every fascicle is ideally disposed to produce posterior sagittal rotation of its vertebra. The right-angle orientation, however, precludes any action as a posterior horizontal translator. Therefore the multifidus can only exert the "rocking" component of extension of the lumbar spine or control this component during flexion.

Knowing that multifidus is primarily a posterior sagittal rotator of the lumbar spine makes it possible to resolve the paradox about its activity during horizontal rotation of the trunk.[6] First, rotation of the lumbar spine is an indirect action. Active rotation of the lumbar spine occurs only if the thorax is first rotated and is therefore secondary to thoracic rotation. Second, it must be realized that a muscle with two vectors of action cannot use these vectors independently. If the muscle contracts, then both vectors are exerted. Thus multifidus cannot exert axial rotation without simultaneously exerting a much larger posterior sagittal rotation.

The principal muscles that produce rotation of the thorax are the oblique abdominal muscles. The horizontal component of their orientation is able to turn the thoracic cage in the horizontal plane and thereby impart axial rotation to the lumbar spine. However, the oblique abdominal muscles also have a vertical component to their orientation. Therefore, if they contract to produce rotation they will also simultaneously cause flexion of the trunk and therefore of the lumbar spine. To counteract this flexion and maintain pure axial rotation, extensors of the lumbar spine must be recruited, and this is how multifidus becomes involved in rotation.

The role of multifidus in rotation is not to produce rotation but to oppose the flexion effect of the abdominal muscles as they produce rotation. The aberrant motion "stabilized" by multifidus during rotation is therefore the unwanted flexion unavoidably produced by the abdominal muscles.[6]

Apart from its action on individual lumbar vertebrae, the multifidus, because of its polysegmental nature, can also exert indirect effects on any interposed vertebrae. Because the line of action of any long fascicle of multifidus lies behind the lordotic curve of the lumbar spine, such fascicles can act like bowstrings on those segments of the curve that intervene between the attachments of the fascicle. The bowstring effect would tend to accentuate the lumbar lordosis, resulting in compression of intervertebral discs posteriorly and strain of the discs and longitudinal ligament anteriorly. Thus a secondary effect of the action of multifidus is to increase the lumbar lordosis and the compressive and tensile loads on any vertebrae and intervertebral discs interposed between its attachments.

Lumbar Erector Spinae

The lumbar erector spinae lies lateral to the multifidus and forms the prominent dorsolateral contour of the back muscles in the lumbar region. It consists of two muscles—the **longissimus thoracis** and the **iliocostalis lumborum.** Furthermore, each of these muscles has two components: a lumbar part, consisting of fascicles arising from lumbar vertebrae, and a thoracic part, consisting of fascicles arising from thoracic vertebrae or ribs.[5,7] These four parts may be referred to respectively as longissimus thoracis *pars lumborum,* iliocostalis lumborum *pars lumborum,* longissimus thoracis *pars thoracis,* and iliocostalis lumborum *pars thoracis.*[7]

In the lumbar region, the longissimus and iliocostalis are separated from each other by the **lumbar intermuscular aponeurosis,** an anteroposterior continuation of the erector spinae aponeurosis.[5,7] It appears as a flat sheet of collagen fibers that extend rostrally from the medial aspect of the posterior superior iliac spine for 6 to 8 cm. It is formed mainly by the caudal tendons of the rostral four fascicles of the lumbar component of longissimus (Fig. 4-5).

Longissimus Thoracis Pars Lumborum

The longissimus thoracis pars lumborum is composed of five fascicles, each arising from the accessory process and the adjacent medial end of the dorsal surface of the transverse process of a lumbar vertebra (see Fig. 4-5).

The fascicle from the L5 vertebra is the deepest and shortest. Its fibers insert directly into the medial aspect of the posterior superior iliac spine. The

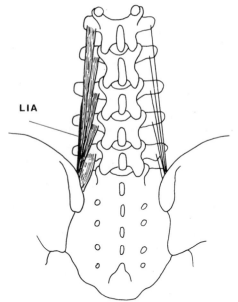

LIA

Fig. 4-5 The lumbar fibers of longissimus (longissimus thoracis pars lumborum). On the left, the five fascicles of the intact muscle are drawn. The formation of the lumbar intermuscular aponeurosis *(LIA)* by the lumbar fascicles of longissimus is depicted. On the right, the lines indicate the attachments and span of the fascicles. (Reproduced, with permission, from Bogduk N: Clinical Anatomy of the Lumbar Spine and Sacrum. (3rd ed.) Churchill Livingstone, Edinburgh, 1997.)

fascicle from L4 also lies deeply, but lateral to that from L5. Succeeding fascicles lie progressively more dorsally so that the L3 fascicle covers those from L4 and L5, but is itself covered by the L2 fascicle, while the L1 fascicle lies most superficially.

The L1 to L4 fascicles all form tendons at their caudal ends, which converge to form the lumbar intermuscular aponeurosis, which eventually attaches to a narrow area on the ilium immediately lateral to the insertion of the L5 fascicle. The lumbar intermuscular aponeurosis thus represents a common tendon of insertion, or the aponeurosis, of the bulk of the lumbar fibers of longissimus.

Each fascicle of the lumbar longissimus has both a dorsoventral and a rostrocaudal orientation.[7] Therefore the action of each fascicle can be resolved into a vertical vector and a horizontal vector, the relative sizes of which differ from L1 to L5 (Fig. 4-6, *A*). Consequently, the relative actions of longissimus differ at each segmental level. Furthermore, the action of longissimus as a whole will differ according to whether the muscle contracts unilaterally or bilaterally.

The large vertical vector of each fascicle lies lateral to the axis of lateral flexion and behind the axis of sagittal rotation of each vertebra. Thus by contracting unilaterally the longissimus can laterally flex the vertebral column, but by acting bilaterally the various fascicles can act, like multifidus, to produce posterior sagittal rotation of their vertebra of origin. However, their attachments to the accessory and transverse processes lie close to the axes of sagittal rotation, and therefore their capacity to produce posterior sagittal rotation is less efficient than that of multifidus, which acts through the long levers of the spinous processes.[7]

The horizontal vectors of the longissimus are directed backward. Therefore when contracting bilaterally the longissimus is capable of drawing the

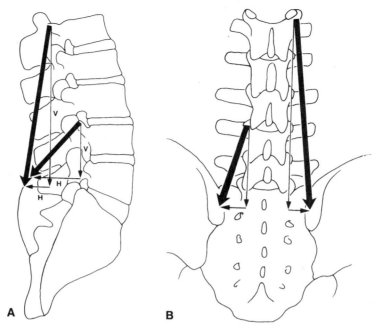

Fig. 4-6   The force vectors of the longissimus thoracis pars lumborum. **A,** In a lateral view, the oblique line of action of each fascicle of longissimus can be resolved into a vertical *(V)* and a horizontal *(H)* vector. The horizontal vectors of lower lumbar fascicles are larger. **B,** In a postero-anterior view, the line of action of the fascicles can be resolved into a major vertical vector and a much smaller horizontal vector. (Reproduced, with permission, from Bogduk N: Clinical Anatomy of the Lumbar Spine and Sacrum. (3rd ed.) Churchill Livingstone, Edinburgh, 1997.)

lumbar vertebrae backward. This action of posterior translation can restore the anterior translation of the lumbar vertebrae that occurs during flexion of the lumbar column. The capacity for posterior translation is greatest at lower lumbar levels where the fascicles of longissimus assume a greater dorsoventral orientation (see Fig. 4-6, *B*).

Reviewing the horizontal and vertical actions of longissimus together, it can be seen that longissimus expresses a continuum of combined actions along the length of the lumbar vertebral column. From below upward, its capacity as a posterior sagittal rotator increases, and from above downward the fascicles are better designed to resist or restore anterior translation. However, the longissimus cannot exert its horizontal and vertical vectors independently. Thus whatever horizontal translation it exerts must occur simultaneously with posterior sagittal rotation. The resolution into vectors simply reveals the relative amounts of simultaneous translation and sagittal rotation exerted at different segmental levels.

It might be deduced that because of the horizontal vector of longissimus, this muscle acting unilaterally could draw the accessory and transverse processes backward and therefore produce axial rotation. However, in this regard the fascicles of longissimus are oriented almost directly toward the axis of axial rotation and so are at a marked mechanical disadvantage to produce axial rotation.

Iliocostalis Lumborum Pars Lumborum

The lumbar component of iliocostalis lumborum consists of four overlying fascicles arising from the L1 through L4 vertebrae. Rostrally, each fascicle attaches to the tip of the transverse process and to an area extending 2 to 3 cm laterally onto the middle layer of the thoracolumbar fascia (Fig. 4-7).

The fascicle from L4 is the deepest, and caudally it is attached directly to the iliac crest just lateral to the posterior superior iliac spine. This fascicle is covered by the fascicle from L3 that has a similar but more dorsolaterally located attachment on the iliac crest. In sequence, L2 covers L3 and L1 covers L2, with insertions on the iliac crest becoming successively more dorsal and lateral. The most lateral fascicles attach to the iliac crest just medial to the attachment of the "lateral raphe" of the thoracolumbar fascia (see below). The most medial fibers of iliocostalis contribute to the lumbar intermuscular aponeurosis, but only to a minor extent.

Although an L5 fascicle of iliocostalis lumborum is not described in the literature, it is represented in the iliolumbar "ligament." In neonates and children this "ligament" is said to be completely muscular in structure.[19] By the third decade of life the muscle fibers are entirely replaced by collagen, giving rise to the familiar iliolumbar ligament.[19] On the basis of sites of attachment and relative orientation the posterior band of the iliolumbar ligament

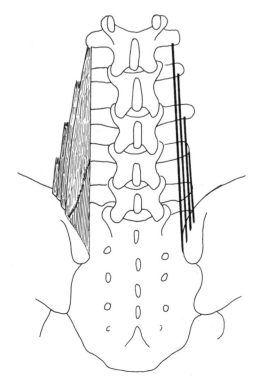

Fig. 4-7 The lumbar fibers of iliocostalis (iliocostalis lumborum pars lumborum). On the left, the four lumbar fascicles of iliocostalis are shown. On the right, their span and attachments are indicated by the lines. (Reproduced, with permission, from Bogduk N: Clinical Anatomy of the Lumbar Spine and Sacrum. (3rd ed.) Churchill Livingstone, Edinburgh, 1997.)

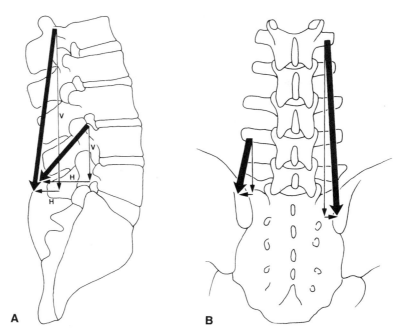

Fig. 4-8 The force vectors of the iliocostalis lumborum pars lumborum. **A,** In a lateral view, the line of action of the fascicles can be resolved into vertical *(V)* and horizontal *(H)* vectors. The horizontal vectors are larger at lower lumbar levels. **B,** In a postero-anterior view, the line of action is resolved into a vertical vector and a very small horizontal vector. (Reproduced, with permission, from Bogduk N: Clinical Anatomy of the Lumbar Spine and Sacrum. (3rd ed.) Churchill Livingstone, Edinburgh, 1997.)

would appear to be derived from the L5 fascicle of iliocostalis, while the anterior band of the ligament is a derivative of the quadratus lumborum.

The disposition of the lumbar fascicles of iliocostalis is similar to that of the lumbar longissimus, except that the fascicles are situated more laterally. Like the action of the lumbar longissimus, the action of the lumbar fascicles of iliocostalis can be resolved into horizontal and vertical vectors (Fig. 4-8, *A*).

The vertical vector is still predominant, and therefore the lumbar fascicles of iliocostalis contracting bilaterally can act as posterior sagittal rotators (Fig. 4-8, *B*), but because of the horizontal vector, a posterior translation will be exerted simultaneously, principally at lower lumbar levels where the fascicles of iliocostalis have a greater forward orientation. Contracting unilaterally, the lumbar fascicles of iliocostalis can act as lateral flexors of the lumbar vertebrae, for which action the transverse processes provide very substantial levers.

Contracting unilaterally, the fibers of iliocostalis are better suited to exert axial rotation than the fascicles of lumbar longissimus, for their attachment to the tips of the transverse processes displaces the fibers of iliocostalis from the axis of horizontal rotation and provides them with substantial levers for this action. Because of this leverage, the lower fascicles of iliocostalis are the only intrinsic muscles of the lumbar spine reasonably disposed to produce horizontal rotation. Their effectiveness as rotators, however, is dwarfed by the oblique abdominal muscles that act on the ribs and produce lumbar rotation indirectly by rotating the thoracic cage. However, because iliocostalis cannot exert axial rotation without simultaneously exerting posterior sagittal rotation, the muscle is well suited to co-operate with multifidus to oppose the flexion effect of the abdominal muscles when they act to rotate the trunk.

Longissimus Thoracis Pars Thoracis

The thoracic fibers of longissimus thoracis typically consist of 11 or 12 pairs of small fascicles arising from the ribs and transverse processes of T1 or T2 down to T12 (Fig. 4-9). At each level, two tendons can usually be recognized, a medial one from the tip of the transverse process and a lateral one from the rib, although in the upper three or four levels the latter may merge medially with the fascicle from the transverse process. Each rostral tendon extends 3 to 4 cm before forming a small muscle belly measuring 7 to 8 cm in length. The muscle bellies from the higher levels overlap those from lower levels. Each muscle belly eventually forms a caudal tendon that extends into the lumbar region. The tendons run in parallel, with those from higher levels being most medial. The fascicles from the T2 level attach to the L3 spinous process, while the fascicles from the remaining levels insert into spinous processes at progressively lower levels. For example, those from T5

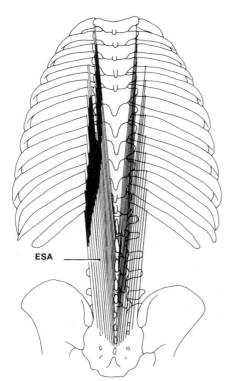

ESA

Fig. 4-9 The thoracic fibers of longissimus (longissimus thoracis pars thoracis). The intact fascicles are shown on the left. The darkened areas represent the short muscle bellies of each fascicle. Note the short rostral tendons of each fascicle, and the long caudal tendons, which collectively constitute most of the erector spinae aponeurosis *(esa)*. The span of the individual fascicles is indicated on the right. (Reproduced, with permission, from Bogduk N: Clinical Anatomy of the Lumbar Spine and Sacrum. (3rd ed.) Churchill Livingstone, Edinburgh, 1997.)

attach to L5 and those from T7 to S2 or S3. Those from T8 to T12 diverge from the midline to find attachment to the sacrum along a line extending from the S3 spinous process to the caudal extent of the posterior superior iliac spine.[19] The lateral edge of the caudal tendon of T12 lies alongside the dorsal edge of the lumbar intermuscular aponeurosis formed by the caudal tendon of the L1 longissimus bundle.

The side-to-side aggregation of the caudal tendons of longissimus thoracis pars thoracis forms much of what is termed the *erector spinae aponeurosis,* which covers the lumbar fibers of longissimus and iliocostalis but affords no attachment to them.

The longissimus thoracis pars thoracis is designed to act on thoracic vertebrae and ribs. Nonetheless, when contracting bilaterally it acts indirectly on the lumbar vertebral column and uses the erector spinae aponeurosis to produce an increase in the lumbar lordosis. However, not all of the fascicles of longissimus thoracis span the entire lumbar vertebral column. Those from the second rib and T2 reach only as far as L3, and only those fascicles arising between the T6 or T7 and the T12 levels actually span the entire lumbar region. Consequently, only a portion of the whole thoracic longissimus acts on all the lumbar vertebrae.

The oblique orientation of the longissimus thoracis pars thoracis also permits it to laterally flex the thoracic vertebral column and thereby indirectly flex the lumbar vertebral column laterally.

Iliocostalis Lumborum Pars Thoracis

The iliocostalis lumborum pars thoracis consists of fascicles from the lower seven or eight ribs that attach caudally to the ilium and sacrum (Fig. 4-10). These fascicles represent the thoracic component of iliocostalis lumborum and should not be confused with the iliocostalis thoracis, which is restricted to the thoracic region between the upper six and lower six ribs.

Each fascicle of the iliocostalis lumborum pars thoracis arises from the angle of the rib via a ribbon-like tendon measuring some 9 to 10 cm in length. It then forms a muscle belly of 8 to 10 cm in length. Thereafter, each fascicle continues as a tendon, contributing to the erector spinae aponeurosis and ultimately attaching to the posterior superior iliac spine. The most medial tendons from the more rostral fascicles often attach more medially, to the dorsal surface of the sacrum caudal to the insertion of multifidus.

The thoracic fascicles of iliocostalis lumborum have no attachment to lumbar vertebrae. They attach to the iliac crest and thereby span the lumbar region. Consequently, by acting bilaterally, it is possible for them to exert an indirect "bowstring" effect on the vertebral column, causing an increase in the lordosis of the lumbar spine. Acting unilaterally, the iliocostalis lumborum pars thoracis can use the leverage afforded by the ribs to laterally flex the thoracic cage and thereby laterally flex the lumbar vertebral column indirectly. The distance between the ribs and ilium does not shorten greatly during rotation of the trunk, and therefore the iliocostalis lumborum pars thoracis can have little action as an axial rotator. However, contralateral ro-

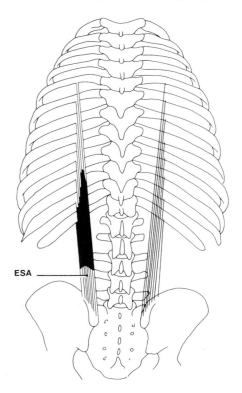

ESA

Fig. 4-10   The thoracic fibers of iliocostalis lumborum (iliocostalis lumborum pars thoracis). The intact fascicles are shown on the left, and their span is shown on the right. The caudal tendons of the fascicles collectively form the lateral parts of the erector spinae aponeurosis (esa). (Reproduced, with permission, from Bogduk N: Clinical Anatomy of the Lumbar Spine and Sacrum. (3rd ed.) Churchill Livingstone, Edinburgh, 1997.)

tation greatly increases this distance, and the iliocostalis lumborum pars thoracis can serve to derotate the thoracic cage and therefore the lumbar spine.

ERECTOR SPINAE APONEUROSIS

One of the cardinal revelations of studies of the lumbar erector spinae[5,7] is that this muscle consists of both lumbar and thoracic fibers. Modern textbook descriptions largely do not recognize the lumbar fibers, especially those of iliocostalis[5]; they also do not note that the lumbar fibers (of both longissimus and iliocostalis) have attachments quite separate to those of the thoracic fibers. The lumbar fibers of the longissimus and iliocostalis pass between the lumbar vertebrae and the ilium. Thus, through these muscles, the lumbar vertebrae are anchored directly to the ilium. They do not gain any attachment to the erector spinae aponeurosis, which is the implication of all modern textbook descriptions that deal with the erector spinae.

The erector spinae aponeurosis is described as a broad sheet of tendinous fibers that is attached to the ilium, the sacrum, and the lumbar and sacral spinous processes and that forms a common origin for the lower part of the erector spinae.[2] However, as described above, the erector spinae aponeurosis is formed almost exclusively by the tendons of the longissimus thoracis pars thoracis and iliocostalis pars thoracis.[5,7] The medial half or so of the aponeurosis is formed by the tendons of longissimus thoracis, and the

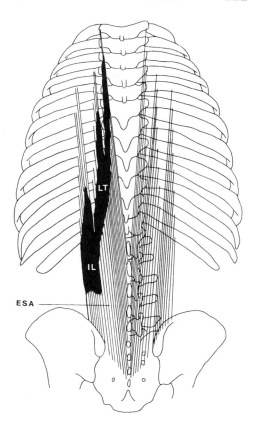

Fig. 4-11 The erector spinae aponeurosis *(ESA).* This broad sheet is formed by the caudal tendons of the thoracic fibers of longissimus thoracis *(LT)* and iliocostalis lumborum *(IL).* (Reproduced, with permission, from Bogduk N: Clinical Anatomy of the Lumbar Spine and Sacrum (3rd ed.) Churchill Livingstone, Edinburgh, 1997.)

lateral half is formed by the iliocostalis lumborum (Fig. 4-11). The only additional contribution comes from the most superficial fibers of multifidus from upper lumbar levels, which contribute a small number of fibers to the aponeurosis[8] (see Figs. 4-9; 4-10). Nonetheless, the erector spinae aponeurosis is essentially formed only by the caudal attachments of muscles acting from thoracic levels.

The lumbar fibers of erector spinae do not attach to the erector spinae aponeurosis. Indeed, the aponeurosis is free to move over the surface of the underlying lumbar fibers, and this suggests that the lumbar fibers, which form the bulk of the lumbar back musculature, can act independently from the rest of the erector spinae.

THORACOLUMBAR FASCIA

The thoracolumbar fascia consists of three layers of fascia that envelop the muscles of the lumbar spine, effectively separating them into three compartments. The **anterior layer** of thoracolumbar fascia is quite thin and is derived from the fascia of quadratus lumborum. It covers the anterior surface of quadratus lumborum and is attached medially to the anterior surfaces of the lumbar transverse processes. In the intertransverse spaces it blends with the intertransverse ligaments and may be viewed as one of the lateral extensions of the intertransverse ligaments. Lateral to the quadratus lumborum, the anterior layer blends with the other layers of the thoracolumbar fascia.

The **middle layer** of thoracolumbar fascia lies behind the quadratus lumborum. Medially, it is attached to the tips of the lumbar transverse processes and is directly continuous with the intertransverse ligaments. Laterally, it gives rise to the aponeurosis of the transversus abdominis. Its actual identity is debatable. It may represent a lateral continuation of the intertransverse ligaments, a medial continuation of the transversus aponeurosis, a thickening of the posterior fascia of the quadratus, or a combination of any or all of these.

The **posterior layer** of thoracolumbar fascia covers the back muscles. It arises from the lumbar spinous processes in the midline posteriorly and wraps around the back muscles to blend with the other layers of the thoracolumbar fascia along the lateral border of the iliocostalis lumborum. The union of the fasciae is quite dense at this site, and the middle and posterior layers in particular form a dense raphe that, for purposes of reference, has been called the **lateral raphe.**[20]

Traditionally, the thoracolumbar fascia has been ascribed no other function than to invest the back muscles and to provide an attachment for the transversus abdominis and the internal oblique muscles.[2] However, in recent years there has been considerable interest in its biomechanical role in the stability of the lumbar spine, particularly in the flexed posture and in lifting. This has resulted in anatomic and biomechanical studies of the anatomy and function of the thoracolumbar fascia, notably its posterior layer.[20,21,22,23]

The posterior layer of thoracolumbar fascia covers the back muscles from the lumbosacral region through to the thoracic region as far rostrally as the splenius muscle. In the lumbar region, it is attached to the tips of the spinous processes in the midline. Lateral to the erector spinae, between the twelfth rib and the iliac crest, it unites with the middle layer of thoracolumbar fascia in the lateral raphe. At sacral levels, the posterior layer extends from the midline to the posterior superior iliac spine and the posterior segment of the iliac crest. Here it fuses with the underlying erector spinae aponeurosis and blends with fibers of the aponeurosis of the gluteus maximus.

On close inspection, the posterior layer exhibits a cross-hatched appearance, manifest because it consists of two laminae: a **superficial lamina** with fibers orientated caudomedially, and a **deep lamina** with fibers oriented caudolaterally.[20,23]

The superficial lamina is formed by the aponeurosis of latissimus dorsi, but the disposition and attachments of its constituent fibers differ according to the portion of latissimus dorsi from which they are derived (Fig. 4-12). Those fibers derived from the most lateral 2 to 3 cm of the muscle are short and insert directly into the iliac crest without contributing to the thoracolumbar fascia. Fibers from the next most lateral 2 cm of the muscle approach the iliac crest near the lateral margin of the erector spinae, but then deflect medially, bypassing the crest to attach to the L5 and sacral spinous processes. These fibers form the sacral portion of the superficial lamina. A third series of fibers become aponeurotic just lateral to the lumbar erector

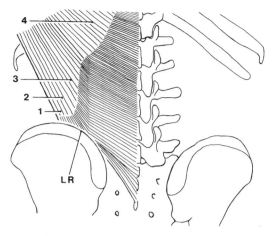

Fig. 4-12 The superficial lamina of the posterior layer of thoracolumbar fascia. *1,* Aponeurotic fibers of the most lateral fascicles of latissimus dorsi insert directly into the iliac crest. *2,* Aponeurotic fibers of the next most lateral part of latissimus dorsi glance past the iliac crest and reach the midline at sacral levels. *3,* Aponeurotic fibers from this portion of the muscle attach to the underlying lateral raphe *(lr),* and then deflect medially to reach the midline at the L3 to L5 levels. *4,* Aponeurotic fibers from the upper portions of latissimus dorsi pass directly to the midline at thoracolumbar levels. (Reproduced, with permission, from Bogduk N: Clinical Anatomy of the Lumbar Spine and Sacrum. (3rd ed.) Churchill Livingstone, Edinburgh, 1997.)

spinae. At the lateral border of the erector spinae they blend with the other layers of thoracolumbar fascia in the lateral raphe, but then they deflect medially, continuing over the back muscles to reach the midline at the levels of the L3, L4, and L5 spinous processes. These fibers form the lumbar portion of the superficial lamina of the posterior layer of thoracolumbar fascia.

The rostral portions of the latissimus dorsi cross the back muscles and do not become aponeurotic until some 5 cm lateral to the midline at the L3 and higher levels. These aponeurotic fibers form the thoracolumbar and thoracic portions of the thoracolumbar fascia.

Beneath the superficial lamina, the deep lamina of the posterior layer consists of bands of collagen fibers emanating from the midline, principally from the lumbar spinous processes (Fig. 4-13). The bands from the L4, L5, and S1 spinous processes pass caudolaterally to the posterior superior iliac spine. Those from the L3 spinous process and L3-L4 interspinous ligament wrap around the lateral margin of the erector spinae to fuse with the middle layer of thoracolumbar fascia in the lateral raphe. Above L3 the deep lamina progressively becomes thinner, consisting of sparse bands of collagen that dissipate laterally over the erector spinae. A deep lamina is not formed at thoracic levels.

Collectively, the superficial and deep laminae of the posterior layer of thoracolumbar fascia form a retinaculum over the back muscles. Attached to the midline medially and the posterior superior iliac spine and lateral raphe laterally, the fascia covers, or ensheaths, the back muscles, preventing their

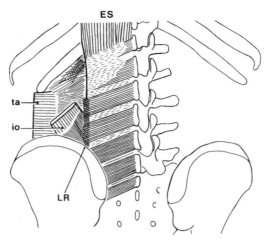

Fig. 4-13 The deep lamina of the posterior layer of thoracolumbar fascia. Bands of collagen fibers pass from the midline to the posterior superior iliac spine and to the lateral raphe *(lr)*. Those bands from the L4 and L5 spinous processes form alar-like ligaments that anchor these processes to the ilium. Attaching to the lateral raphe laterally are the aponeurosis of transversus abdominis *(ta)*, and a variable number of the most posterior fibers of internal oblique *(io)*. (Reproduced, with permission, from Bogduk N: Clinical Anatomy of the Lumbar Spine and Sacrum. (3rd ed.) Churchill Livingstone, Edinburgh, 1997.)

displacement dorsally. Additionally, the deep lamina alone forms a series of distinct ligaments. When viewed bilaterally, the bands of fibers from the L4 and L5 spinous processes appear like alar ligaments, anchoring these spinous processes to the ilia. The band from the L3 spinous process anchors this process indirectly to the ilium via the lateral raphe. Finally, the lateral raphe forms a site where the two laminae of the posterior layer fuse not only with the middle layer of thoracolumbar fascia but also with the transversus abdominis, whose middle fibers arise from the lateral raphe (Fig. 4-13). The posterior layer of thoracolumbar fascia thereby provides an indirect attachment for the transversus abdominis to the lumbar spinous processes. The mechanical significance of these three morphologic features is explored below in the section on functions of the back muscles and their fascia.

FUNCTIONS OF THE BACK MUSCLES AND THEIR FASCIA

Each of the lumbar back muscles is capable of several possible actions. No action is unique to a muscle, and no muscle has a single action. Instead, the back muscles provide a pool of possible actions that may be recruited to suit the needs of the vertebral column. Therefore the functions of the back muscles need to be considered in terms of the observed movements of the vertebral column. Three types of movements can be addressed: (1) minor active movements of the vertebral column, (2) postural movements, and (3) major movements in forward bending and lifting. In this context "postural movements" refers to movements, usually subconscious, that occur to adjust and maintain a desired posture when this is disturbed, usually by the influence of gravity.

MINOR ACTIVE MOVEMENTS

In the upright position the lumbar back muscles play little or no active role in executing movement because gravity provides the necessary force. During extension the back muscles contribute to the initial tilt, drawing the line of gravity backward,[24, 25] but are unnecessary for further extension. Muscle activity is recruited when the movement is forced or resisted[26] but is restricted to muscles acting on the thorax. The lumbar multifidus, for example, shows little or no involvement.[27]

The lateral flexors can bend the lumbar spine sideways but once the center of gravity of the trunk is displaced, lateral flexion can continue under the influence of gravity. However, the ipsilateral lateral flexors are used to direct the movement, and the contralateral muscles are required to balance the action of gravity and control the rate and extent of movement. Consequently, lateral flexion is accompanied by bilateral activity of the lumbar back muscles, but the contralateral muscles are relatively more active because they must balance the load of the laterally flexing spine.[24, 25, 28, 29, 30, 31] If a weight is held in the hand on the side to which the spine is laterally flexed, a greater load is applied to the spine, and the contralateral back muscles show greater activity to balance this load.[28, 30]

MAINTENANCE OF POSTURE

The upright vertebral column is well stabilized by its joints and ligaments, but it is still liable to displacement by gravity or when subject to asymmetric weightbearing. The back muscles serve to correct such displacements and, depending on the direction of any displacement, the appropriate back muscles will be recruited.

During standing at ease, the back muscles may show slight continuous activity,[18, 24, 25, 26, 29, 31–41] intermittent activity,[24, 26, 31, 41, 42] or no activity,[35, 38, 39, 40, 41] and the amount of activity can be influenced by changing the position of the head or allowing the trunk to sway.[24]

The explanation for these differences probably lies in the location of the line of gravity in relation to the lumbar spine in different individuals.[26, 35, 40, 41, 43] In about 75% of individuals the line of gravity passes in front of the center of the L4 vertebra and therefore essentially in front of the lumbar spine.[35, 40] Consequently, gravity will exert a constant tendency to pull the thorax and lumbar spine into flexion. To preserve an upright posture, a constant level of activity in the posterior sagittal rotators of the lumbar spine will be needed to oppose the tendency to flexion. Conversely, when the line of gravity passes behind the lumbar spine, gravity tends to extend it, and back muscle activity is not required. Instead abdominal muscle activity is recruited to prevent the spine extending under gravity.[35, 40]

Activities that displace the center of gravity of the trunk sideways will tend to cause lateral flexion. To prevent undesired lateral flexion, the contralateral lateral flexors will contract. This occurs when weights are carried in one hand.[24,38] Carrying equal weights in both hands does not displace the line of gravity, and back muscle activity is not increased substantially on either side of the body.[24,38]

During sitting the activity of the back muscles is similar to that during standing,[33,34,44,45] but in supported sitting, as with the elbows resting on the knees, there is no activity in the lumbar back muscles,[24,31] and with arms resting on a desk, back muscle activity is substantially decreased.[33,34,44] In reclined sitting the back rest supports the weight of the thorax, lessening the need for muscular support. Consequently, increasing the declination of the back rest of a seat decreases lumbar back muscle activity.[33,44,46,47]

MAJOR ACTIVE MOVEMENTS

Forward flexion and extension of the spine from the flexed position are movements during which the back muscles have their most important function. As the spine bends forward, there is an increase in the activity of the back muscles,[18,24,25,27,28,29,31,32,42,48,49,50,51] and this increase is proportional to the angle of flexion and the size of any load carried.[28,30,52,53] The movement of forward flexion is produced by gravity, but the extent and the rate at which it proceeds is controlled by the eccentric contraction of the back muscles. Movement of the thorax on the lumbar spine is controlled by the long thoracic fibers of longissimus and iliocostalis. The long tendons of insertion allow these muscles to act around the convexity of the increasing thoracic kyphosis and anchor the thorax to the ilium and sacrum. In the lumbar region, the multifidus and the lumbar fascicles of longissimus and iliocostalis act to control the anterior sagittal rotation of the lumbar vertebrae. At the same time the lumbar fascicles of longissimus and iliocostalis also act to control the associated anterior translation of the lumbar vertebrae.

At a certain point during forward flexion, the activity in the back muscles ceases, and the vertebral column is braced by the locking of the zygapophysial joints and tension in its posterior ligaments (see Chapter 7). This phenomenon is known as "critical point."[25,42,43,54] However, critical point does not occur in all individuals nor in all muscles.[18,24,31,41] When it does occur, it does so when the spine has reached about 90% maximum flexion, even though at this stage the hip flexion that occurs in forward bending is still only 60% complete.[43,54] Carrying weights during flexion causes the critical point to occur later in the range of vertebral flexion.[43,54]

The physiologic basis for critical point is still obscure. It may be due to reflex inhibition initiated by proprioceptors in the lumbar joints and ligaments, or in muscle stretch and length receptors.[54] Whatever the mechanism, the significance of critical point is that it marks the transition of spinal loadbearing from muscles to the ligamentous system.

Extension of the trunk from the flexed position is characterized by high levels of back muscle activity.[18,24,25,42,51] In the thoracic region the iliocostalis and longissimus, acting around the thoracic kyphosis, lift the thorax by rotating it backward. The lumbar vertebrae are rotated backward principally by the lumbar multifidus, causing their superior surfaces to be progressively tilted upward to support the rising thorax.

COMPRESSIVE LOADS OF THE BACK MUSCLES

Because of the downward direction of their action, as the back muscles contract they exert a longitudinal compression of the lumbar vertebral column, and this compression raises the pressure in the lumbar intervertebral discs. Any activity that involves the back muscles therefore is associated with a rise in nuclear pressure. As measured in the L3-L4 intervertebral disc, the nuclear pressure correlates with the degree of myoelectric activity in the back muscles.[28,30,47,55,56] As muscle activity increases, disc pressure rises.

Disc pressures and myoelectric activity of the back muscles have been used extensively to quantify the stresses applied to the lumbar spine in various postures and by various activities.[33,45,46,47,57-62] From the standing position, forward bending causes the greatest increase in disc pressure. Lifting a weight in this position raises disc pressure even further, and the pressure is greatly increased if a load is lifted with the lumbar spine both flexed and rotated. Throughout these various maneuvers, back muscle activity increases in proportion to the disc pressure.

One of the prime revelations of combined discometric and electromyographic studies of the lumbar spine during lifting relates to the comparative stresses applied to the lumbar spine by different lifting tactics. In essence, it has been shown that, on the basis of changes in disc pressure and back muscle activity, there are no differences between using a "stoop" lift or a "leg" lift, i.e., lifting a weight with a bent back versus lifting with a straight back.[28,46,47,63] The critical factor is the distance of the load from the body. The further the load is from the chest the greater the stresses on the lumbar spine, and the greater the disc pressure and back muscle activity.[63] Performing a "leg" lift with a straight back as opposed to maintaining a lordosis involves about 5% less electromyographic activity in the back muscles early in the lift but little difference thereafter.[64]

Strength of the Back Muscles

The strength of the back muscles has been determined in experiments on normal volunteers.[65] Two measures of strength are available: the absolute maximum force of contraction in the upright posture and the moment generated on the lumbar spine. The absolute maximum strength of the back muscles as a whole is about 4000N. Acting on the short moment arms provided by the spinous processes and pedicles of the lumbar vertebrae, this force converts to an extensor moment of 200 Nm. These figures apply to average males under the age of 30; young females exhibit about 60% of this strength, while individuals over the age of 30 are about 10% to 30% weaker, respectively.[65] Easy standing involves some 2% to 5% of maximum isometric strength; manual handling of heavy loads involves between 75% and 100%; sitting involves between 3% and 15% of maximum activity.[66]

Detailed dissection studies have allowed the strength of contraction to be apportioned to individual components of the back muscles.[67] Of the total extensor moment, the thoracic fibers of iliocostalis and longissimus account for some 50%. Thus half of the extensor moment on the lumbar spine is exerted through the erector spinae aponeurosis. The other half is exerted by the muscles that act directly on the lumbar vertebrae, with multifidus providing half of that 50% and longissimus thoracis pars lumborum and iliocostalis lumborum pars lumborum providing the remainder. The compression loads exerted by the lumbar back muscles differ from segment to segment because of the different spans and attachments of the various muscles. However, at L5-S1 the thoracic fibers of the lumbar erector spinae exert about 42% of the total compression load, the lumbar fibers of this muscle contribute 36%, and the multifidus contributes 22%.[67] At higher lumbar levels, relatively more of the total compression load on the segment is exerted by the thoracic fibers of the lumbar erector spinae.

With respect to shear forces, in the upright position the various lumbar back muscles exert forces that differ in magnitude and in direction at different levels.[67] This arises because of the different orientation of particular fascicles of the various muscles and because of the different orientation of particular vertebrae in the lumbar lordosis. As a result, multifidus exerts mainly anterior shear forces at upper lumbar levels but either anterior or posterior shear forces at lower levels; the lumbar fibers of erector spinae exert posterior shear forces on the vertebrae to which they are attached, but anterior shear forces on vertebrae below these; the thoracic fibers of lumbar erector spinae exert posterior shear forces on upper lumbar segments but anterior shear forces on L4 and L5.[67] The net effect is that the back muscles exert posterior shear forces on upper lumbar segments in the upright spine but, paradoxically, they exert a net anterior shear force on L5.

Intriguingly, flexion of the lumbar spine does not compromise the strength of the back muscles.[68] The moment arms of some fascicles are reduced by flexion but those of others are increased, resulting in no significant change in the total capacity to generate moments. All fascicles, however, are elongated; but although this reduces their maximum force on active contraction, it increases the passive tension in the muscles, resulting in no reduction in total tension. Consequently, upon flexion, the total extensor moment of the back muscles and the compression load that they exert change little from those in the upright position. However, the shear forces change appreciably. The posterior shear forces on upper lumbar segments are reduced by flexion, but the shear force on L5 reverses from an anterior shear force in the upright position to a posterior shear force in full flexion.[68]

With respect to axial rotation, although the back muscles have reasonable moment arms, they are compromised by their longitudinal orientation.[69] Only their horizontal vectors can exert axial rotation, but these are very small components of the action of any of the muscles. As a result the total, maximal possible torque exerted by all the back muscles is next to trivial, and that exerted by any one muscle is negligible.[69] Consequently, the back muscles afford no stability to the lumbar spine in axial rotation. For that the lumbar spine is reliant on the abdominal muscles.[69]

Histochemistry

As postural muscles, the back muscles are dominated by slow-twitch fibers. Furthermore, the density of slow-twitch and fast-twitch fibers differs from muscle to muscle.

Slow-twitch fibers constitute some 70% of the fibers of longissimus.[66] They constitute about 55% of the iliocostalis and multifidus. Reciprocally, fast-twitch type A fibers constitute 20% of the fibres of multifidus, iliocostalis, and longissimus, and fast-twitch type B constitute 25% of the fibers of multifidus and iliocostalis but only 11% of longissimus.[66]

These histochemical profiles seem to correlate with the fatigue resistance of the back muscles and their endurance times, which are higher than most human muscles.[66] However, individuals exhibit a large variance in fatigue resistance.[66] It is possible that endurance may be a direct function of the density of slow-twitch fibers in the back muscles, that lack of resistance to fatigue is a risk factor for back injury, and that conditioning can change the histochemical profile of an individual to overcome this risk. These possibilities, however, remain to be explored.

Lifting

In biomechanical terms, the act of lifting constitutes a problem in balancing moments. When an individual bends forward to execute a lift, flexion occurs at the hip joint and in the lumbar spine. Indeed, most of the forward movement seen during trunk flexion occurs at the hip joint.[54] The flexion forces are generated by gravity acting on the mass of the object to be lifted and on the mass of the trunk above the level of the hip joint and lumbar spine (Fig. 4-14). These forces exert flexion moments on both the hip joint and the lumbar spine. In each case the moment will be the product of the force and its perpendicular distance from the joint in question. The total flexion moment acting on each joint will be the sum of the moments exerted by the mass to be lifted and the mass of the trunk. For a lift to be executed these flexion moments have to be overcome by a moment acting in the opposite direction. This could be exerted by longitudinal forces acting downward behind the hip joint and vertebral column or by forces acting upward in front of the joints pushing the trunk upward.

There are no doubts as to the capacity of the hip extensors to generate large moments and overcome the flexion moments exerted on the hip joint even by the heaviest of loads that might be lifted.[70,71] However, the hip extensors are able to rotate only the pelvis backward on the femurs; they do not act on the lumbar spine. Thus, regardless of what happens at the hip joint, the lumbar spine still remains subject to a flexion moment that must be

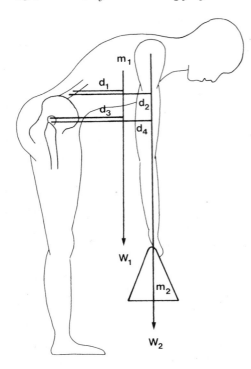

Fig. 4-14 The flexion moments exerted on a flexed trunk. Forces generated by the weight of the trunk and the load to be lifted act vertically in front of the lumbar spine and hip joint. The moments they exert on each joint are proportional to the distance between the line of action of each force and the joint in question. The mass of the trunk (m_1) exerts a force (W_1) that acts a measurable distance in front of the lumbar spine (d_1) and the hip joint (d_3). The mass to be lifted (m_2) exerts a force (W_2) that acts a measurable distance from the lumbar spine (d_2) and the hip joint (d_4). The respective moments acting on the lumbar spine will be W_1d_1 and W_1d_3; those on the hip joint will be W_2d_2 and W_2d_4. (Reproduced, with permission, from Bogduk N: Clinical Anatomy of the Lumbar Spine and Sacrum (3rd ed.) Churchill Livingstone, Edinburgh, 1997.)

overcome in some other way. Without an appropriate mechanism the lumbar spine would stay flexed as the hips extended; indeed as the pelvis rotated backward, flexion of the lumbar spine would be accentuated as its bottom end was pulled backward with the pelvis while its top end remained stationary under the load of the flexion moment. A mechanism is required to allow the lumbar spine to resist this deformation or to cause it to extend in unison with the hip joint.

Despite much investigation and debate, the exact nature of this mechanism remains unresolved. In various ways the back muscles, intra-abdominal pressure, the thoracolumbar fascia, and the posterior ligamentous system have been believed to participate.

For light lifts the flexion moments generated are relatively small. In the case of a 70 kg man lifting a 10 kg mass in a fully stooped position, the upper trunk weighs about 40 kg and acts about 30 cm in front of the lumbar spine while the arms holding the mass to be lifted lie about 45 cm in front of the lumbar spine. The respective flexion moments are, therefore: $40 \times 9.8 \times 0.30 = 117.6$ Nm, and $10 \times 9.8 \times 0.45 = 44.1$ Nm, a total of 161.7 Nm. This load is well within the capacity of the back muscles (200 Nm, see above). Thus, as the hips extend, the lumbar back muscles are capable of resisting further flexion of the lumbar spine, and indeed could even actively extend it, and the weight would be lifted.

Increasing the load to be lifted to over 30 kg increases the flexion moment to 132.2 Nm, which, when added to the flexion moment of the upper trunk, exceeds the capacity of the back muscles. To remain within the capacity of the back muscles such loads must be carried closer to the lumbar spine; i.e., they must be borne with a much shorter moment arm. Even so, decreasing the moment arm to about 15 cm limits the load to be carried to about 90 kg. The back muscles are simply not strong enough to raise greater loads. Such realizations have generated concepts of several additional mechanisms that serve to aid the back muscles in overcoming large flexion moments.

In 1957 Bartelink[72] raised the proposition that intra-abdominal pressure could aid the lumbar spine in resisting flexion by acting upward on the diaphragm—the so-called intra-abdominal balloon mechanism. Bartelink himself was circumspect and reserved in raising this conjecture, but the concept was rapidly popularized, particularly among physiotherapists. Even though it was never validated, the concept seemed to be treated as fact. It received early endorsement in orthopedic circles,[27] and intra-abdominal pressure was adopted by ergonomists and others as a measure of spinal stress and safe-lifting standards.[73–80] In more contemporary studies, intra-abdominal pressure has been monitored during various spinal movements and lifting tasks.[28,63,81]

Reservations about the validity of the abdominal balloon mechanism have arisen from several quarters. Studies of lifting tasks reveal that, unlike myoelectric activity, intra-abdominal pressure does not correlate well with the size of the load being lifted or the applied stress on the vertebral column as measured by intradiscal pressure.[55,56,82] Indeed, deliberately increasing intra-abdominal pressure by a Valsalva maneuver does not relieve the load on the lumbar spine but actually increases it.[83] Clinical studies have shown that although abdominal muscles are weaker than normal in patients with back pain, intra-abdominal pressure is not different.[84] Furthermore, strengthening the abdominal muscles both in normal individuals[85] and in patients with back pain[86] does not influence intra-abdominal pressure during lifting.

The most strident criticism of the intra-abdominal balloon theory comes from bioengineers and others who maintain that (1) to generate any significant antiflexion moment the pressure required would exceed the maximum hoop tension of the abdominal muscles[87,88,89]; (2) such a pressure would be so high as to obstruct the abdominal aorta[87] (a reservation raised by Bartelink himself[72]); and (3) because the abdominal muscles lie in front of the lumbar spine and connect the thorax to the pelvis, whenever they contract to generate pressure they must also exert a flexion moment on the trunk, which would negate any antiflexion value of the intra-abdominal pressure.[70,71,89,90]

These reservations inspired an alternative explanation of the role of the abdominal muscles during lifting. Farfan, Gracovetsky, and colleagues[22,70,89,91] noted the criss-cross arrangement of the fibers in the posterior layer of thoracolumbar fascia and surmised that if lateral tension was applied to this fascia it would result in an extension moment being exerted on the lumbar spinous processes. Such tension could be exerted by the abdominal muscles that arise from the thoracolumbar fascia, and the trigonometry of the fibers in the thoracolumbar fascia was such that they could convert lateral tension into an appreciable extension moment—the so-called "gain" of the thoracolumbar fascia.[89] The role of the abdominal muscles during lifting was thus to brace, if not actually extend, the lumbar spine by pulling on the thoracolumbar fascia. Any rises in intra-abdominal pressure were thereby only coincidental, occurring because of the contraction of the abdominal muscles acting on the thoracolumbar fascia.

Subsequent anatomic studies revealed several liabilities of this model.[20] First, the posterior layer of thoracolumbar fascia is well developed only in the lower lumbar region, but nevertheless its fibers are appropriately orientated to enable lateral tension exerted on the fascia to produce extension moments at least on the L2 to L5 spinous processes (Fig. 4-15). However, dissection reveals that of the abdominal muscles, internal oblique offers only a few fibers that irregularly attach to the thoracolumbar fascia; transversus abdominis is the only muscle that consistently attaches to the thoracolumbar fascia, but only its very middle fibers do so. The size of these fibers is such that even on maximum contraction the force they exert is very small. Calculations revealed that the extensor moment they could exert on the lumbar spine amounted to less than 6 Nm.[92] Thus the contribution that abdominal muscles might make to antiflexion moments is trivial, a conclusion also borne out by subsequent, independent modeling studies.[81]

A totally different model of lifting was elaborated by Farfan and Gracovetsky.[22,70,89] Noting the weakness of the back muscles, these authors pro-

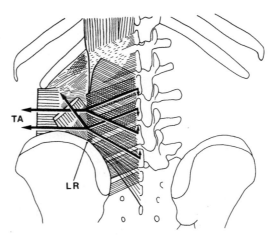

Fig. 4-15 The mechanics of the thoracolumbar fascia. From any point in the lateral raphe *(lr)*, lateral tension in the posterior layer of the thoracolumbar fascia is transmitted upward through the deep lamina of the posterior layer, and downward through the superficial layer. Because of the obliquity of these lines of tension, a small downward vector is generated at the midline attachment of the deep lamina, and a small upward vector is generated at the midline attachment of the superficial lamina. These mutually opposite vectors tend to approximate or oppose the separation the L2 and L4, and L3 and L5 spinous processes. Lateral tension on the fascia can be exerted by the transversus abdominis (TA), and to a lesser extent by the few fibers of internal oblique when they attach to the lateral raphe. (Reproduced, with permission, from Bogduk N: Clinical Anatomy of the Lumbar Spine and Sacrum. (3rd ed.) Churchill Livingstone, Edinburgh, 1997.)

posed that extension of the lumbar spine was not required to lift heavy loads or loads with long moment arms. They proposed that the lumbar spine should remain fully flexed in order to engage, i.e., maximally stretch, what they referred to as the "posterior ligamentous system," namely the capsules of the zygapophysial joints, the interspinous and supraspinous ligaments, and the posterior layer of thoracolumbar fascia, the latter acting passively to transmit tension between the lumbar spinous processes and ilium.

Under such conditions the active energy for a lift was provided by the powerful hip extensor muscles. These rotated the pelvis backward. Meanwhile, the external load acting on the upper trunk kept the lumbar spine flexed. Tension would develop in the posterior ligamentous system, which bridged the thorax and pelvis. With the posterior ligamentous system so engaged, as the pelvis rotated backward the lumbar spine would be passively raised while remaining in a fully flexed position. In essence, the posterior sagittal rotation of the pelvis would be transmitted through the posterior ligaments first to the L5 vertebra, then to L4 and so on, up through the lumbar spine into the thorax. All that was required was that the posterior ligamentous system be sufficiently strong to withstand the passive tension generated in it by the movement of the pelvis at one end and the weight of the trunk and external load at the other. The lumbar spine would thereby be raised like a long, rigid arm rotating on the pelvis and raising the external load with it.

Contraction of the back muscles was not required if the ligaments could take the load. Indeed, muscle contraction was distinctly undesirable because any active extension of the lumbar spine would disengage the posterior ligaments and preclude them from transmitting tension. The back muscles could be recruited only once the trunk had been raised sufficiently to shorten the moment arm of the external load, reducing its flexion moment to within the capacity of the back muscles.

The attraction of this model was that it overcame the problem of the relative weakness of the back muscles by dispensing with their need to act, which in turn was consistent with the myoelectric silence of the back muscles at full flexion of the trunk and the recruitment of muscle activity only once the trunk had been elevated and the flexion moment arm had been reduced. Support for the model also came from surgical studies, which reported that if the midline ligaments and thoracolumbar fascia were conscientiously reconstructed after multilevel laminectomies, the postoperative recovery and rehabilitation of patients were enhanced.[93]

However, while attractive in a qualitative sense, the mechanism of the posterior ligamentous system was not validated quantitatively. The model requires that the ligaments be strong enough to sustain the loads applied. In this regard, data on the strength of the posterior ligaments is scant and irregular, but sufficient data are available to permit an initial appraisal of the feasibility of the posterior ligament model.

The strength of spinal ligaments varies considerably, but average values can be calculated. Table 4-1 summarizes some of the available data. It is evident that the strongest posterior "ligaments" of the lumbar spine are the zy-

| Table 4-1 | Strength of the Posterior Ligamentous System. Average Force at Failure has been Calculated Using Raw Data Provided in the References Cited. The Moment Arms are Estimates Based on Inspection of a Representative Vertebra Measuring the Perpendicular Distance Between the Location of the Axes of Rotation of the Lumbar Spine and the Sites of Attachment of the Various Ligaments. | | | |

Ligament	Reference	Average Force at Failure (N)	Moment Arm (m)	Maximum Moment (Nm)
Posterior longitudinal	94	90	0.02	1.8
Ligamentum flavum	94	244	0.03	7.3
Zygapophysial joint	94	680	0.04	27.2
capsule	95	672		
Interspinous	94	107	0.05	5.4
Thoracolumbar fascia	94	500	0.06	30.0
Total				51.7

gapophysial joint capsules and the thoracolumbar fascia forming the midline "supraspinous ligament." However, when the relatively short moment arms over which these ligaments act are considered, it is found that the maximum moment they can sustain is relatively small. Even the sum total of all their moments is considerably less than that required for heavy lifting and is four times less than the maximum strength of the back muscles. Of course, it is possible that the data quoted may not be representative of the true mean values of the strength of these ligaments, but it does not seem likely that the literature quoted underestimated their strength by a factor of four or more. Under these conditions, it is evident that the posterior ligamentous system alone is not strong enough to perform the role required of it in heavy lifting. The posterior ligamentous system is not strong enough to replace the back muscles as a mechanism to prevent flexion of the lumbar spine during lifting. Some other mechanism must operate.

One such mechanism is that of the **hydraulic amplifier** effect.[91] It was originally proposed by Farfan, Gracovetsky, and Lamy[91] that because the thoracolumbar fascia surrounded the back muscles as a retinaculum it could serve to brace these muscles and enhance their power. The engineering basis for this effect is complicated, and the concept remained unexplored until very recently. A mathematical proof has been published that suggests that by investing the back muscles the thoracolumbar fascia enhances the strength of the back muscles by some 30%.[96] This is an appreciable increase and an attractive mechanism for enhancing the antiflexion capacity of the back muscles. However, the validity of this proof is still being questioned on the grounds that the principles used, while applicable to the behavior of solids, may not be applicable to muscles. Thus the concept of the hydraulic amplifier mechanism still remains under scrutiny.

A contrasting model has been proposed to explain the mechanics of the lumbar spine in lifting. It is based on arch theory and maintains that the behavior, stability, and strength of the lumbar spine during lifting can be explained by viewing the lumbar spine as an arch braced by intra-abdominal pressure.[97,98] However, this intriguing concept has not met with any degree of acceptance and has been challenged from some quarters.[99]

In summary, despite much effort over recent years the exact mechanism of heavy lifting remains unexplained. The back muscles are too weak to extend the lumbar spine against large flexion moments; the intra-abdominal balloon has been refuted; the abdominal mechanism and thoracolumbar fascia have been refuted, and the posterior ligamentous system appears too weak to replace the back muscles. Engineering models of the hydraulic amplifier effect and the arch model are still subject to debate.

Two questions remain to be answered: (1) What provides the missing force to sustain heavy loads? (2) Why is intra-abdominal pressure so consistently generated during lifts if it neither braces the thoracolumbar fascia nor provides an intra-abdominal balloon? At present these questions can only be addressed by conjecture, but certain concepts are worthy of consideration.

With regard to intra-abdominal pressure, one concept that has been overlooked in studies of lifting is the role of the abdominal muscles in controlling axial rotation of the trunk. Investigators have focused their attention on movements in the sagittal plane during lifting and have ignored the fact that when bent forward to grasp an object to be lifted the trunk is liable to axial rotation. Unless the external load is perfectly balanced and lies exactly in the midline, it will cause the trunk to twist to the left or the right. Thus, to keep the weight in the midline and in the sagittal plane, the lifter must control any twisting effect. The oblique abdominal muscles are the principal rotators of the trunk and would be responsible for this bracing. In contracting to control axial rotation, the abdominal muscles would secondarily raise intra-abdominal pressure. This pressure rise is therefore an epiphenomenon and would reflect not the size of any external load but its tendency to twist the flexed trunk.

With regard to loads in the sagittal plane, the passive strength of the back muscles has been neglected in discussions of lifting. From the behavior of isolated muscle fibers it is known that as a muscle elongates its maximum contractile force diminishes, but its passive elastic tension rises; so much so that in an elongated muscle the total passive and active tension generated is at least equal to the maximum contractile capacity of the muscle at resting length. Thus, although they become electrically silent at full flexion, the back muscles are still capable of providing passive tension equal to their maximum contractile strength. This would allow the silent muscles to supplement the engaged posterior ligamentous system. With the back muscles providing some 200 Nm and the ligaments some 50 Nm or more, the total antiflexion capacity of the lumbar spine rises to about 250 Nm, which would allow some 30 kg to be safely lifted at 90 degrees trunk flexion. Larger loads could be sustained by proportionally shortening the moment arm. Consequently, the mechanism of lifting may well be essentially as proposed by Farfan and Gracovetsky,[22,70,91] except that the passive tension in the back muscles constitutes the major component of the "posterior ligamentous system."

REFERENCES

1. Bogduk N, Pearcy M, Hadfield G: Anatomy and biomechanics of psoas major. Clin Biomech 7:109–119, 1992
2. Williams PL, et al (Eds.): Gray's Anatomy. (38th ed.) Churchill Livingstone, Edinburgh. 1995
3. Cave AJE: The innervation and morphology of the cervical intertransverse muscles. J Anat 71:497–515, 1937
4. Poirier P: Myologie. In Poirier P, Charpy A: Traite d'Anatomie Humaine. (3rd ed.) Vol. 2. Fasc 1. Masson, Paris, 1912
5. Bogduk N: A reappraisal of the anatomy of the human lumbar erector spinae. J Anat 131:525–540, 1980
6. Macintosh JE, Bogduk N: The biomechanics of the lumbar multifidus. Clin Biomech 1:205–213, 1986
7. Macintosh JE, Bogduk N: The morphology of the lumbar erector spinae. Spine 12:658–668, 1986
8. Macintosh JE, Valencia F, Bogduk N, Munro RR: The morphology of the lumbar multifidus muscles. Clin Biomech 1:196–204, 1986
9. Bogduk N, Wilson AS, Tynan W: The human lumbar dorsal rami. J Anat 134:383–397, 1982
10. Bogduk N: The lumbar mamillo-accessory ligament. Its anatomical and neurosurgical significance. Spine 6:162–167, 1981
11. Abrahams VC: The physiology of neck muscles; their role in head movement and maintenance of posture. Can J Physiol Pharmacol 55:332–338, 1977
12. Abrahams VC: Sensory and motor specialization in some muscles of the neck. TINS 4:24–27, 1981
13. Cooper S, Danial PM: Muscles spindles in man, their morphology in the lumbricals and the deep muscles of the neck. Brain 86:563–594, 1963
14. Bastide G, Zadeh J, Lefebvre D: Are the "little muscles" what we think they are? Surg Radiol Anat 11:255–256, 1989
15. Nitz AJ, Peck D: Comparison of muscle spindle concentrations in large and small human epaxial muscles acting in parallel combinations. Am Surg 52:273–277, 1986
16. Peck D, Buxton DF, Nitz A: A comparison of spindle concentrations in large and small muscles acting in parallel combinations. J Morphol 180:243–252, 1984
17. Lewin T, Moffet B, Viidik A: The morphology of the lumbar synovial intervertebral joints. Acta Morphol Neerlando-Scandinav 4:299–319, 1962
18. Donisch EW, Basmajian JV: Electromyography of deep back muscles in man. Am J Anat 133:25–36, 1972
19. Luk KDK, Ho HC, Leong JCY: The iliolumbar ligament. A study of its anatomy, development and clinical significance. J Bone Joint Surg 68B:197–200, 1986
20. Bogduk N, Macintosh J: The applied anatomy of the thoracolumbar fascia. Spine 9:164–170, 1984
21. Fairbank JCT, O'Brien JP: The abdominal cavity and thoracolumbar fascia as stabilisers of the lumbar spine in patients with low back pain. Engineering Aspects of the Spine. Mechanical Engineering Publications, 2:83–88, 1980
22. Gracovetsky S, Farfan HF, Lamy C: The mechanism of the lumbar spine. Spine 6:249–262, 1981

23. Vleeming A, Pool-Goudzwaard AL, Stoeckart R, et al: The posterior layer of the thoracolumbar fascia: its function in load transfer from spine to legs. Spine 20:753–758, 1995
24. Floyd WF, Silver PHS: The function of the erectores spinae muscles in certain movements and postures in man. J Physiol 129:184–203, 1955
25. Morris JM, Benner G, Lucas DB: An electromyographic study of the intrinsic muscles of the back in man. J Anat 96:509–520, 1962
26. Ortengren R, Andersson GBJ: Electromyographic studies of trunk muscles with special reference to the functional anatomy of the lumbar spine. Spine 2:44–52, 1977
27. Morris JM, Lucas DB, Bresler B: Role of the trunk in stability of the spine. J Bone Joint Surg 43A:327–351, 1961
28. Andersson GBJ, Ortengren R, Nachemson A: Intradiscal pressure, intra-abdominal pressure and myoelectric back muscle activity related to posture and loading. Clin Orthop 129:156–164, 1977
29. Carlsoo S: The static muscle load in different work positions: an electromyographic study. Ergonomics 4:193–211, 1961
30. Ortengren R, Andersson G, Nachemson A: Lumbar loads in fixed working postures during flexion and rotation. In Asmussen E, Jorgensen K (Eds.): Biomechanics VI-B, International Series on Biomechanics. Vol 2B. Human Kinetics, Champaign, Illinois, 1978
31. Portnoy H, Morin F: Electromyographic study of the postural muscles in various positions and movements. Am J Physiol 186:122–126, 1956
32. Allen CEL: Muscle action potentials used in the study of dynamic anatomy. Br J Phys Med 11:66–73, 1948
33. Andersson BJG, Ortengren R: Myoelectric activity during sitting. Scand J Rehabil Med Suppl 3:73–90, 1974
34. Andersson BJG, Jonsson B, Ortengren R: Myoelectric activity in individual lumbar erector spinae muscles in sitting: a study with surface and wire electrodes. Scand J Rehabil Med Suppl 3:91–108, 1974
35. Asmussen E, Klausen K: Form and function of the erect human spine. Clin Orthop 25:55–63, 1962
36. Carlsoo S: Influence of frontal and dorsal loads on muscle activity and on the weight distribution in the feet. Acta Orthop Scand 34:299–309, 1964
37. De Vries HA: Muscle tonus in postural muscles. Am J Phys Med 44:275–291, 1965
38. Jonsson B: The functions of the individual muscles in the lumbar part of the spinae muscle. Electromyography 10:5–21, 1970
39. Joseph J, McColl I: Electromyography of muscles of posture: posterior vertebral muscles in males. J Physiol 157:33–37, 1961
40. Klausen K: The form and function of the loaded human spine. Acta Physiol Scand 65:176–190, 1965
41. Valencia FP, Munro RR: An electromyographic study of the lumbar multifidus in man. Electromyogr Clin Neurophysiol 25:205–221, 1985
42. Floyd WF, Silver PHS: Function of erectores spinae in flexion of the trunk. Lancet 1:133–134, 1951
43. Kippers V, Parker AW: Electromyographic studies of erectores spinae: symmetrical postures and sagittal trunk motion. Aust J Physiother 31:95–105, 1985
44. Andersson BJG, Ortengren R: Lumbar disc pressure and myoelectric back muscle activity during sitting. II. Studies of an office chair. Scand J Rehabil Med 6:115–121, 1974

45. Andersson BJG, Ortengren R, Nachemson AL, et al: The sitting posture: an electromyographic and discometric study. Orthop Clin North Am 6:105–120, 1975
46. Nachemson AL: The lumbar spine. An orthopaedic challenge. Spine 1:59–71, 1976
47. Nachemson A: Lumbar intradiscal pressure. In Jayson MIV (Ed.): The Lumbar Spine and Backache. (2nd ed.) Pitman, London, 1980
48. Golding JSR: Electromyography of the erector spinae in low back pain. Postgrad Med J 28:401–406, 1952
49. Koreska J, Robertson D, Mills RH: Biomechanics of the lumbar spine and its clinical significance. Orthop Clin North Am 8:121–123, 1977
50. Okada M: Electromyographic assessment of the muscular load in forward bending postures. J Fac Sci Univ Tokyo 8:311–336, 1970
51. Pauly JE: An electromyographic analysis of certain movements and exercises. I. Some deep muscles of the back. Anat Rec 155:223–234, 1966
52. Andersson GBJ, Ortengren R, Herberts P: Quantitative electromyographic studies of back muscle activity related to posture and loading. Orthop Clin North Am 8:85–96, 1977
53. Schulz A, Andersson GBJ, Ortengren R, et al: Analysis and quantitative myoelectric measurements of loads on the lumbar spine when holding weights in standing postures. Spine 7:390–397, 1982
54. Kippers V, Parker AW: Posture related to myoelectric silence of erectores spinae during trunk flexion. Spine 7:740–745, 1984
55. Ortengren R, Andersson GBJ, Nachemson AL: Studies of relationships between lumbar disc pressure, myoelectric back muscle activity, and intra-abdominal (intragastric) pressure. Spine 6:98–103, 1981
56. Andersson GBJ: Loads on the lumbar spine: in vivo measurements and biomechanical analyses. In Winter DA, Norman RW, Wells RP, Hayes KC, Patla AE (Eds.) Biomechanics IX-B, International Series on Biomechanics. Human Kinetics, Champaign, Illinois, 1983
57. Nachemson A, Morris JM: In vivo measurements of intradiscal pressure. J Bone Joint Surg 46:1077–1092, 1964
58. Nachemson AL, Elfstrom G: Intravital dynamic pressure measurements in lumbar discs. A study of common movements, maneuvers and exercises. Scand J Rehabil Med 2 Supp 1:1–40, 1970
59. Nachemson A: The load on lumbar disks in different positions of the body. Clin Orthop 45:107–122, 1966
60. Andersson GBJ, Ortengren R, Nachemson A: Quantitative studies of the back in different working postures. Scand J Rehabil Med Supp 6:173–181, 1978
61. Andersson BJG, Ortengren R, Nachemson A, Elfstrom G: Lumbar disc pressure and myoelectric activity during sitting. I. Studies on an experimental chair. Scand J Rehabil Med 6:104–114, 1974
62. Andersson BJG, Ortengren R, Nachemson A, Elfstrom G: Lumbar disc pressure and myoelectric back muscle activity during sitting. IV. Studies on a car driver's seat. Scand J Rehabil Med 6:128–133, 1974
63. Andersson GBJ, Ortengren R, Nachemson A: Quantitative studies of back loads in lifting. Spine 1:178–184, 1976
64. Vakos JP, Nitz AJ, Threlkeld AJ, Shapiro R: Electromyographic activity of selected trunk and hip muscles during a squat lift: effect of varying the lumbar posture. Spine 19:687–695, 1994
65. McNeill T, Warwick D, Andersson G, Schultz A: Trunk strengths in attempted

flexion, extension, and lateral bending in healthy subjects and patients with low-back disorders. Spine 5:529–538, 1980

66. Jorgensen K, Nicholaisen T, Kato M: Muscle fiber distribution, capillary density, and enzymatic activities in the lumbar paravertebral muscles of young men: significance for isometric endurance. Spine 18:1439–1450, 1993

67. Bogduk N, Macintosh JE, Pearcy MJ: A universal model of the lumbar back muscles in the upright position. Spine 17:897–913, 1992

68. Macintosh JE, Bogduk N, Pearcy MJ: The effects of flexion on the geometry and actions of the lumbar erector spinae. Spine 18:884–893, 1993

69. Macintosh JE, Pearcy MJ, Bogduk N: The axial torque of the lumbar back muscles: torsion strength of the back muscles. Aust N Z J Surg 63:205–212, 1993

70. Farfan HF: Muscular mechanism of the lumbar spine and the position of power and efficiency. Orthop Clin North Am 6:135–144, 1975

71. Farfan HF: The biomechanical advantage of lordosis and hip extension for upright activity. Man as compared with other anthropoids. Spine 3:336–342, 1978

72. Bartelink DL: The role of abdominal pressure in relieving the pressure on the lumbar intervertebral discs. J Bone Joint Surg 39B:718–725, 1957

73. Davis PR: Posture of the trunk during the lifting of weights. Br Med J 1:87–89, 1959

74. Davis PR: The use of intra-abdominal pressure in evaluating stresses on the lumbar spine. Spine 6:90–92, 1981

75. Davis PR, Stubbs DA: Safe levels of manual forces for young males (1). Appl Ergon 8:141–150, 1977

76. Davis PR, Troup JDG: Pressures in the trunk cavities when pulling, pushing, and lifting. Ergonomics 7:465–474, 1964

77. Stubbs DA: Trunk stresses in construction and other industrial workers. Spine 6:83–89, 1981

78. Troup JDG: Relation of lumbar spine disorders to heavy manual work and lifting. Lancet 1:857–861, 1965

79. Troup JDG: Dynamic factors in the analysis of stoop and crouch lifting methods: a methodological approach to the development of safe materials handling standards. Orthop Clin North Am 8:201–209, 1977

80. Troup JDG: Biomechanics of the vertebral column. Physiotherapy 65:238–244, 1979

81. McGill SM, Norman RW: Potential of lumbodorsal fascia forces to generate back extension moments during squat lifts. J Biomed Eng 10:312–318, 1988

82. Leskinen TPJ, Stalhammar HR, Kuorinka IAA, Troup JDG: Hip torque, lumbosacral compression, and intraabdominal pressure in lifting and lowering tasks. In Winter DA, Norman RW, Wells RP, et al (Eds.): Biomechanics IXB, International Series on Biomechanics. Human Kinetics, Champaign, Illinois, 1983

83. Nachemson AL, Andersson GBJ, Schultz AB: Valsalva maneuver biomechanics. Effects on trunk load of elevated intraabdominal pressure. Spine 11:476–479, 1986

84. Hemborg B, Moritz U: Intra-abdominal pressure and trunk muscle activity during lifting II: chronic low-back patients. Scand J Rehabil Med 17:5–13, 1985

85. Hemborg B, Moritz, Hamberg J, Lowing H, Akesson I: Intra-abdominal pressure and trunk muscle activity during lifting—effect of abdominal muscle training in healthy subjects. Scand J Rehabil Med 15:183–196, 1983

86. Hemborg B, Moritz U, Hamberg J, Holmstrom E, et al: Intra-abdominal pressure and trunk muscle activity during lifting. III: effects of abdominal muscle training in chronic low-back patients. Scand J Rehabil Med 17:15–24, 1985

87. Farfan HF, Gracovetsky S: The abdominal mechanism. Paper presented at the International Society for the Study of the Lumbar Spine Meeting, Paris, 1981

88. Farfan HF, Gracovetsky S, Helleur C: The role of mathematical models in the assessment of task in the workplace. In Winter DA, Norman RW, Wells RP, et al (Eds.): Biomechanics IXB, International Series on Biomechanics. Human Kinetics, Champaign, Illinois, 1983

89. Gracovetsky S, Farfan HF, Helleur C: The abdominal mechanism. Spine 10:317–324, 1985

90. Bearn JG: The significance of the activity of the abdominal muscles in weight lifting. Acta Anat 45:83–89, 1961

91. Gracovetsky S, Farfan HF, Lamy C: A mathematical model of the lumbar spine using an optimal system to control muscles and ligaments. Orthop Clin North Am 8:135–153, 1977

92. Macintosh JE, Bogduk N, Gracovetsky S: The biomechanics of the thoracolumbar fascia. Clin Biomech 2:78–83, 1987

93. Crock HV, Crock MC: A technique for decompression of the lumbar spinal canal. Neuro-Orthopaedics 5:96–99, 1988

94. Mykelbust JB, Pintar F, Yoganandan N, et al: Tensile strength of spinal ligaments. Spine 13:526–531, 1988

95. Cyron BM, Hutton WC: The tensile strength of the capsular ligaments of the apophyseal joints. J Anat 132:145–150, 1981

96. Hukins DWL, Aspden RM, Hickey DS: Thoracolumbar fascia can increase the efficiency of the erector spinae muscles. Clin Biomech 5:30–34, 1990

97. Aspden RM: Intra-abdominal pressure and its role in spinal mechanics. Clin Biomech 2:168–174, 1987

98. Aspden RM: The spine as an arch. A new mathematical model. Spine 14:266–274, 1989

99. Adams M: Letter to the editor. Spine 14:1272, 1989

5

Mechanical Diagnosis and Therapy for Disorders of the Low Back

Robin A. McKenzie

In the first edition of *Physical Therapy of the Low Back*[1] I suggested that over the next few years, physical therapists would have the opportunity to become the key professionals within medicine responsible for the delivery of conservative care for mechanical disorders of the spine. It was my view that if appropriate steps were not taken we may never have another opportunity to achieve this goal.

I suspect the opportunity is almost lost. Since 1987 the practice by physiotherapists of diagnosis and assessment of mechanical disorders affecting the low back has changed little. The belief that symmetry is normal and asymmetry a likely cause of musculoskeletal disorder is widespread. Diagnostic systems based on the detection of asymmetry by observation and palpation abound. Palpation of joint motion to detect hyper- or hypomobility is still one of the mainstays of therapists specializing in manual therapy. Instability is another common diagnosis among therapists. In my view there is no credible support in the scientific literature for these assessment systems or the resulting diagnostic conclusions.[2]

Current physical therapies also remain unchanged, although the underlying philosophies may have been altered to fit new theories. The scientific literature in the past decade reveals no new developments in the treatment of low back pain and, if we are to believe the guidelines, no evidence that any one treatment in common use is better than awaiting the resolution of natural history. Physiotherapists, it could be said, are no further ahead than they were in 1987 in their quest for acceptance as the main carers of the problem back.

Chiropractic, on the other hand is flourishing. In 1993, the British Medical Association published a report[3] officially endorsing chiropractic and stated "A profession such as chiropractic which now has a discrete and established education and research base should practice alongside orthodox medical care and be regulated on a similar basis."

Chiropractors in the United States already see more patients with mechanical back pain than the combined total of patients seen by all other back health providers. Political and scientific support and recognition for chiropractic is growing steadily.

Chiropractic is now supported by the World Health Organization. The Foundation for Chiropractic Research has produced credible studies supporting the use of spinal manipulation. Guidelines for the treatment of acute low back pain issued in the United States, New Zealand, and the United Kingdom recommend spinal manipulation at least in the first few days following onset, and the Danish government funds chiropractic manipulation without the requirement of medical referral. Chiropractors have been quick to make capital from these developments.

Chiropractors are continually adding to their treatment protocols the useless trappings of physiotherapy in the form of modalities such as heat, ultrasound, ice, laser therapy, transcutaneous electrical stimulation, infrared, short-wave diathermy, interferential therapy, or magnetic therapy.[4,5,6,7] In doing so they may well damage the image that has been slowly improving with the scientific validation of manipulation.

Since the study by Meade, et al[8] chiropractic is taking on a new and confident profile. Education of chiropractors is moving toward the traditional medical training model, and more medical professionals are involved in their education. Through their political lobbying chiropractors have succeeded in having legislation bar physical therapists from practicing spinal manipulation in some states in the United States.

Chiropractors usually make a diagnosis based on palpation of intersegmental motion or from radiologic screening. However, neither palpation nor radiographs are helpful in determining diagnosis in nonspecific mechanical low back pain. Magnetic resonance imaging (MRI) and computed tomography (CT) are also unreliable because of the frequency of false-positive reporting. Chiropractic diagnosis and therapy in general have remained unchanged in the past decade but have flourished because of a carefully orchestrated and executed program of improved education, research, marketing, and publicity. The physiotherapy profession has failed to follow suit. Chiropractic has taken advantage of the many studies complementary to spinal manipulation.[8-14] Chiropractors emerging from the colleges today are well educated, are not claiming to treat all manner of diseases, and are genuinely interested in seeking better ways of managing and caring for their patients. I suspect that worldwide, doctors of chiropractic have made great advances.

The "evidence-based guidelines" issued in the United States, New Zealand, Australia, Denmark, and Great Britain for the treatment of mechanical back disorders recommend that active care replace passive care; that modalities are out; and that exercise, activity, and movement are the means by which we are most likely to improve the health of injured spinal structures. Methods of treatment that create dependency should be discouraged.

PATHOLOGY

Modern medicine has advanced with such rapidity that it can be fairly stated that in the past 30 years we have learned more of the precise nature of the causes of spinal pain than in all of previous recorded history, and the search has narrowed to the two structures most likely to be involved in the production of most mechanical back pain.[15]

The intervertebral disc, with its strong annulus fibrosus retaining the gel-like nucleus, is probably the most common source of back pain.[16–23] Mooney[24] has stated that "In summary, where is the pain coming from in the chronic low back pain patient? I believe its source ultimately, is in the disc."

The journal *Spine* has published the results of many studies aimed at the examination of intervertebral disc structure, function, pathology, and treatment. The other mobile structures to capture the attention of those investigating back pain are the zygapophyseal joints. These are also probable sources of pain, but the precise pathologic process causing the pain is unknown, and the frequency of "facet" joint pain, however, has been challenged in at least two studies.[25, 26]

Undoubtedly, disorders of the sacroiliac joint occur, but most are inflammatory. That true mechanical lesions occur is also recognized. However, they are uncommon and usually only occur following pregnancy.[27] Physical therapists, especially in the United States[2] or wherever therapists are receiving instruction from osteopaths, are "rediscovering" sacroiliac pathology in large numbers of patients. If so, either the proponents are mistaken or the literature is in error.

There is a mistaken belief among some physical therapists that articular asymmetry is a contributing factor to the onset of backache. Although orthopedic opinion does not support the proposal,[28] muscle imbalance as well as muscle strain are also regarded by many to be common causes of persistent back pain. If articular asymmetry or muscle imbalance were causative factors in back pain, patients with scoliosis could be expected to have a higher incidence of pain than that experienced by the general population. They do not. Kostuik[29] and Dieck[30] found that postural asymmetry had no effect in back pain causation.

It is now generally accepted that most low back problems are mechanical, probably arising in the intervertebral disc early in adult life and in the zygapophyseal joints much later in life.[31–34] Therefore the treatment for these particular problems should mainly be mechanical. Mechanical treatments have been applied for 3000 years of recorded history,[35] and most treatments today for the alleviation of back pain contain mechanical components.[24, 36]

We still cannot, in many cases, positively identify the cause or the source of the pain. Even with sophisticated imaging tools such as CT scans and MRI, the rate of reporting of false positives reduces their reliability.

MECHANICAL TREATMENT

By adopting active mechanical procedures for treating mechanical low back pain, physical therapists have much to gain. In the 1950s physiotherapists, especially in British Commonwealth countries, began incorporating manipulative procedures in their treatments. Prior to this, mechanical therapy within physiotherapy consisted of techniques of massage and exercise in which the proponents were particularly adept. Then along came spinal manipulative therapy (SMT), but there was no amalgamation between the exercise of physiotherapy and the manipulation of the osteopath and chiropractor. The conceptual model for the dispensing of exercise was completely different from the conceptual model for the use of manipulative therapy. There was no marriage between patient-generated and therapist-generated force. The two partners were incompatible.

Presently all over the world enthusiastic physiotherapists, frustrated and stifled by years of control by medicine or disillusioned by the use of ineffectual methods of physiotherapy, are "discovering" mobilization and manipulation and are delivering SMT as the treatment of choice for most patients with spinal pain. This initial enthusiasm, although understandable, must be tempered and brought into perspective. Those of us well experienced in the use of manipulative therapy still derive that unique satisfaction whenever a spectacular improvement is obtained. There is no doubt that many patients benefit from SMT. Several studies demonstrate that there is a short-term benefit obtained from SMT.[9-14]

SMT has a particular and important part to play in the treatment of spinal pain. But not everyone will benefit from the procedure. Those in the profession who, due to long experience with SMT, are fully aware of the limitations as well as the benefits of this form of treatment, must utilize this experience to moderate the excesses that accompany the overuse of manipulative techniques.

Until we learn to distinguish between improvement that occurs directly as a result of treatment and improvement that results from spontaneous healing or the natural history, our credibility is at risk. When our patients improve over a period of 3 to 4 months, can we seriously attribute their recovery to our manipulative or mechanical prowess applied over this period? Failure to recognize and understand the natural history and self-limiting characteristics of "nonspecific" spinal disorders will perpetuate the inability of so many to critically review their treatment methods and results.

We must always be aware that most currently prescribed manual therapies for mechanical spinal disorders create patient dependence. Wherever we do something to or for the patient, the patient, and very often the therapist, attribute any improvement to the treatment dispensed. Ignorance or disregard of the natural history of mechanical back disorders allows all health providers to claim a success rate of over 90%.

If there is the slightest chance that patients can be educated in a method of treatment that enables them to reduce their own pain and disability using their own understanding and resources, they should receive that education. Every patient is entitled to this information, and every therapist should be obliged to provide it.

THE USE OF PAIN PATTERNS IN ASSESSMENT AND DIAGNOSIS

The Quebec Task Force (QTF) on activity-related low back pain published its report in 1987.[15] The report stated that the cause of pain in 90% of cases was unknown. The authors, in recommending the use of pain patterns to classify nonspecific mechanical disorders, attempted to avoid the perpetuation of diagnoses that are more likely to be wrong than right.

The pain patterns described in the first four categories of the QTF represent 90% of activity-related low back disorders. They also represent progressively complex pathologies. As the symptoms radiate further from the midline, a pathologic process evolves that is more likely to be resistant to simple treatment methods. Thus category 1 is the least complex disorder and category 4, representing compression or interference of the conductivity of spinal nerves, is the most complex and potentially disabling condition.

1. Pain in the lumbar, dorsal, or cervical areas, without radiation below the gluteal fold or beyond the shoulder, respectively, and in the absence of neurologic signs.

2. Pain in the lumbar dorsal or cervical areas, with radiation proximally (i.e., to an upper or lower limb but not beyond the elbow or the knee, respectively) and not accompanied by neurologic signs.

3. Pain in the lumbar, dorsal, or cervical areas, with radiation distally (i.e., beyond the knee or the elbow, respectively) but without neurologic signs.

4. Pain in the lumbar, dorsal, or cervical areas, with radiation to a limb and with the presence of neurologic signs (e.g., focal muscular weakness, asymmetry of reflexes, sensory loss in a dermatome, or specific loss of intestinal, bladder, or sexual function).

This category includes the radicular syndromes, which are well described in classic textbooks. These radicular syndromes may be due to various pathologies, the most frequent one being the discal hernia. However, other mechanical distortions of the spine, such as facet hypertrophy, may trigger an irritation or a radicular deficit.

The use of pain patterns to identify progressively complex mechanical disorders of the low back has been described in my text published in 1981.[36] The classification by pain patterns, as contained in the QTF report, is remarkably similar to my own. Indeed, the McKenzie system of assessment and treatment originally evolved from an ability to systematically alter pain location by applying repeated movements, or static end-range loading, which caused pain to move from a distal to a more central location (centralization). When this occurs, a QTF classification can be changed from a more-complex to a less-complex category.

"Centralization of pain" is indicative of good outcome and when present provides a prognostic indicator in all patients with radiating or referred symptoms.[37] Donelson, April, et al[41] have linked the centralization of pain to discogenic pathology in a study reporting a highly significant relationship.[38] The authors reported that centralization can reliably distinguish between discogenic and nondiscogenic pain and provides considerable help in distinguishing between a competent and noncompetent annulus. Donelson, Werneke, et al[39] have reported the reliability of centralization as a predictor of good outcome in both acute and chronic populations with back pain. Conversely, noncentralizers are highly likely to have poor outcomes. The ability to predict at an early stage those patients likely to have long-term problems is an important step in the evolution of improved spinal care.

Mechanical pain arises from trauma, (with pain of limited duration), internal derangement of the intervertebral disc, (which may often appear as recurring and episodic pain) or contracture or adaptive shortening (with persisting pain long after repair is complete). A further simple and uncomplicated cause of mechanical pain is prolonged static loading in the absence of injury. Each disorder causes pain to behave in a characteristic fashion.

Centralization or peripheralization of pain occurs most commonly in the case of decreasing or increasing internal disruption of the intervertebral disc.[40] It is also reported that pain expands, usually distally, with increasing mechanical deformation of soft tissues and retreats with the reduction of deformation. Zucherman et al[18] have reported that thermal stimulation of the internal annulus can cause pain to be referred to the lower limb, and the greater the stimulation the further the pain can extend, even below the knee. This is consistent with the findings of Donelson and Aprill.[41]

STATIC AND DYNAMIC MECHANICAL EVALUATION

The identification of movements that produce, increase, or cause pain to peripheralize is an important step in the management and prevention of further injury. Conversely, movements that abolish, decrease, or centralize symptoms can be used to develop the therapeutic program. Repeated movements also enable the identification of problems arising from contractures and fibrosis. This differentiation is necessary because the former require different treatment from the latter.

The most appropriate mechanical procedure, (patient-applied static or repeated end-range loading, therapist-applied loading, or therapist-applied mobilization or manipulation), the preferred direction for delivery of the procedure, and the need for progression of loading forces may be determined from the static and dynamic mechanical evaluation.

Alterations in pain intensity and location following static loading in flexed or extended postures are correlated with pain responses obtained from repetitive end-range sagittal and frontal plane movements performed in loaded and unloaded positions. Following the performance of these movements, a subdivision of patients within the nonspecific spectrum of back pain is possible. The movements that in the assessment cause pain to cease, reduce, or centralize are then applied as a therapy, in most cases as self-applied therapy.

SYNDROMES IN NONSPECIFIC LOW BACK PAIN

Three different responses may be found from the dynamic assessment and allow the identification of three syndromes: postural, dysfunction, and derangement. Patients in the derangement group are by far the most frequently encountered. The precise means of identification and the concepts and methods of treatment of these syndromes are described in detail else-where.[36]

Postural Syndrome

Patients with the postural syndrome are usually under 30 years of age, have sedentary occupations, and frequently are under-exercised. As a result of prolonged end-range static loading, such as occurs in sitting and bending, they develop pain locally, adjacent to the midline of the spinal column. Such patients frequently complain of pain felt separately or simultaneously in the cervical, thoracic, and lumbar areas. The pain arises from prolonged stress of normal tissue. The pain ceases on release of stress. Pain in this syndrome is never induced by movement, is rarely referred, and is never constant. There is no pathologic process and no pain on or loss of movement and symptoms are entirely subjective.[36]

Dysfunction Syndrome

Pain in the dysfunction syndrome usually develops insidiously, appearing locally, adjacent to the midline of the spinal column, and is provoked on attempting full movement that deforms adaptively shortened or contracted soft tissues. Pain is always felt at end-range limitation and does not occur during movement. With the exception of a patient with nerve-root adherence, pain from dysfunction is never referred.

Loss of movement in this syndrome can arise over time because of poor postural habits and lack of exercise. Poor postural habits allow adaptive shortening of certain structures. The result is a gradual reduction of mobility with aging. The movements reduced are usually those extension movements essential for the maintenance of the very erect posture.

Contracture or adherence of soft tissues following trauma also causes painful restricted motion. Should lack of movement following injury allow the formation of an inextensible scar within or adjacent to otherwise healthy structures, restriction of movement and pain will persist long after repair is complete. The pain resulting from stretching of this inextensible scar appears only on attempting full end-range movements. The pain does not occur during the movement or before the scar is stretched. Surrounding healthy structures capable of further extensibility are restricted by the scar tissue itself. Thus the persisting pain results directly from imperfect repair. The patient believes he is still injured because the pain is felt at the site of the original injury.

It is not possible to identify the structure causing the pain of dysfunction, but any of the soft tissues adjacent to the vertebral column may adaptively shorten or may be damaged. Thus the pain may result from injury to any of the ligamentous structures in the segment from the intervertebral disc, the zygapophyseal joints, or the superficial or deep muscles or their attachments. The pain may also result from adherence of the spinal nerve root or dura following intervertebral disc prolapse or herniation. Described simply, the pain of dysfunction is produced immediately when adherent or contracted tissues are stretched. The pain stops immediately when stretching ceases.[36]

Derangement Syndrome

The derangement syndrome mostly affects those age 20 to 55, and onset is often without apparent cause. Pain can appear quite rapidly, that is, in a matter of a few hours, or over a day or two those affected change from completely normal to significantly disabled persons. The pain of internal "derangement" or disruption of the intervertebral disc can be extreme. Acute deformity of scoliosis, kyphosis, and fixation in extension are common. The symptoms may be felt locally, in the midline or adjacent to the spinal column, and may radiate or be referred to the leg distally in the form of pain, paresthesia, or numbness. The symptoms are produced or resolved, increased or reduced, may centralize or peripheralize, or remain better or worse following the repetition of certain movements or the maintenance of certain positions.

Pain from the derangement syndrome may alter and change in regard to both the location of the pain and the extent of the area affected, which may increase or decrease. Pain from the derangement syndrome may cross the midline and for no apparent reason move from the right of the low back to the left.

Discogenic pathology should always be suspected when the patient describes that symptoms change location with repeated movements or prolonged positioning. Change in the distribution or location of the fluid nucleus or sequestrum within the intact annulus may alter the location of pain according to the site of annular deformation.[42] Posterocentral bulging will cause central or bilateral pain, whereas posterolateral bulging will cause unilateral pain.[43,44]

Pain from the derangement syndrome will be constant as long as tissue within the intact annulus remains displaced. There may be no position in which the patient can find relief. The pain may be present whether movement is performed or not, and this pain is usually described as an ache. That ache is then made worse by movement in certain directions and reduced by movement in other directions.

In the derangement syndrome, especially in severe cases, gross loss of movement may occur. Displaced tissue obstructs movement in the direction of the displacement. In severe cases the degree of displacement is such that postural deformities, such as kyphosis and scoliosis, are forced. Sudden loss of spinal mobility and the sudden appearance of postural deformity in acute low back and neck pain may be compared to the sudden locking that may occur in the knee joint, where internal derangement of the meniscus is common.

The mechanism of internal derangement of the intervertebral disc is not fully understood. That the nucleus pulposus can herniate through a torn annular wall in a young adult is established.[45, 46] It is highly likely that this will occur as a consequence of sudden or violent movement, or with sustained postures in younger patients. Older patients have a stiffer, less-fluid nucleus,[47] which is much more difficult to displace from within its annular envelope.[45, 46, 48] It is hypothesized that prior to a frank annular lesion with nuclear herniation, incomplete tears exist into which nuclear material may be displaced. This may alter the joint mechanics and may be responsible for the postural deformities (e.g., localized scoliosis) observed.

Creep within the disc from prolonged loading in a sustained posture will change its shape and disturb the normal alignment of adjacent vertebrae.[48, 49] This change of shape will also affect the ability of the joint surface to move in its normal pathway,[49] and movement deviation to the right or left of the sagittal plan will result on attempting flexion or extension.

Described simply, the pain of derangement occurs as a consequence of a change in disc shape with related misalignment of the mobile segment and its associated abnormal stresses.[36]

Identification of the different syndromes is based on the effects of repeated movements on the initiation of the pain: the point in the movement pathway where pain is first perceived; the site of the pain and subsequent change of location of the pain; the increasing or decreasing intensity of the pain; and finally abolition of the pain. Mechanical pain can arise from a limited number of events or combination of events causing force to be applied to innervated soft tissues. Those soft tissues may be in a normal state, a contracted state, or an anatomically altered state with a change in the shape of the disc. Any of these events can be identified by the response of the patient's pain to the deliberate application of certain mechanical stresses.

Atypical Responses to Mechanical Evaluation

When, over a period of 3 or 4 days of mechanical assessment, no repeated end-range movement or positional loading can be found to reduce or centralize symptoms, the patient's condition is probably unsuited for mechanical therapy. The patient should be referred for further investigation. Using the mechanical model of assessment, it is unusual to find that this recommendation is unwarranted.

In the presence of any inflammation, pain or aching will be constant. Repeated movements will increase the pain, which will remain worse for some time afterward, even at rest. No movement or position will be found that reduces or centralizes the symptoms. The same response is often seen in the presence of an irreducible derangement of the intervertebral disc, causing nerve root compression.

It is not uncommon for exercise, mobilization, and even spinal manipulation to be applied unwittingly to conditions with an inflammatory component. This most commonly occurs following trauma before the resolution of the inflammatory response. The resulting exacerbation of pain is not surprising. Yet therapists, believing the condition to be mechanical, attribute the response to an "irritable" joint condition.

The "irritable" tag is also often applied when mobilization or manipulation is given in the wrong direction in the presence of derangement. This will cause an exacerbation of the symptoms. If the procedures are applied in the direction that reduces the derangement, using centralization of the symptoms as the guide, the symptoms will respond to the correction.

Patients with inflammatory disorders, such as ankylosing spondylitis with spondylolisthesis or other undetected minor fracture, will all have increased levels of pain from the mechanical evaluation described above. The increased level of pain will rarely remain for more than 24 hours and will then subside to its former level.

In the presence of spinal tumors or infections, or vertebral body fractures, responses to mechanical evaluation will differ, but whenever significant erosion of the bone has occurred, very severe pain will result from even gentle pressure in the vicinity of the affected segments. The patients will react by rigidly splinting the whole spine and will cry out in great pain. In 40 years I have seen less than 20 such cases, but the lasting impressions from each have been the same.

In summary, pathologic processes unsuited to mechanical therapies will behave atypically and be quickly exposed and recognized when tested in the manner described.

MECHANICAL THERAPY FOR NONSPECIFIC SYNDROMES

The term *patient management* means the organization, supervision, and implementation of the strategies to be applied for the successful education and treatment of the patient. Clinicians will already have their own systems in place for patient management. These systems vary, of course, but the broad principles outlined below remain the same for all. The message I wish to convey is that every patient needs education, but not every patient needs treatment.

Once the patient has been questioned regarding the history of his or her complaint and an examination of the appearance and function of the affected region has been performed, a diagnosis can be made. From this diagnosis the therapeutic management can be structured to suit the patient's requirements. The therapeutic management should consist, first and most important, of an educational component. Second, and only if necessary, an active mechanical therapy component may follow. The majority of patients will only require the educational component during their management.

Education Component of Management

All patients require education. Education consists first of a description of the natural history of the disorder. The patient must understand the nature of the environment necessary for the creation of good quality repair. He or she must also be given a brief description of the healing process and learn to cooperate fully in the prevention of events that may disrupt or delay healing.

The likely outcome of various interventions should be explained so that the patient may decide whether or not to wait for the natural history to run its course or to proceed with one or more of the treatment options. In the event that the patient decides to proceed with therapy, he or she must then be acquainted with the techniques of self-treatment and told why, in the event that this fails to provide benefit within the specified time, therapist intervention will need to follow. The recovery of full, pain-free movement must be the ultimate aim of the treatment; therefore all patients must learn the progressions of exercise necessary to achieve total functional recovery.

Finally, the patient must be instructed sufficiently so that he or she can avoid recurrence of the problem, and in the event of recurrence, minimize the consequences. Thus the patient can play a major role in his or her own rehabilitation.

Active Mechanical Therapy Component

Soon after injury, education in procedures designed to stimulate good quality tissue repair is necessary. Cross linkage of collagen occurs during repair and may result in the development of an inextensible or adherent scar. The developing repair tissue should retain the qualities of extensibility whenever possible. This is best achieved by applying gentle natural tension, which stimulates the repair process and at the same time prevents cross linkage of collagen. Once repair is established, procedures are applied to restore any restriction of motion and recover any lost function.

The therapist's role is to gently guide the patient through and beyond the healing process to the point where recovery of function calls for and allows more vigorous measures. The management will first consist of self-treatment procedures and, in the event that these fail to provide improvement, procedures that require the assistance of the therapist will be added.

The therapist will identify the direction of functional impairment and provide mechanical techniques that restore full range of pain-free movement. The therapist may be required to aid in the reduction of internal derangement. Reduction by self-applied procedures is sometimes difficult, and it may be necessary for the therapist to mobilize or manipulate to achieve reduction. The therapist must also identify postural forces that, if not removed, may delay recovery following trauma.

Strengthening exercises are necessary in cases where loss of power is affecting the patient at either work or play. These can be introduced once pain permits where strength loss is apparent at an early stage.

To Treat or Not to Treat?

Whether the problem is post-traumatic, nontraumatic, inflammatory, or degenerative, it should never be assumed that treatment by physical therapy is always necessary. There can be no justification for applying physical treatment unless that treatment is known to accelerate the natural history or will assist in the recovery of function. This does not mean, however, that the patient should not be given comprehensive guidance and education in the avoidance of activities or postures that may delay recovery or disrupt the healing process. All patients are entitled to that guidance and any educational tools that may be relevant to their problem. Furthermore, all therapists should be obliged to provide the relevant information to secure the best response in the manner best suited to the patient's physical, social, and financial well being.

At the time of the first interview, and mainly from the patient's history, we can usually identify whether or not the patient will require education or treatment or a combination of both. Where the onset of pain is very recent, it may be necessary to reduce activity or avoid the painful movement so that healing may proceed without disruption. Education and instruction alone will usually ensure an uneventful recovery. Further education to prevent loss of function will complete the management. A follow-up telephone call to the patient should be made a few days later to determine if a further consultation is necessary. There is as yet no evidence that physical treatment accelerates the time required for recovery from such minor problems.

If, at the first interview, the patient reports that following an initial period of rest the symptoms showed little or no improvement, advice or assistance of some sort will be necessary. We should determine whether or not the period of rest was sufficient. A few days of rest following the onset of pain should have given some indication of the need for further advice. If the patient has already rested for 10 days with no appreciable benefit resulting, assistance is certainly indicated. The nature and extent of the assistance required will be determined following the mechanical evaluation. If applied too soon after injury, movement may further delay repair. On the other hand, if the commencement of active movement is unduly delayed, the stimulus to repair that is provided by early movement does not occur.

Before deciding the management plan it is useful to consider the status of the patient's condition.

Condition Improving

When the patient reports that his or her condition is improving, a review of the problem and its prognosis is all that is required. Avoid the inclination to embark on a program of exercise; advice should suffice. Whatever the origin of the symptoms, whether inflammatory, degenerative, or post-traumatic, improvement in the patient's condition is the ultimate aim of treatment. If that process is already under way, continuing at a steady rate, and accompanied at the same time by improvement in function, there is little justification for any intervention other than education and assurance. Provide guidelines for the progression of activity and exercise where necessary, but such patients do not need to attend a clinic for regular "treatment."

Condition Unchanging

When the patient reports that a slow, insidious onset of pain with movement has developed over time and is now unchanging, a routine approach to the assessment can proceed, and education and instruction for a suspected dysfunction can be provided immediately.

If the patient describes that symptoms resulting from trauma 2 to 3 weeks ago are unchanged since onset, it could mean that healing has not occurred or is suffering frequent disruption. It is uncommon but not impossible for healing to take longer than 3 or 4 weeks, especially if the patient is overactive and disrupts the process of repair. Athletes, sportsmen, and women are frequently guilty of returning prematurely to full activity.

If healing has not occurred following injury, the patient will report that he or she experiences a constant ache, and no movement or position can be found to reduce or stop it. This will be determined following the mechanical assessment. However, in the case described above, there is a strong possibility that derangement of some intra-articular component has occurred. Derangement will also cause constant aching and pain that may continue unabated for weeks, until reduction occurs either spontaneously as a result of a chance event or by manipulation. Unlike pain from the inflammatory process, certain repeated movements or sustained positions will reduce the pain when derangement is causative. This will be clarified after the mechanical assessment.

When the patient reports unchanging pain over several weeks or months, and rest has failed to provide improvement, the condition must be tolerant of the existing level of exercise and therefore is unlikely to be aggravated by controlled mechanical therapy. Unless findings emerge from the assessment process to suggest that further tests or more caution are required, education and instruction in a vigorous self-treatment program is indicated. Therapist intervention at this point is unnecessary but may follow shortly should self-treatment and guidance fail to provide recovery.

Condition Worsening

In the event that the patient describes that his or her symptoms are worsening since onset, it will be necessary to investigate the cause of deterioration. Should the symptoms be localized, it may be that inadequate avoidance of the causative activity is all that has worsened the condition. However, the possibility of the presence of an underlying inflammatory or more serious disease process should always be considered. If the patient has been or looks unwell, or if the reactions to mechanical evaluation are atypical or fail to affect the symptoms, the patient should be referred for further investigation. Appropriate blood tests or radiologic assessment may shed light on the origin of the symptoms in such cases.

Having excluded the possibility of serious pathology, a rather gentle approach to the mechanical evaluation is always required if the patient describes that their pain is progressively increasing. Increasing pain intensity could indicate that early movement is not immediately appropriate. Under these circumstances a purely educational approach is indicated, certainly for the first 24 to 48 hours.

Patients whose symptoms are worsening should be seen on a daily basis until stability or improvement occurs, or until it becomes obvious that referral for further investigation is necessary.

CONCLUSIONS

Following an analysis of the history and the mechanical assessment, it will be possible to classify the patient into at least one of the categories outlined below. The patient may describe symptoms of more than one syndrome. It is possible for the patient to intermittently experience localized postural symptoms resulting from prolonged loading, and at the same time to experience constant referred pain from internal derangement.

From the classification it should be possible to determine the required management program for the patient, or to refer him or her to a more appropriate source of care in the event that the condition is unsuited to the mechanical approach.

It should also be possible at this stage to decide whether or not the patient is likely to require therapist intervention or a purely educational and self-treatment program. If there is any doubt regarding the patient's ability to comprehend and comply with the program, the details should be provided in writing.

After excluding the patient with an inflammatory condition or other disorders unsuitable for mechanical therapy, the patient should fit one of the following diagnostic categories:

Trauma/repair incomplete/inflammatory—Rest/movement
Postural—Re-educate
Dysfunction—Remodel end range
Derangement—Reduce

Postural Syndrome

Normal tissues can become painful in everyday life by the application of prolonged stresses commonly appearing during static postural loading conditions, such as prolonged sitting, standing, or bending.

Correction of faulty postural habits removes inappropriate causative stresses. No other treatment is required. In order to remove the cause of pain, the therapist must educate the patient.

Dysfunction Syndrome

Shortened structures cause limited movement and simultaneously cause pain when the shortened structure is stretched.

Treatment should be provided to remodel contracted or adherent structures. The dysfunction is not rapidly reversible; weeks are required to remodel and lengthen the structures. Structures that have adaptively shortened over weeks and months cannot suddenly lengthen by the application of high-velocity thrusts without incurring damage. Regular end-range exercise must be considered as the most likely therapy to influence shortened structures. Remodeling by continuous passive motion (Salter) has been found to assist in the regeneration of cartilage in the knee. Matsumoto[50] has reported that collagen synthesis of nucleus pulposus cells was promoted and the population of cells significantly increased as a result of cyclic mechanical stretch carried out over a period of 2 to 4 days. These studies suggest that repeated end-range movements carried out by the patient or by continuous passive motion (CPM) equipment could accelerate remodeling in patients with this syndrome.

Derangement Syndrome

An example of derangement syndrome is a frank tear of the annulus fibrosis with nuclear displacement or annular bulging. The patient experiences aching without movement, increased pain with movement in certain directions as displacement increases, and reduced pain in other directions as displacement decreases.

In the event that the annulus remains intact this syndrome is subject to mostly rapid reversal. The use of patient self-treatment methods using repeated end-range movement has been successful in the reduction of derangement within the lower lumbar segments. The rate of reduction of derangement can be accelerated significantly in a large number of cases with the use of repeated end-range passive exercise (REPEX) CPM associated with appropriate self-treatment protocols; maintaining reduction by correcting posture and avoiding inappropriate positions; restoring function before adaptive changes are established; and teaching prevention of recurrence and self-treatment. Mobilization and SMT now become important and may be required if self-treatment provides insufficient reductive pressures.

Mechanical forces used to treat mechanical disorders of the low back should be applied in a graduated form, first using patient self-treatment repeated movements, progressing through mobilization, and ending with the application of manipulative procedures.

The time to apply our special techniques of mobilization and manipulation arrives when the patient, having exhausted all possibilities of self-treatment, requires an increase in the degree of pressure in the appropriate direction; that direction, having already been determined during exercises, allows mobilizing procedures to commence. Manipulation is indicated only when there is no improvement with the use of mobilization. Thus the gradual development of increasing force to bring about change is a logical and safe method of applying mechanical therapies, assuming that vertebral and vascular pathology are excluded. The ultimate weapon we have is the manipulative thrust technique. Why use that weapon on day 1 when it may well be that the patient, without being approached by the therapist, is capable of causing the change himself (and learning an important self-management lesson)?

We should postpone or avoid mobilization and manipulation until we have determined that resolution of the problem is impossible using the patient's own positions and movements. This concept offers up to 70% of people referred to physical therapists with mechanical low back pain the opportunity to treat and manage their own problem and thus become independent of therapists.[51,52]

Some patients are unable to self-treat with lasting benefit and will always require the special skills of the manipulative therapist. The manual correction of acute lumbar or sciatic scoliosis or the reduction of acute lumbar pain with kyphosis are two examples of this requirement. Others will require techniques in the form of mobilization, and some of those will additionally require manipulative thrust procedures.

Spinal manipulative therapy has a particular and important part to play in the treatment of mechanical spinal pain but its dispensation is greatly misused. It is now possible to determine within 4 days from commencement of assessment whether manipulative therapy will be necessary at all. It is not necessary to apply the technique in order to find out retrospectively if the procedure was indicated. Spinal mobilization and manipulation should not be dispensed to the entire population with back pain in order to ensure that the very few who really need it actually receive it.

When all mechanical therapies fail to improve the patient's condition, and modulation of pain is considered necessary, physical therapists must ask whether modulating pain with physical therapy "gadgetry" is better for the patient and society as a whole than dispensation of rather inexpensive medication.

REPEATED END-RANGE PASSIVE EXERCISE (REPEX) AND REMODELING

To assist with the remodeling required in the treatment of dysfunction, a CPM motion device was developed that enables unlimited cycles of progressive end-range exercise to be applied to the lumbar spine. Several hundred cycles per day can be applied if necessary. REPEX has now been in use in many countries since 1992. Findings indicate that REPEX is as effective as the exercise protocols in resolving certain mechanical disorders of the lower back and is superior to exercise in certain other categories (Fig. 5-1).

REPEX enables fine incremental progressions to be made in the applied range of flexion or extension. The equipment delivers 10 cycles/min of end-range motion, which in the case of patients with derangement syndrome is progressively increased as reduction of the derangement is achieved. Differentiation between dysfunction and derangement is imperative, and such differentiation must be made prior to the application of REPEX. The patient should be assessed therefore and the nature of the derangement determined using the McKenzie assessment protocol.

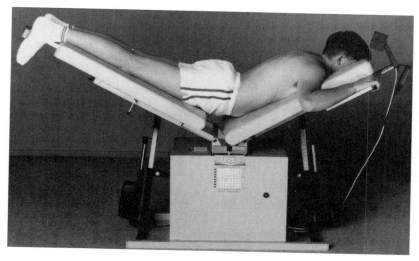

Fig. 5-1 REPEX: repeated end-range passive movements.

The fine control of REPEX and the unlimited number of delivery cycles provide a remodeling process previously unobtainable by patient self-treatment exercises. It is important that spinal segments restricted by contracture or fibrosis are not overstretched. REPEX has the capacity to overstretch, and treatment of dysfunction should be progressed slowly in comparison with the rapid progressions applied to patients with the derangement syndrome.

REPEX is a potent tool for the alleviation of pain and the recovery of function in mechanical spinal disorders. As such it also has the potential to cause harm if used improperly.

REHABILITATION FOR CHRONIC LOW BACK PAIN

The McKenzie Institute International established a residential spinal therapy and rehabilitation center in 1990 for the treatment of chronic and recurrent mechanical spine disorders. The results of a study comparing four rehabilitation programs conducted by the New Zealand Accident Compensation Corporation showed that the Institute program was successful in restoring 63% of patients to workability as measured by the corporation's own medical assessors. Patients were referred to the program from throughout New Zealand. The average length of time off work was 26 months.

The rehabilitation program required patient participation 7 hours daily for 14 days. The procedures provided consisted first of several hundred cycles on REPEX equipment for the first 3 or 4 days. Fear of movement in many cases was dispelled by this procedure. Patients were then taught customized exercises, the intensity being progressively increased during the first week. Gymnasium activities and "play hardening" were introduced from the commencement of the program. Play hardening consisted of twice-daily table tennis, basketball, tennis, competitive jogging, and golf.

The patients attending the McKenzie Institute program had been off work longer, the duration of the current symptoms was longer, and more patients had been hospitalized for nonoperative treatment. The Institute program was superior to the other three programs in comparing pre- and post-treatment fitness to work, pre- and post-treatment work capacity test, pre- and post-test functional limitation profile score, the psychosocial profile score, and the depression score. Range of motion recovery in the Institute program was significantly superior than any of the other programs.[53]

LITERATURE REVIEW

The scientific literature in the field of low back pain remains sadly lacking in well-designed and controlled randomized studies evaluating the effectiveness of treatments for low back and neck pain. Clinicians worldwide are justifiably indignant when poorly designed, poorly controlled, and statistically manipulated studies are produced each year by nonclinical investigators poorly equipped to deal with the complexities that abound in this field. Are clinicians destined to live with the continuous flow of studies that either apologize for the limitations and interpret with caution or are subsequently criticized as being seriously flawed by investigators providing contradictory findings?

In the various arenas of scientific endeavor, it is customary to have a thorough understanding of the subject under investigation. For example, oceanographers are expected to know something about the seas, the constitution of salt water, the living organisms, both plant and animal, to be found in the deep, and certainly the nature of the tides and currents that flow about the surface. Similarly, geologists are expected to know and understand the age, origin, and composition of the various strata of the earth and in the learning process spend many years studying in the field. However, when it comes to the study of back pain, surprisingly, no knowledge of the affliction itself or its treatment is necessarily required. When investigating a particular treatment method it seems there is no great need to become even slightly familiar with its practical implementation.

Clinicians must demand better from the investigators. This especially applies to those who have never been involved in the management of a wide variety of the patients with back problems.

The McKenzie protocols for both diagnosis and treatment of the low back have been subject to various investigations in many parts of the world. The investigations of the treatment methods have produced varied results. Few of the studies have been methodologically strong. Studies of the assessment leading to diagnosis have been investigated with stronger and more positive results. In particular, the value of the techniques that can achieve centralization have been confirmed, and the importance of centralization itself has been established.[41, 54–63]

Following publication of my observations on centralization, Donelson[41] was the first to report centralization of pain as a reliable predictor of outcome in patients with low back and referred pain. Patients with acute, subacute, and chronic back and leg pain were evaluated using repeated end-range sagittal flexion and extension. A significant majority of the centralizers had good to excellent outcomes. Of those who peripheralized, the majority had poor outcome.

Since that time several other studies have confirmed the value of centralization of pain as a predictor of outcome in acute, subacute, and chronic patient populations.[41, 54–63]

In a later study[56] in applying repeated sagittal movement testing to end range, it was found that most patients consistently demonstrated a directional preference, the majority centralizing or reducing pain with extension movements. In those same patients flexion was found to increase pain.

A further study on centralization of pain[57] found that a similar directional preference was shown in a majority of patients tested in the frontal plane, most experiencing centralization or reduction of symptoms when laterally flexing toward the painful side.[41, 54–63] More recently, Werneke[64] confirmed the value of centralization in predicting good and poor outcomes in patients with back and referred pain.

Protocols for the mechanical assessment of the lumbar spine have also been shown to be effective in diagnosing intervertebral disc pathology. Donelson, Aprill, et al[41] found that centralizing pain was reliable in differentiating between contained and uncontained lumbar intervertebral disc protrusion. The relationship between pain centralization and the intervertebral disc as the pain generator has also been established in this study.

Several studies, although not well designed, have shown beneficial patient outcomes from self-treatment exercise. Studies by Ponte,[65] Nwuga and Nwuga,[66] Kopp,[67] Williams,[68] Donelson[41, 55, 57, 58] Alexander,[69] Stankovic,[70] and McKinney[71] have all demonstrated the benefits of this approach to the assessment and treatment of mechanical spinal disorders.

Razmjou[72] found that qualified McKenzie-trained therapists were highly reliable in intertester assessment of the McKenzie diagnostic categories. At the first assessment substantial agreement was reached, and in the second follow-up assessment almost perfect agreement was made in identifying the syndrome category.

In a randomized, blind study comparing the use of McKenzie with two other treatments (back school and 90/90 traction) 97% of the patients treated with McKenzie had improved after 1 week, whereas less than 50% improved with either of the other two methods, or fewer than would be expected with no treatment at all.

Stankovitch[70] compared the McKenzie system with a mini–back school program in treating acute low back pain in a working population. The McKenzie-treated workers had a median sick leave of 10 days versus 17.5 days in the comparison group and a mean sick-listing for recurrences the first year of 27 days versus 40 days with mini–back school. Only 45% of the McKenzie-treated workers had first-year relapses versus 80% of the comparison group. The average number of McKenzie treatments during the acute episode was only 5.5. It would appear that the McKenzie patients resolved their acute episode and disability faster, were better able to prevent recurrences, and were able to minimize disability when symptoms did recur.

Williams et al[68] found that the adoption of extended lumbar sitting postures reduced or centralized pain in patients with nonspecific low back and referred pain. The effects were most marked in those with leg symptoms. Flexed postures, on the other hand, showed no similar reduction in pain intensity or location change.

Roberts[73] compared McKenzie treatment with nonsteroidal anti-inflammatory drug therapy. His patients were recruited prospectively and were treated within 3 weeks of onset of an attack of low back pain. Both groups of patients were encouraged to mobilize actively. Rest, after the first 2 days, was discouraged. The major measure of outcome was a widely used disability questionnaire. At 7 weeks after onset of the attack, the McKenzie-treated patients were less disabled compared with the drug treatment patients.

Psychologic assessment was performed on all patients in connection with their personal responsibility for pain control. Patients undergoing McKenzie therapy were significantly more responsible for personal pain control than the drug-treatment patients 7 weeks after the onset of the low back pain. This responsibility alteration was still significantly different when measured 6 months later. McKenzie therapy alters the way patients think about pain.

Roberts' study also found that those who centralized showed better responses than the patients in whom the syndrome was unclear. Scores of pain intensity matched a score for peripheralization with a very significant degree of correlation.

In 1986 Kopp et al[67] reported that of 67 patients with herniated nucleus pulposus (HNP) treated with the McKenzie extension protocol, 35 patients were able to achieve normal lumbar extension within 3 days of admission to the hospital. The remaining 32 patients all required surgery, and of these only two were able to achieve extension before surgery. All 67 had failed 6 weeks of conservative treatment prior to being treated by the McKenzie protocol. Kopp and co-workers concluded that the ability of patients with HNP and radiculopathy to achieve full passive lumbar extension is a useful predictor to select patients who can be expected to respond favorably to conservative management.

Alexander et al[69] reported on a follow-up of the patients in the Kopp study. it was found that after an average of almost 6 years from onset, 33 of the 35 patients who did not require surgery were satisfied with the result, and 82% had been able to resume their old jobs. At long-term follow-up, Alexander and co-workers found that a negative extension sign was confirmed as a predictor of a favorable response to nonoperative treatment of HNP in 91% of the nonsurgical group in Kopp's study.

Cherkin[74] compared a modified McKenzie treatment protocol with chiropractic manipulation and an educational booklet. The McKenzie protocol normally includes spinal manipulation as the last in the list of progressions of force applied to end range. Manipulation by physiotherapists is not permitted under law in the State of Washington and in this study was omitted from the usual McKenzie protocol.

The results demonstrated that McKenzie individualized end-range movements chosen on the basis of centralization were as effective as manipulation and required fewer treatments to achieve the same result. At 1-year follow-up there was no difference between the groups.

Only one study has assessed the long-term value of this treatment approach for mechanical problems in the cervical spine. In a single-blind randomized prospective study, McKinney[71] found that advice to exercise and correct posture in the early phase after injury was superior to outpatient physiotherapy consisting of hot and cold applications, pulsed short-wave diathermy, hydrotherapy, traction, and active and passive movements. At 2-year follow-up fewer patients in the exercise group had persisting symptoms. McKinney suggested that the reason for the superior results in the exercise groups was that patients given responsibility for their own treatment may become self-sufficient at managing minor episodes, and there may be psychologic advantages to making patients responsible for their own treatment rather than victims of their own symptoms.

In guidelines for the treatment of back pain issued by the Danish Ministry of Health in 1998[75] the McKenzie treatment protocol is recommended for both acute and chronic back pain problems with or without radiation. The McKenzie technology as a diagnostic method is strongly recommended for patients when the pain source is the intervertebral disc, and the method has value as a prognostic indicator.

CONCLUSIONS

In my text published in 1981, I described the disc model to explain the causes of many back problems, especially recurrent problems.[36] I predicted that internal derangement of the intervertebral disc was caused by posterior displacement of the nucleus during flexion; that compensatory movements toward extension would reverse that process and reduce the symptoms. The validity of that model has been substantially established. It is now known that the nucleus moves posteriorly in flexion and anteriorly with extension. The relationship between centralizing symptoms and disc pathology has also been recognized. I described also that if patients' symptoms could be centralized, the prognosis was excellent. That has also been confirmed. I indicated that acute attacks of back pain were likely to occur more frequently in the first hours of the day as a result of flexion activities affecting the hydrated disc. That also has since been confirmed.

The McKenzie approach to the diagnosis of spinal pain is often misunderstood. It does not treat all patients with extension as though it were the opposite of Williams' flexion exercises. It is also a much more complex discipline to carry out than this brief description can convey. The McKenzie system is based primarily on symptomatic response to various loading strategies. The symptomatic response will be related to the increasing or decreasing acute spinal deformity, and obstruction to active motion, these factors being the only direct links we have with the obscure underlying pathology.

The success of the McKenzie system is dependent on the training and expertise of the physician and therapist especially. Typically, 2 years of clinical experience with assessment and treatment of mechanical spinal disorder, coupled with appropriate education and certification, are minimum requirements for effective education in this method.

REFERENCES

1. McKenzie RA: Mechanical diagnosis and therapy for low back pain: toward a better understanding. In Twomey LT, Taylor JR (Eds.): Clinics in Physical Therapy. Physical Therapy of the Low Back. Churchill Livingstone, New York, 1987
2. Potter NA, Rothstein JM: Intertester reliability for selected clinical tests of the sacroiliac joint. Phys Ther 65:1671, 1985
3. BMA: Complementary Medicine—New Approaches to Good Practice, BMA Oxford University Press, Oxford, 1993
4. Landen BR: Heat and cold for the relief of low back pain? Phys Ter 47:1126, 1967
5. Klein RG, Eek BC: Low energy laser and exercise for chronic low back pain: double-blind controlled trial. Arch Phys Med Rehabil 71:34, 1990
6. Deyo RA, Walsh N, Martin D, et al: A controlled trial of transcutaneous electronic nerve stimulation (TENS) and exercise for chronic low back pain. N Engl J Med 322:1627, 1990
7. Gnatz SM: Increased radicular pain due to therapeutic ultrasound applied to the back. Arch Phys Med Rehabil 70:493, 1989
8. Meade TW, Dyer S, Browne W, et al: Low back pain of mechanical origin: randomized comparison of chiropractic and hospital outpatient treatment. Br Med J 300:1431, 1990
9. Brunarski DJ: Clinical trials of spinal manipulation. J Manip Phys Ter 7:4, 1984
10. Doran DML, Newell DJ: Manipulation in treatment of low back pain: a multicenter study. Br Med J 2:161, 1975
11. Farrell JB, Twomey LT: Acute low back pain. Comparison of two conservative treatment approaches. Proceedings of Manipulative Therapists Association of Australia, Perth, Western Australia, 1983
12. Hadler NM, Curtis P, Gillings DB, Stinnett S: A benefit of spinal manipulation as adjunctive therapy for acute low back pain: a stratified, controlled trial. Spine 12:7, 1987
13. Hoehler FK, Tobis JS, Buerger AA: Spinal manipulation for low back pain. JAMA 245:1835, 1981
14. Sims-Williams H, Jayson MIV, Young SMS: Controlled trial of mobilization and manipulation for patients with low back pain in general practice. Br Med J 2:1338, 1978
15. Spitzer WO, LeBlanc FE, Dupuis M, et al: Scientific approach to the assessment and management of activity-related spinal disorders. A monograph for clinicians. Report of the Quebec Task Force on spinal disorders. Spine 12:75, 1987
16. Vanharanta H, Sachs BL, Spivey MA, et al: The relationship of pain provocation to lumbar disc deterioration as seen by CT/discography study. Spine 12:295, 1987
17. Vanharanta H, Guyer RD, Ohnmeiss DD, et al: Disc deterioration in low back syndromes: a prospective, multicenter CT/discography study. Spine 13:1345, 1988
18. Zucherman J, Derby R, Hsu K, et al: Normal magnetic resonance imaging with abnormal discography. Spine 13:1355, 1988
19. Kornberg M: Discography and magnetic resonance imaging in the diagnosis of lumbar disc disruption. Spine 14:1368, 1989

20. Butler D, Trafimow JH, Anderson GBJ, et al: Discs degenerate before facets. Spine 15:111, 1990
21. Kuslich SD, Ulstrom RN, Michael CJ: The tissue origin of low back pain and sciatica: a report of pain response to tissue stimulation during operations on the lumbar spine using local anesthesia. Orthop Clin North Am 22:181, 1991
22. Smyth MJ, Wright V: Sciatica and the intervertebral disc. An experimental study. J Bone Joint Surg 40A:1401, 1958
23. Hirsch C: The anatomical basis for low back pain. Acta Orthop Scand 33:1, 1963
24. Mooney V: University of Arizona Symposium on Back Pain: The present and the future, Tucson, Arizona, March 11–14, 1992
25. Jackson RP, Jacobs RR, Montesano PX: 1988 Volvo Award in Clinical Sciences. Facet join injection in low-back pain. A prospective statistical study. Spine 13:966, 1988
26. Luilius G, Laasoner EM, Myllynen P, et al: Lumbar facet joint syndrome. A randomised clinical trial. J Bone Joint Surg 77B:1108, 1989
27. Dixon A: Diagnosis of low back pain. In Jayson M (Ed.): The Lumbar Spine and Back Pain. Pitman Medical, Tunbridge Wells, England, 1980
28. Suzuki N, Seiichi E: A quantitative study of trunk muscle strength and fatigability in the low back pain syndrome. Spine 8:1, 1983
29. Kostuik J: Adult scoliosis. In Frymoyer JW (Ed.): The Adult Spine. Raven Press, New York, 1997
30. Dieck GS: An epidemiological study of the relationship between postural asymmetry in the teen years and subsequent back and neck pain. Spine 10:872, 1985
31. Twomey L, Taylor J: Age changes in the lumbar intervertebral discs. Acta Orthop Scand 56:496, 1985
32. Coventry MB, Ghormley RK, Kernohan JW: The intervetebral disc: part II. Changes in the intervertebral disc concomitant with age. J Bone Joint Surg 27:233, 1945
33. Coventry MB, Ghormley RK, Kernohan JW: The intervertebral disc: part III. Pathological changes in the intervertebral disc. J Bone Joint Surg 27:460, 1945
34. Vernon-Roberts B: The pathology and interrelation of intervertebral disc lesions. In Jayson M (Ed.): The Lumbar Spine and Back Pain. (2nd Ed.) Pitman Medical, Tunbridge Wells, England, 1980
35. Schiotz EH, Cyriax J: Manipulation past and present. Heinemann, London, 1975
36. McKenzie RA: The Lumbar Spine. Mechanical Diagnosis and Therapy. Spinal Publications, Waikanae, New Zealand, 1981
37. Donelson R, Murphy K, Silva G: Centralisation phenomenon: its usefulness in evaluating and treating referred pain. Spine 14:3, 1990
38. Donelson R, Aprill C, Medcalf R, Grant W: A prospective study of centralisation of lumbar and referred pain. Spine 22:1115, 1997
39. Werneke M, Hart D, Cook D: A descriptive study of the centralisation phenomenon. Spine 24:676, 1999
40. Kellgren JH: The anatomical source of back pain. Rheumatol Rehab 16:3–12, 1997
41. Donelson R, Aprill C, Medcalf R, Grant W: A prospective study of centralisation of lumbar and referred pain: a predictor of symptomatic discs and anular competence. Spine 22:1115–1122, 1997

42. Shepperd JAN: Patterns of internal disc dynamics, cadaver motion studies. Video presented at the International Society for the Study of the Lumbar Spine Meeting, Boston, June 13–14, 1990

43. Cloward RB: Cervical diskography: a contribution to the etiology and mechanism of neck, shoulder and arm pain. Ann Surg 150:1052, 1959

44. Murphey F: Sources and patterns of pain in disc disease. Clin Neurosurg 15:343, 1968

45. Adams MA, Hutton WC: Prolapsed intervertebral disc: a hyperflexion injury. Spine 7:3, 1982

46. Adams MA, Hutton WC: Gradual disc prolapse. Spine 10:6, 1985

47. Taylor JR, Twomey LT: The lumbar spine from infancy to old age. In Twomey LT, Taylor JR (eds): Clinics in Physical Therapy. Physical Therapy of the Low Back. Churchill Livingstone, New York, 1987

48. Farfan HF: Mechanical Disorders of the Low Back. Lea & Febiger, Philadelphia, 1973

49. Panjabi M, Drag MH, Chung TQ: Effects of disc injury on mechanical behaviour of the human spine. Spine 9:7, 1984

50. Matsumoto T, Kawakami M, Kuribayashi K, Takenaka T, Tamaki T. Cyclic mechanical stretch stress increases the growth rate and collagen synthesis of nucleus pulposus cells in vitro. Spine 24:315, 1999

51. McKenzie RA: Treat Your Own Back. Spinal Publications, Waikanae, New Zealand, 1981

52. McKenzie RA: Prophylaxis in recurrent low back pain. NZ Med J 89:627, 1979

53. New Zealand Accident Compensation Corporation: Chronic Backs Study. Wellington, New Zealand, 1994

54. Delitto A, Cibulka MT, Erhanrd RE, et al: Evidence for an extension-mobilization category in acute low back syndrome: a prescriptive validation pilot study. Phys Ther 73(4):216, 1993

55. Donelson R, Silva G, Murphy K: The centralisation phenomenon: its usefulness in evaluating and treating referred pain. Spine 15(3):211–213, 1990

56. Donelson R, Grant W, et al: Pain response to sagittal end-range spinal motion: a multi-centred, prospective, randomised trial. Spine 16:S206–212, 1991

57. Donelson R, Grant W, et al: Pain response to end-range spinal motion in the frontal plane: A multi-centred, prospective trial. Presented at the International Society for the Study of the Lumbar Spine, Heidelberg, Germany, May 1991

58. Donelson R, Grant W, Kamps C, Richman P: Clinical analysis of symptom response to sagittal end-range cervical test movements. Cervical Spine Research Society, New York, NY, December 2–4, 1993

59. Erhard RE, Delitto A, Cibulka MT: Relative effectiveness of an extension program and a combined program of manipulation and flexion and extension exercises in patients with acute low back syndrome. Phys Ther 74:1093–1100, 1994

60. Karas R, McIntosh G, Hall H, et al: The relationship between nonorganic signs and centralisation of symptoms in the prediction of return to work for patients with low back pain. Phys Ther 77:354–360, 1997

61. Long A: The centralisation phenomenon: its usefulness as a predictor of outcome in conservative treatment of chronic low back pain. Joint Congress of American Physical Therapy Association and Canadian Physical Therapy, Toronto, Canada, June 1994

62. Sufka A, Hauger B, Trenary M, et al: Centralisation of low back pain and perceived functional outcome. J Orthop Sports Phys Ther 27:205–212, 1998

63. Williams MM, Hawley JA, McKenzie RA, et al: A comparison of the effects of two sitting postures on back and referred pain. Spine 16:1185–1191, 1991

64. Werneke M, Hart D, Cook D: Centralisation phenomenon as a prognostic factor for chronic low back pain and disability. Spine Impress, 1999

65. Ponte DJ, Jensen GJ, Kent BE: A preliminary report on the use of the McKenzie protocol versus Williams protocol in the treatment of low back pain. J Orthop Sports Phys Ther 6:130, 1984

66. Nwuga G, Nwuga V: Relative therapeutic efficacy of the Williams and McKenzie protocols in back pain management. Physiother Pract 1:99, 1985

67. Kopp JR, Alexander AH, Turocy RH, et al: The use of lumbar extension in the evaluation and treatment of patients with acute herniated nucleus pulposus. A preliminary report. Clin Orthop 202:211, 1986

68. Williams MM, Hawley JA, McKenzie RA, Van Wijmen PM: A comparison of the effects of two sitting postures on back and referred pain. Spine 16:1185, 1991

69. Alexander AH, Jones AM, Rosenbaum Jr DH: Nonoperative management of herniated nucleus pulposus: patient selection by the extension sign—long term follow-up. Presented to The North American Spine Society Annual Meeting, Monterey, California, August 8–11, 1990.

70. Stankovic R, Johnell O: Conservative treatment of acute low-back pain. A prospective randomised trial: McKenzie method of treatment versus patient education in Mini Back School. Spine 15:2, 1990

71. McKinney LA: Early mobilisation and outcome in acute sprains of the neck. Br Med J 299:1006, 1989

72. Razmjou H, Cramer J, Yamada R: Intertester Reliability of the McKenzie Evaluation of Mechanical Low Back Pain. North American Pain Society, Chicago, 1999

73. Roberts AP: The conservative treatment of low back pain. Thesis, Nottingham, England, 1990

74. Cherkin D: Pilot randomised trials of physical and educational interventions for low back pain. BOAT Newsletter. Vol. 2. University of Washington, Seattle, Washington, June 1992

75. Danish Ministry of Health: Low back pain treatment and prevention, Danish Ministry of Health, August 1998

6

Manipulative Physical Therapy in the Management of Selected Low Lumbar Syndromes

Patricia H. Trott
Ruth Grant

In recent years there have been considerable advances in the understanding of spinal pain mechanisms,[1] but as Gifford and Butler[2] point out, knowledge of pain mechanisms has not been embraced by clinicians and integrated into their clinical practice.

Clinicians must have good clinical reasoning skills.[3] A thorough patient examination includes consideration of the stage of tissue healing and identification of the predominant pain mechanisms in operation,[2] whether nociceptive, peripheral neurogenic, central, affective/cognitive, or autonomic/motor mechanisms.

Musculoskeletal tissue injuries and inflammation involve nociception from the damaged target tissues of a nerve (muscles, joints, ligaments, tendons, and fascia) and peripheral neurogenic pain from damage to a nerve root or a peripheral nerve.[4] These pain mechanisms are relatively easy to recognize because the pain follows known anatomic pathways and has a mechanical behavior in that stressing the tissue source aggravates the pain and rest eases it.

Repeated peripheral nociception has been shown to sensitize cells in the dorsal horn. This, together with altered descending pain control systems from higher centers, results in ongoing pain long after healing of the original peripheral injuries.[5,6] These pains do not necessarily follow a known anatomic pain pattern, nor do they have a clear response to mechanical examination or treatment. This chronic pain has been shown to be more closely related to changes in spinal and supraspinal circuitry and central processing.[7,8,9] In general, cognitive and emotional dimensions of pain become more involved the longer a problem exists. Thus management of chronic pain states should not be directed toward the original site(s) of tissue injury but instead toward improved function through patient education and understanding of the pain mechanisms involved.[10] Clinicians must take

167

into account the affective side to pain experiences and through education, and with the help of clinical psychologists, help patients to focus on improving all dimensions of their dysfunction. The sympathetic nervous system is involved in all injuries and pain states. The way one thinks and feels powerfully influences sympathetic activity, and clinicians should make use of the beneficial effects of lessening a patient's fear and anxiety as a strategy for pain management.[11]

In this chapter, the authors present pain patterns of peripheral nociception where the patients can be divided into two groups according to the history. Patients in the first group have a *history of injury,* such as fall or direct blow, or are referred following surgery. The tissues that are injured depend on the direction and force of the injury, and thus the therapist cannot predict the pattern of the symptoms and signs or the response to treatment. The second group includes patients who have a *history of symptoms occurring spontaneously* or following some trivial incident such as sneezing or bending to pick up a light object. Patients in this second group have symptoms, signs, and histories that are easily recognized, and these conditions respond in a predictable way to manipulative physical therapy.

This chapter is predicated on a recognition and understanding of the pathology and patterns of pain presentation discussed in previous chapters and is therefore specifically directed to technique selection and application in the management of some common syndromes (clinical presentations) of the low lumbar spine (L4-S1) seen in physical therapy practice. Although discussion is restricted to the use of passive movement techniques, the need for a detailed assessment of the soft-tissue components and the muscular control of the spine and pelvis is stressed, and these aspects together with ergonomic advice are included in the overall management of low lumbar problems (these aspects are covered in other chapters of this book).

Before describing such lumbar conditions, discussion of the factors that govern the selection of passive movement techniques is necessary.

SELECTION OF TECHNIQUES

Diagnosis

A definitive diagnosis is not always possible in the clinical setting. This is particularly the case for low lumbar disorders and is related to the following factors.

1. In many cases the etiology is multifactorial and includes both an inflammatory and a mechanical cause.
2. Pain arising from certain tissues does not follow a specific anatomic pattern.
3. A particular pathologic process can give differing patterns of symptoms and signs.

For example, patients with a diagnosis of disc herniation with nerve root irritation can exhibit differing clinical presentations; that is, the symptoms may be acute and severe, or chronic. The distribution of pain may vary, being worse either proximally or distally, with or without neurologic changes. The pattern of limitation of movements may vary from gross restriction of flexion and straight-leg raising (SLR) due to pain, to full range and pain-free flexion but with marked restriction of extension.

Clearly, a diagnostic label alone is of limited help when choosing physical treatment modalities, especially when selecting passive movement techniques. Rather, treatment selection is based on the way the condition presents in terms of pathobiologic pain mechanisms, abnormalities of movement, and the history of the disorder. Knowing which structures can cause pain and the different patterns of pain response that can occur during test movements is fundamental to the selection of passive movement techniques.

Physical therapists, and in particular manipulative physical therapists, are skilled in the diagnosis of mechanical disorders of the neuromusculoskeletal system. They are also trained to recognize when symptoms do not have a mechanical basis, such as in cases of chronic pain with central sensitization,[2] and when to suspect an inflammatory component. In many cases radiologic and hematologic tests are required to exclude other pathologic processes.

Pain-Sensitive Structures and Their Pain Patterns

In the lumbar spine the common structures that cause symptoms are the joints[12, 13] and their supportive tissues,[13] and the pain-sensitive structures in the vertebral and foraminal canals.[14–18]

Intervertebral Joints

Intervertebral Disc. Pain from disorders of the intervertebral disc is commonly deep and ill defined, presenting as a wide area across the low back or as a vague buttock pain. This pain may spread to the upper posterior thigh or lower abdomen; some authorities claim that pain originating in the disc itself is not referred into the lower leg.[19] The pain may be central, to one side, or bilateral (symmetric or asymmetric). A damaged disc may impinge against the posterior longitudinal ligament or the dura or, as it herniates, disc material can impinge on or irritate the nerve root sleeve or the nerve root, causing referred pain.[13, 20]

Discogenic pain behaves differently from pain arising from other structures, in that (1) following a sustained posture, rapid reversal of that posture is both painful and stiff (e.g., standing up quickly after prolonged sitting), and (2) speed of movement will vary the position at which pain is experienced (i.e., with increased speed, pain is experienced earlier in the range of motion). Discogenic pain may be aggravated by either compressive or stretching movements.[21]

Zygapophyseal Joint. Like other synovial joints, the zygapophyseal joint may present with an intraarticular disorder (which is made more painful when the articular surfaces are compressed) or a periarticular disorder (which is worsened by movements that place stress on the capsule).

Commonly, zygapophyseal joint pain is felt locally as a unilateral back pain, which when severe can spread down the entire limb.[13,22] The site of pain is not exclusive to one zygapophyseal joint; therefore the source of pain must be confirmed by clinical examination. In its chronic form, there may be no local pain over the affected joint, but a distal localized patch of pain. This is a common phenomenon in the thoracolumbar region; similar clinical findings for the lower lumbar area have not been substantiated by research.

Ligamentous and Capsular Structures.   Referred pain from specific spinal ligamentous structures follows no known neurologic pattern.[13,23] Based on clinical experience, Maitland[21] reported that ligamentous and capsular pain is felt maximally over the ligament and that the pain may spread into the lower limb. Movements that stretch the ligament/capsule may produce sharp local pain or a stretched sensation at the symptomatic site.

Structures in the Vertebral and Foraminal Canals

The pain-sensitive structures in the vertebral and foraminal canals are the dura anteriorly,[16,17] the nerve-root sleeves, the nerve roots, and the blood vessels of the epidural space.[18,24]

The structures comprising the vertebral canal that are pain sensitive are the posterior longitudinal ligament, posterior portions of the annuli fibrosi, and the anterior aspect of the lamina.[12] The pain-sensitive components of the foraminal canals are the posterolateral aspect of the intervertebral disc and the zygapophyseal joint.[13] Passive-movement tests will implicate a loss of mobility and/or increase in tension of the neuromeningeal tissues.

Dura and Nerve-Root Sleeve.   Dural pain does not have a segmental pattern of reference.[14] However, stimulation of the nerve root sleeve gives rise to symptoms of similar distribution to those arising from stimulation of that nerve root. The only reported difference is that the nerve root frequently gives rise to symptoms that are more severe distally, and the pain is often associated with paresthesia. These phenomena are not seen with irritation of the nerve root sleeve.[25]

Radicular Pain.   Mechanical or chemical irritation of the sensory nerve root causes pain and/or paresthesia in the distal part of a dermatome. If felt throughout a dermatome, these symptoms are often worse distally.[26] Movements that narrow the intervertebral canal and foramen (extension, rotation, and lateral flexion to the affected side) are likely to reproduce or aggravate the nerve root pain or paresthesia. Clinically, pain can be conclusively attributed to the nerve root only if there are neurologic changes indicating a loss of conduction along that nerve root. Passive movement tests that specifically test the neuromeningeal structures are straight leg raise (SLR), prone knee flexion (PKF), passive neck flexion (PNF), and the slump test. These tests are described in major textbooks on manipulative therapy.[20,21,27,28] They are used not only as examination techniques but also in treatment.

Range/Pain Response to Movement

Test movements of the low lumbar intervertebral joints and the neuromeningeal tissues produce common patterns.

Stretching or Compressing Pain

Unilateral back pain may be reproduced by either stretching (e.g., lateral flexion away from the painful side) or compressing the faulty tissues (e.g., lateral flexion toward the painful side).

End-of-Range or Through-Range Pain

Pain may be reproduced at the limit of a particular movement (i.e., when the soft tissue restraints are put on stretch) or during the performance of a movement, increasing near the limit of the movement. Through-range pain is common in joints in which there is a constant ache.

Local and Referred Pain

In patients who have referred pain, the pain response to test movements influences the selection of passive movement techniques. For example, test movements, even when firmly applied, may elicit only local back pain. In these patients the movement may be applied firmly without risk of exacerbation of symptoms. In cases where the test movement has to be sustained at the end of the range of motion to reproduce the referred pain, a treatment technique that is sustained will be required. In contrast to this, test movements that immediately cause distal leg symptoms require very gentle treatment in a manner that does not reproduce the distal symptoms. Test movements that cause latent referred pain or that cause the referred pain to linger also indicate the need for caution in treatment.

History

Any history taken should include the onset and progression of the disorder. Conditions that have a spontaneous (nontraumatic) onset have a characteristic progressive history; that is, there is a pattern that is typical of a degenerating disc or of postural ligamentous pain. Knowing the history that is typical for these conditions helps the clinician to recognize the present stage of the disorder and to match this with the symptoms and signs to form a syndrome. Typical histories are presented in the case studies at the end of this chapter.

A detailed history provides information as to the stability or progressive nature of the disorder. This will guide the extent and strength of techniques used and may contraindicate certain techniques. This is particularly important in cases of a progressive disc disorder, when injudicious treatment may convert a potential disc protrusion into a herniated disc with neurologic changes.

The progression of the disorder allows the prediction of the outcome of treatment, number of treatment sessions needed, and long-term prognosis.

The following case history illustrates these aspects of history taking.

> A 25-year-old gardener presented with a 10-year history of low back pain, which started one school vacation when he worked as a builder's laborer. He then remained symptom-free until he began work as a gardener 7 years ago. Prolonged digging caused low back pain, which initially would be gone by the next morning, but this slowly worsened to the extent that the pain spread to his left buttock and posterior thigh and took longer to settle. In the last 6 months he has required treatment; two or three treatments of heat and extension exercises have completely relieved his symptoms. Two weeks ago, he tripped over a stone and experienced sharp pain in his left calf and paresthesia of his left fifth toe. This has not responded to heat and exercises, but he has been able to continue his gardening.

This history is typical of a progressive and worsening disc disorder, and the patient is now at a stage where he has nerve root irritation. Although a trivial incident provoked this episode, the disorder is relatively stable in that he can continue gardening without worsening his symptoms.

More specific treatment will be required and can be performed firmly without risk of exacerbation of his symptoms. The goal of treatment is to make him symptom-free while anticipating that there may be further episodes due to the progressive nature of his disorder.

Symptoms

The area in which a patient feels the symptoms and the manner in which they vary in relation to posture and movement assist in the recognition of syndromes with a peripheral pain mechanism, and if they match the response to physical examination, can assist in the selection of passive movement techniques. A movement or combination of movements that simulate a position or movement described by the patient as one that causes the pain, can be used as the treatment technique. The following case history illustrates this.

> A right-handed tennis player complains of right-side low back pain as he commences serving. In this position his low lumbar spine is extended, laterally flexed, and rotated to the right. Examination confirms that this combined position reproduces his pain, and testing of intervertebral movement reveals hypomobility at the L5-S1 joint.

An effective treatment would consist of placing his low lumbar spine into this combined position and then passively stretching one of these movements, carefully localizing the movement to the L5-S1 joint.

Two other important aspects of the patient's symptoms are the *severity* of the pain and the *irritability* of the disorder. Severity relates to the examiner's interpretation of the severity of the pain based on the patient's description and functional limitations resulting from the pain. Irritability (or touchiness) of the disorder is based on three things: (1) how much activity the patient can perform before being stopped by pain; (2) the degree and distribution of pain provoked by that activity; and (3) how long the pain takes to subside to its original level. (This is the most informative part and serves as a guide to the probable response of the symptoms to examination and treatment.)

In the previous example of the tennis player, a nonirritable disorder would be one in which he experiences momentary pain each time he serves (in this case the treatment described previously would be applicable). In contrast to this, an irritable disorder would be one in which his back pain lasts for several minutes after serving a ball, and this pain increases to the extent that after serving one game his back is so painful that he cannot continue to play and has to rest for 1 hour to ease his pain. In this example, a technique that reproduced his symptoms would not be the initial choice of treatment. Instead, his lumbar spine would be positioned in the most comfortable position and a pain-free technique would be performed.

Signs

Signs refer to physical examination findings. Physical examination tests are used to identify or exclude certain structures as the source of a patient's symptoms. In particular, the tests determine the involvement of the intervertebral joints and neuromeningeal tissues and whether conduction of the spinal cord and cauda equina is altered. They help indicate the degree of irritability of the disorder and demonstrate whether symptoms have a stretch or compression component.

The physical examination of movements includes the following three sections.

1. The gross physiologic movements of the lumbar spine (flexion, extension, lateral flexion, and rotation). It may be necessary to examine these movements in different combinations and in varied sequences, to sustain these positions, or to perform them with distraction or compression
2. Passive physiologic and accessory movements at each intervertebral segment
3. The neuromeningeal tissues in the vertebral and foraminal canals (using SLR, PNF, PKF, and the slump test)

Reaching a diagnosis of a mechanical disorder of the neuromusculoskeletal tissues is important, to isolate the structures at fault by knowing the symptom distribution and the response to physical tests. Knowledge of the movements that increase or decrease the symptom response, not the diagnostic title, is the main determinant of how to apply passive movement in treatment.

Selection of Technique Based on Effect

Mobilization/Manipulation

Passive movement as a treatment technique can be broadly divided into its use as mobilization (passive oscillatory movements) or manipulation (small amplitude thrust/stretch performed at speed at the limit of a range of movement).

Mobilization is the method of choice for most lumbar disorders because it can be used as a treatment for pain or for restoring movement in a hypomobile joint. It can be adapted to suit the severity of the pain, the irritability of the disorder, and the stages and stability of the pathologic process.

Manipulation is the treatment of choice when an intervertebral joint is locked. To regain mobility in cases of an irritable joint condition, a single, localized manipulation may be less aggravating than repeated stretching by mobilization.

Position of the Intervertebral Joint and Direction of the Movement Technique

Treatment by passive movement involves careful postioning of the particular intervertebral segment and the selection of the most effective direction of movement. These are based on a knowledge of spinal biomechanics and the desired symptom response.

Manipulation. Manipulation is applied in the direction of limitation in order to stretch the tissues in that particular direction. For example, using biomechanical principles, the lumbar spine can be positioned (in lateral flexion and contralateral rotation) to isolate movement to the desired intervertebral segment, and a rotary thrust can then be applied in the appropriate direction.

Passive Mobilization. When using passive mobilization, both the position of the intervertebral joint and the direction of movement are varied according to the desired effect of the technique. Some examples are:

1. *To avoid any discomfort or pain:* In cases where the pain is severe or the disorder is irritable, the symptoms should not be provoked or aggravated. The lumbar spine should be positioned so that the painful intervertebral segment is pain free, and the movement technique performed must also be pain free.

2. *To cause or to avoid reproduction of referred pain:* Provocation of referred pain is safe when the condition is nonirritable and when it is not an acute radicular pain disorder. In these cases it may be necessary to cause some leg pain to gain improvement; thus the spine should be positioned to either provoke some symptoms or to enable the treatment technique to provoke the referred symptoms. Findings indicating radicular pain (i.e., pain

worse distally and the presence of neurologic changes), when the examination of movements reproduces the distal pain, should warn the clinician against using a technique that provoked the referred pain.

3. *To open one side of the intervertebral joint* (i.e., to stretch the disc, distract the zygapophyseal joint, and widen the foraminal canal on one side): This should be the choice in cases of nerve root irritation or compression or in cases of a progressive unilateral disc disorder. For example, to widen the right side of the L4-L5 intervertebral space, the spine should be positioned in the combined position of flexion, lateral flexion, and rotation to the left. Which of these movements to emphasize as the treatment technique depends on the pain response.

4. *To stretch tissues that are contracted:* Joints that are both painful and hypomobile can respond differently to passive mobilization, depending to a large extent on the irritability. The pain response during the performance of a technique, and its effect over the next 24 hours, will guide the clinician in the choice of which direction to move the joint and how firmly to stretch the contracted tissues. A favorable response to gentle oscillatory stretches is that the pain experienced during the technique decreases, thus allowing the movement to be performed more strongly. A worsening of the pain response indicates that this direction of movement is aggravating the condition.

5. *To move the intervertebral joints or the canal structures:* If movements of the intervertebral joints and of the neuromeningeal structures in the canal both reproduce the patient's leg symptoms during the physical assessment, a technique directed at altering the intervertebral joint movements should be the first choice of treatment. The effect on the intervertebral joint signs and the canal signs is noted and, if the latter are not improving, movement of the neuromeningeal tissues is added or substituted. In cases of only back and/or buttock pain and where the canal tests more effectively reproduce this pain, the first choice would be to use movement of the canal structures (e.g., PNF, SLR, PKF, or the slump test).

Manner of Movement Technique Performance

Selection of a treatment technique relates not only to the direction of movement but also to the manner in which it is applied. The amplitude can be varied from a barely perceptible movement to one that makes use of the total available range. The rhythm can be varied from a smooth, evenly applied movement to one that is staccato. Similarly, the speed and the position in range in which the movement is performed can be altered.

Passive movement techniques must be modified according to the intention of the technique, and this is based on the symptoms experienced by the patient during the technique, the quality of the movement, the presence of spasm, and the end feel. It is not possible to discuss these details in any depth in this chapter, but only to present the two ends of the symptom spectrum, which ranges from a constant ache with pain experienced through range, to stiffness with mild discomfort felt only at the end of range of certain movements as presented below. For a full description, see Maitland.[21]

Constant Aching with Pain Through Range.   The lumbar spine must be placed in a position of maximal comfort (usually one of slight flexion and midposition for the other movements). The treatment technique will be of small amplitude and performed slowly and smoothly (so that there is no discomfort produced or, where discomfort is constant, with no increase in the level of aching). The movement technique may be a physiologic or an accessory movement, and its performance should result in an immediate lessening of pain. In some patients there may be an immediate effect, but in others the effect should be noted over 24 hours.

Stiffness with Mild Discomfort Felt Only at the End of Range of Certain Movements.   The lumbar spine is carefully positioned at or near the limit of the stiff directions of movement (i.e., in the position that best reproduces the stiffness and discomfort). The treatment technique will be one that places maximal stretch on the hypomobile intervertebral segment. The technique should be firmly applied, of small amplitude, and either sustained or staccato in rhythm. If the level of discomfort increases with the firm stretching, large-amplitude movements can be interspersed every 40 to 60 seconds.

CASE STUDIES

This section presents some clinical syndromes that have a clearly recognizable peripheral pain mechanism. Each syndrome has a history of spontaneous onset of symptoms, and management is restricted to treatment by passive movement. The syndromes are presented as case histories.

Acute Back Pain (Discogenic)

History

A 35-year-old man experienced a mild central backache after pushing a car one morning. This ache intensified during a 40-minute drive to work, and he was unable to get out of the car unaided due to severe low back pain. He had no previous history of backache, and radiographs of his lumbosacral region were normal. After 2 days in bed without any improvement in his symptoms, physical therapy was requested by his doctor.

Symptoms

There was a constant dull backache centered over the L4 to L5 region. The patient was unable to move in bed due to sharp jabs of pain. His most comfortable position was supine with hips and knees flexed over two pillows in crook lying or side lying with his legs (and lumbar spine) flexed.

Signs

The patient was supine for the examination. SLR was almost full range, as was PNF, but both tests slightly increased his back pain. Spreading and compression of the ilia were pain free, and there was no abnormality in lower limb reflexes or sensation (testing muscle strength was not undertaken due to back pain). In crook lying, lumbar rotation to each side was reduced to half range due to pain.

Interpretation

The history suggests discogenic pain—pushing a heavy car would raise intradiscal pressure—with pain worsened by sitting followed by inability to extend the spine. The physical examination was too restricted by pain to be helpful in confirming the source of the patient's symptoms.

Management

Day 1 (Treatment 1). Because SLR was of good range, both legs were comfortably flexed at the hips to 50 degrees, and gentle manual traction was applied by pulling on the patient's legs (Fig. 6-1). During traction his backache decreased. A series of four gentle but sharp tugs were applied to his legs. With each tug, a jab of back pain was experienced, but there was no increase in his constant backache. On reassessment, PNF was full and painless but SLR remained unchanged. The treatment was repeated, resulting in a slight improvement in the patient's SLR on both sides and in his range of lumbar rotations performed in a supine position.

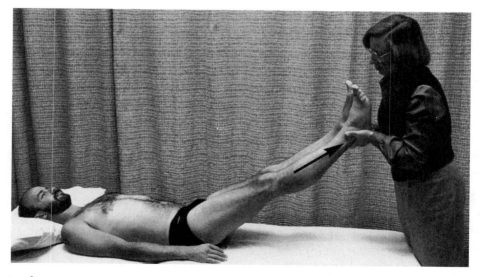

Fig. 6-1 Longitudinal caudad mobilization of the lower lumbar spine, produced by manual traction to the lower limbs.

Day 2 (Treatment 2). The patient reported greater freedom of movements in bed and had been out of bed twice for a hot shower. Examination of his lumbar mobility in standing showed marked limitation of flexion by pain centered over L5, and there was obvious spasm in his erector spinae. Extension was half range, and he had a full range of lateral flexion to each side. Bilateral SLR was full and painless. Manual traction effected no change in his mobility, so he was placed in a prone position with two pillows under his abdomen. From this position of comfort, he was asked to gently and passively extend his spine using a modified push-up technique.[29] This technique was repeated 10 times, with the position sustained for 5 seconds. The patient was encouraged to extend his lumbar spine to his comfortable limit. However, particular care was taken to avoid development of a backache. On reassessment in standing, flexion had improved so that he could reach fingertips to his patellae, and extension was three-quarters of his usual range of motion.

The technique was repeated but this time with the patient lying over only one pillow. After two more applications the patient could lie comfortably prone without a pillow, and in weightbearing there was a further slight increase in his ranges of flexion and extension.

The patient was asked to repeat this technique hourly (3 sets of 10 push-ups, at the end of which he allowed his back to sag into sustained extension for 1 minute, providing there was no reproduction of backache). He was allowed out of bed for short periods but was instructed to avoid sitting.

Day 3 (Treatment 3). The patient was pain free when moving in bed and could be ambulant for more than 1 hour before his ache returned. His range of flexion was such that he was able to reach his fingertips to mid-shin level (normally he could reach his ankles) and to fully extend his lumbar spine with only a mild ache.

The extension push-ups were repeated, with the manipulative therapist stabilizing the patient's pelvis flat on the floor. As this was pain free, the patient was asked to sustain the position and allow his lumbar spine to sag fully into extension. In this extended position, gentle posteroanterior pressures were applied to L5, taking care to cause only mild discomfort. On resuming the flat prone position, sharp, deep pain was felt over L5, but this quickly subsided with repeated gentle extension.

The above regimen was repeated prior to reassessing his mobility in standing. Flexion and extension were now at full range. Gentle overpressure to extension reproduced the same deep, sharp pain.

Days 4, 6, and 10 (Treatments 4, 5, and 6). Subsequent treatments were conducted at the manipulative therapist's clinic and consisted of restoration of full pain-free range of lumbar extension using posteroanterior pressure on L5 with the patient's lumbar spine in extension. By day 6 the patient was symptom free, but experienced a deep ache with firm sustained posteroanterior pressure on L5. When the patient was examined 4 days later, no pain could be elicited by sustained or staccato posteroanterior oscillatory movement.

The patient was discharged with advice regarding lifting and care of his back during sustained postures (especially flexion).

Severe Nerve-Root (Peripheral Neurogenic) Pain

History

A 35-year-old man had suffered from recurrent attacks of low back pain over the last 5 years. These were associated with lifting strains. This present episode commenced 4 days ago when he bent to move the garden hose. He experienced only mild aching in his low back, but over the next few hours his back pain disappeared and he felt strong pain in his left buttock and calf. His calf pain had worsened in the last 24 hours and spread into his left foot.

Symptoms

The patient had constant severe pain in the lateral aspect of his left calf and foot and numbness of the lateral aspect of his left foot. Less severe aching was experienced in his left buttock. Weightbearing and sitting aggravated his back pain. He could gain some relief of symptoms by lying on his right side with his legs (and lumbar spine) flexed.

Signs

The following movements aggravated his buttock and calf/foot pain: flexion to touch his patellae, extension and left lateral flexion to half range, and left SLR limited to 25 degrees. Neurologic examination revealed a reduced left ankle jerk, reduced sensation over the lateral border of the foot, and weak toe flexors (calf power could not be tested due to pain on weightbearing).

Interpretation

There was evidence of S1 nerve root compression. The history of a trivial incident causing this episode and the presence of worsening symptoms indicated that the disorder is both unstable and progressive, requiring care with treatment so as not to worsen the condition.

Management

Day 1 (Treatment 1).   In position of comfort (i.e., lying on right side with lumbar spine comfortably flexed), the pelvis was gently rotated to the right, taking care not to aggravate calf/foot or buttock pain. The technique was performed as far as possible into range without aggravating symptoms; SLR was used as reassessment. After two applications of rotation, flexion was also reassessed. The patient reported easing of his calf symptoms, and both flexion and left SLR had minimally improved; however, extension range remained unaltered. The patient was advised to rest in bed as much as possible and to avoid sitting.

Day 2 (Treatment 2).   The patient reported that his symptoms were unchanged, and his physical signs and neurologic status were found to be unaltered. Rotary mobilization was repeated (as on day 1) with a similar response.

Day 3 (Treatment 3).   No alteration in symptoms or signs. As his symptoms were aggravated by weightbearing, lumbar traction was given (15 lb for 10 minutes). During traction his calf/foot pain was eased, and afterward his SLR improved by 10 degrees.

Day 4 (Treatment 4).   Definite reduction in calf/foot pain and improvement in all physical signs. Traction was repeated (15 lb for 20 minutes). At subsequent treatments both the time and the strength of the traction were increased.

Day 10 (Treatment 8).   There were no leg symptoms, but buttock pain was experienced with prolonged sitting. Physical examination revealed full recovery of neurologic function. The extreme range of flexion, with the addition of neck flexion, reproduced buttock pain; the other spinal movements were full range and pain free. On passive overpressure left SLR lacked 20 degrees and also reproduced left buttock pain.

Interpretation

At this stage, spinal mobility was full and painless, but movement of the neuromeningeal tissues was restricted and reproduced the patient's only remaining symptom. A gentle technique to stretch the neuromeningeal tissues should be used, but reproduction of nerve root symptoms would contraindicate its use at this stage.

Treatment 8 (Continued).   A gentle stretch was applied to left SLR, causing only buttock pain. Following this, flexion plus neck flexion were pain free.

Day 12 (Treatment 9).   The patient was now symptom free, but left SLR still caused buttock pain at 75 degrees.

Interpretation

Despite an excellent response to treatment, in view of the progressive disorder, a decision not to stretch his SLR more firmly was taken. It was decided to review his progress in 2 weeks.

When seen 2 weeks later he had remained symptom free, but his left SLR had not improved. Now that his disorder had stabilized, his SLR was strongly stretched, restoring full range with no return of symptoms.

Chronic Nerve-Root (Radicular) Aching

This may present as either (1) residual symptoms from an acute episode of nerve root pain or (2) chronic aching (not pain) with signs of nerve root compression.

In both cases, the disorder is nonirritable and does not restrict the patient's activities; however, sitting causes an increase in leg symptoms that is consistent with most low lumbar nerve root problems of discogenic origin. The disorder is stable and permits stronger techniques to be applied safely. The following case history illustrates the second type of chronic aching.

History

A 40-year-old housewife presented with a past history of recurrent low back pain for 7 years. One year ago she noticed a dull ache in her left leg. At that time, two or three treatments of passive mobilization completely relieved her symptoms. The current episode began 3 weeks ago, following paving of the garden path with bricks. While stooping to lay the bricks she was conscious of aching in her buttock and down the posterior aspect of her left leg. Rotary mobilization had not helped.

Symptoms

A constant dull ache spread from her left sacroiliac area, down the posterior aspect of her buttock to the heel, together with paresthesia of the lateral aspect of her foot. The ache in her calf and the paresthesia were worsened if she sustained a flexed posture (e.g., vacuuming carpets) for more than 30 minutes or sat for more than 60 minutes.

Signs

There was a full range of pain-free spinal movements, even when these were sustained. Poor intervertebral movement was noted below L3 on extension and on left lateral flexion. Buttock aching was reproduced by adding left lateral flexion to the fully extended position. The addition of left and right rotation made no change in the symptoms. Testing of intervertebral movement confirmed hypomobility at both L4-L5 and L5-S1 motion segments, and posteroanterior pressure over L5 (performed with her spine in extension/left lateral flexion) caused buttock pain.

Tests for the neuromeningeal tissues revealed full SLR, but the left leg had a tighter end feel; the slump test was positive (i.e., left knee extension lacked 30 degrees and caused calf pain, which was eased by releasing cervical flexion). She had slight weakness of her left calf, but otherwise showed no neurologic deficit.

Interpretation

The history implicated a disc disorder that was slowly progressing to interfere with nerve root function. The disorder was stable in that the patient could continue with her daily activities as a housewife. Treatment to change both her intervertebral joint signs and neuromeningeal signs was necessary, using techniques that would temporarily aggravate her leg ache. Treating the intervertebral joint hypomobility first, while observing its effect on both the joint and neuromeningeal signs, was safer.

Management

Day 1 (Treatment 1).   With the patient's low lumbar spine positioned in extension and left lateral flexion, firm posteroanterior pressures were applied to L4 and L5 spinous processes for 60 to 90 seconds, causing local pain and a mild increase in left buttock aching (Fig. 6-2). On reassessment, lumbar extension/left lateral flexion no longer reproduced an increase in buttock ache and low lumbar mobility had improved. The slump test had improved (left knee extension improved by 10 degrees). Treatment was repeated with no further gain in mobility; neurologic function was unchanged.

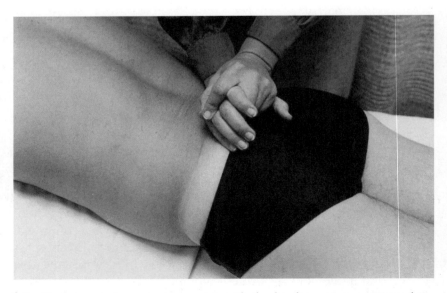

Fig. 6-2   Posteroanterior pressure on L5 with the lumbar spine positioned in extension/left lateral flexion.

Day 3 (Treatment 2). The patient reported no ill effects from treatment and a lessening of her left leg aching. Physical examination showed that she had maintained the improvement gained on day 1. Neurologic function was unchanged. The above treatment was repeated even more strongly and sustained to stretch the tight tissues. The reproduction of only local pain (no referred buttock pain) supported the safety of using a strong stretch. The result of this stretch was that extension/left lateral flexion was painful only when sustained, and in the slump position, knee extension improved by another 10 degrees. Repeating the technique twice gained no further change to the slump test.

Day 5 (Treatment 3). The patient was delighted with her progress. She no longer had a constant ache down her left leg. The ache and paresthesia returned only if she sat for more than 1 hour. On examination, her left calf had regained full strength. Left SLR was no longer tighter than on the right; however, in the slump position, left knee extension still lacked 10 degrees and caused buttock pain.

Treatment was changed to restore mobility in the neuromeningeal tissues. In the slump position, her left knee was stretched into full extension, causing sharp buttock pain (Fig. 6-3). This technique was not repeated until

Fig. 6-3 Passive extension of the left knee performed while in the slump position.

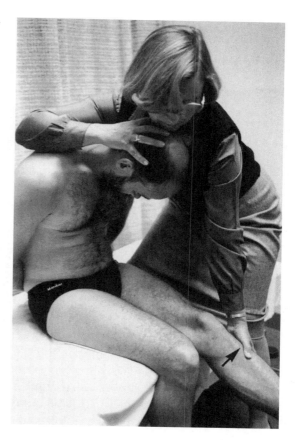

its effect on nerve root conduction was known. This can only be assessed over 24 to 48 hours.

Day 7 (Treatment 4).   There was no return of symptoms following the last treatment. The patient's calf strength and ankle reflex were normal. In the slump position, knee extension still reproduced sharp buttock pain. The stretch to the neuromeningeal tissues was increased by stretching the knee into full extension and stretching the ankle into full dorsiflexion in the slump position. This again caused sharp buttock pain. Reassessment of knee extension in the slump position showed it to be full range with minimal buttock pain. The technique was repeated once more. The patient was asked to experiment with activities such as sustained flexion and sitting for long periods during the next week.

Day 14 (Treatment 5).   The patient reported that she experienced no leg symptoms but that her back ached after activities involving sustained flexion for more than 45 minutes and after sitting more than 90 minutes. She considered this better than she had been for several years. Examination of the slump test revealed full mobility but caused slight buttock pain. The patient was discharged with a home exercise program to maintain the mobility of both her lower lumbar spine and her neuromeningeal tissues.

Mechanical Locking

History

A 20-year-old man complained of a sudden onset of unilateral back pain, which prevented him from standing upright. He had bent forward quickly to catch a ball near his left foot and was unable to straighten because of sharp back pain. He had no past history of back pain, and no spinal radiographs had been taken.

Symptoms

There was no pain when his back was held in slight flexion, but on standing upright pain was experienced to the right of the L5 spinous process.

Signs

The patient was prevented by pain from extending, laterally flexing, or rotating his low lumbar spine to the right. The other movements were full and painless. Passive testing of intersegmental movement revealed an inability to produce the above painful movements at L4-L5, with marked spasm on attempting to do so. Unilaterally, posteroanterior pressures over the right L4-L5 zygapophyseal joint produced marked pain and spasm.

Interpretation

A rapid, unguarded movement in flexion/left lateral flexion gapped the right lumbar zygapophyseal joints, following which there was mechanical blocking of the movements that normally appose the articular surfaces (extension, lateral flexion, and rotation of the trunk to the right). The mechanism of mechanical locking remains a contentious issue.[30,31,32]

A manipulation, localized to the affected intervertebral level, to gap in this case the right L4-L5 zygapophyseal joint, will restore normal joint function.

Management

A rotary manipulation was performed to gap the right L4-L5 zygapophyseal joint. The patient was positioned on his left side with his low lumbar spine flexed and laterally flexed to the right until movement could be palpated at the L4-L5 intervertebral level (Fig. 6-4). In this position, with thumb pressure against the right side of the spinous process of L4 (to stabilize L4), a quick left rotary thrust was applied through the pelvis and to L5 by finger pressure against the left side of the L5 spinous process (to pull L5 into left rotation).

Immediately afterward the patient could fully extend, laterally flex, and rotate his trunk to the right with only soreness experienced at the extreme of these movements. This soreness was lessened by gentle, large-amplitude posteroanterior pressure performed unilaterally over the right L4-L5 zygapophyseal joint. The next day the patient reported by telephone that he was symptom free.

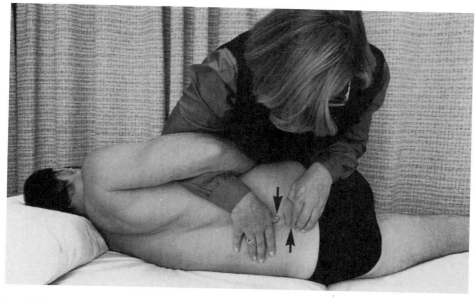

Fig. 6-4 Rotary manipulation is used to open the right L4-L5 zygapophyseal joint.

Zygapophyseal Joint Arthropathy (Causing Only Referred Symptoms)

History

A 50-year-old man described a gradual onset, over 3 days, of aching in the right trochanteric area. This had been present for 1 month. He could not recall any injury to his back, hip, or leg, and he had not experienced pain in any other area. He had no history of back or lower extremity symptoms.

Radiographs of the lumbar spine and hip were normal. He was diagnosed by the referring doctor as suffering from trochanteric bursitis.

Symptoms

The patient experienced a constant deep ache over his right greater trochanter, which was unaltered by posture or activity.

Signs

Lumbar movements were full and pain free with overpressure. Tests for the neuromeningeal tissues, hip, and trochanteric bursitis were negative.

Deep palpation (through the erector spinae) over the right L4-L5 zygapophyseal joint revealed stiffness, local spasm, and tenderness, and there was an area of thickening at the right side of the interspinous space between L4 and L5. These signs were absent on the left side. Reproduction of referred pain was not possible.

Interpretation

Anatomically, pathology of the L4-L5 zygapophyseal joint could give rise to referred pain at the trochanteric area. In the absence of other physical signs, it would be appropriate to mobilize the hypomobile L4-L5 zygapophyseal joint and note any effect on his trochanteric aching. An association between the hypomobile L4-L5 zygapophyseal joint and the trochanteric pain can be made only in retrospect.

Management

The hypomobility was localized to the L4-L5 right zygapophyseal joint; therefore, passive stretching was localized to this joint.

Day 1 (Treatment 1).   Posteroanterior oscillatory pressure was applied firmly for 60 seconds to the spinous processes of L4 and L5, and unilaterally over the painful joint. The patient reported no change in his constant trochanteric ache.

Day 2 (Treatment 2). The patient reported that his right trochanteric pain was now intermittent (and continued unrelated to movement or to changes of posture of his trunk). The treatment was repeated, giving three applications of posteroanterior pressure lasting 60 seconds each. These were interspersed with gentle, large-amplitude oscillations to ease the local soreness.

Days 4, 6, and 8 (Treatments 3, 4, and 5). The patient reported continued improvement of his symptoms, and the mobilization of L4-L5 was progressed in strength and sustained for longer periods to achieve a better stretch on the tight soft tissues (capsule and ligaments). At the last visit, it was necessary to place his lower lumbar spine into full extension and direct the posteroanterior pressures more caudally to detect any residual hypomobility. By this stage, he experienced only occasional transient aching in his thigh, so treatment was stopped, with a review in 2 weeks.

Day 22 (Treatment 6). When reassessed 2 weeks later the patient reported that he was symptom free. Passive mobility tests showed no hypomobility or thickening of soft tissues on the right of the L4-L5 joint.

Zygapophyseal Joint Arthropathy (Intra-articular Problem)

History

A 75-year-old woman complained of a sharp pain to the right of L5 following stepping awkwardly with her right foot into a shallow depression in the pavement 1 week previously. She had become aware of aching in her back, which worsened with each step until it became constant. Because her back was both painful and stiff the following morning, she consulted her doctor. He ordered radiographs to be taken, which revealed narrowing of her lumbosacral disc space and osteoarthritic changes in her lumbosacral zygapophyseal joints. She was given anti-inflammatory medication and advised to rest as much as possible. Five days later her pain was no longer constant, but certain spinal movements still caused considerable pain, and she was referred for physical therapy. She had a past history of low backache for many years if she stood for long periods.

Symptoms

Sharp pain just lateral to the spinous process of L5 on the right was provoked by turning in bed from a supine position onto her right side, and on bending to the right when standing.

Signs

All movements of her low lumbar spine were hypomobile. Lumbar extension and lateral flexion to the right reproduced her pain. Pain was experienced at half range, increasing at the limit of these movements.

Palpation of passive accessory movements revealed marked hypomobility of the L4-L5 and L5-S1 segments, and posteroanterior pressure and transverse pressure to the left reproduced her back pain. Tests for neural mobility and conduction were negative.

Interpretation

This was an elderly woman with a degenerative, stiff lower lumbar spine. A trivial injury (i.e., a sudden jarring up through her right leg) caused the hypomobile joint to become painful.

This was thought to be an intra-articular problem because pain was experienced with movements that closed the right side of the intervertebral joint and because pain was felt early and throughout these movements. Such articular problems respond well to large-amplitude passive mobilization, performed carefully to avoid compression of the articular surfaces. Later, when pain is minimal, treatment may progress to mobilization with the surfaces compressed.

Management

Day 1 (Treatment 1). With the patient lying comfortably on her right side in slight flexion, gentle, large-amplitude left lateral flexion oscillations were produced by moving the pelvis (Fig. 6-5). Care was taken not to cause any discomfort. Following this, extension and right lateral flexion were reassessed. A favorable response was noted in that pain started later in the range of both of these movements. The technique was repeated but no further improvement was noted.

Day 3 (Treatment 2). The patient reported no change in her symptoms, but the improvement in the signs gained with the first treatment had been maintained. The day 1 treatment was repeated twice, after which the pain response to right lateral flexion improved, but extension was unchanged. The technique was changed to accessory posteroanterior central pressure to L4 and L5, again employing large-amplitude movements. This achieved an immediate improvement in the range of extension and a reduction in the pain response.

Day 5 (Treatment 3). The patient was delighted with her progress in that she had no pain turning in bed and her daily movements were painless. Mild pain was experienced at the limit of both extension and right lateral flexion. By adding extension to right lateral flexion, sharp pain was produced. For treatment, her lumbar spine was placed in the position of slight

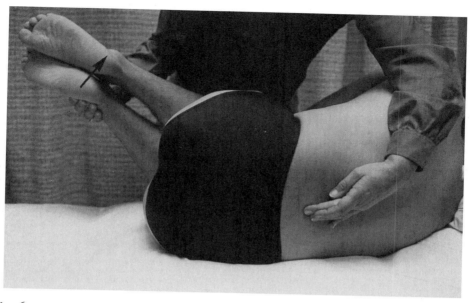

Fig. 6-5   Passive left lateral flexion mobilization of the lower lumbar spine, produced by moving the lower limbs and pelvis.

right lateral flexion combined with extension. In this position, posteroanterior pressure was applied for 30 seconds as a large-amplitude movement, causing slight pain at first. The pain disappeared during performance of this technique, so the spine was placed further into extension and right lateral flexion. Slight pain was again experienced, and again this disappeared with another application of the mobilization. On reassessment, combined right lateral flexion with extension was pain free. Slight pain was experienced only on overpressure.

Day 7 (Treatment 4).   The patient was still symptom free, and right lateral flexion with extension was no longer painful when performed with overpressure. However, slight pain was experienced when right lateral flexion was added to extension.

The spine was placed in this combined position in the same order (full extension and then full right lateral flexion), and posteroanterior central pressure was applied as a strong stretching technique. This caused marked pain and required gentle, large-amplitude posteroanterior pressure to ease the soreness. Following this the patient complained of aching across her lower lumbar area. Pulsed short-wave diathermy for 15 minutes (on a low frequency and low dosage) eased her ache.

Days 10 and 24 (Treatments 5 and 6).   The patient remained symptom free, but extension plus right lateral flexion still reproduced slight pain to the right of L5. By combining these movements on the left side, a similar pain was produced. This was considered likely to be her normal response, and no further treatment was given. This was verified by finding the same signs 2 weeks later, during which time she had remained symptom free.

Postural Pain

History

A 28-year-old mother of three children presented with a 6-month history of gradual onset of low back pain. She could not recall an incident that had caused her symptoms. During her third pregnancy 2 years ago, she had experienced the same pain, but this had settled after the birth. There was no history of trauma, and her radiographs were normal.

Symptoms

The patient was asymptomatic in the morning, but by midafternoon her low back began to ache. This ache worsened as the day progressed, especially during activities requiring her lumbar spine to be held in sustained flexion (bathing the children, making beds, sweeping, vacuuming) and when lifting the children. Sitting and lying eased the pain.

Signs

The patient stood with an increased lumbar lordosis; she had a full range of pain-free movements. Overpressure into full extension was painful, and by combining this with lateral flexion to either side the pain was made worse on that side. Testing of intervertebral movements revealed excellent mobility with the exception of posteroanterior gliding of L5 on the sacrum, which was slightly hypomobile. Tests for neuromeningeal tissues were normal. Her lower abdominal and gluteal muscles were slack and weak.

Interpretation

This was a patient with a young, mobile spine that became painful when the tissues restraining flexion were stressed (posterior ligamentous structures and zygapophyseal joints). There was poor support by the abdominal muscles, which co-contract with the erector spinae and gluteals to stabilize the spine during flexion. Pain was relieved by rest (when stress was taken off the painful tissues).

Management

Day 1 (Treatment 1).   An explanation of the cause of the symptoms was given, and the need to strengthen the abdominals, gluteals, and erector spinae was stressed. Large-amplitude accessory posteroanterior mobilization of her L5-S1 joint to restore her normal mobility at this segment would help this joint to become pain free, but the primary objective was to strengthen the abdominal,[33] gluteal, and erector spinae muscle groups. This was complemented by postural correction (pelvic tilting) and by giving advice on correct lifting techniques and how to restore the lumbar lordosis after periods of sustained flexion (discussed in more detail in other chapters).

Day 5 (Treatment 2).   The patient was seen again to check that she was performing her exercises correctly and regularly. The exercises were progressively increased in difficulty as her muscular control improved. Her lumbosacral joint was again mobilized. She reported no change in her symptoms and was urged to continue her exercises regularly.

Day 21 (Treatment 3).   The patient reported that she was virtually symptom free, experiencing slight aching if she was excessively busy and tired. On examination, lumbar extension combined with lateral flexion to each side was full and painless, as was posteroanterior accessory gliding of L5. The patient was discharged with the advice to maintain good muscle support of her spine by regular exercise.

Coccygeal Pain

History

A 22-year-old female bank clerk complained of a gradual onset over 3 days of localized coccygeal pain. There was no history of lumbar or pelvic symptoms, trauma, or childbirth.

Symptoms

The patient's coccygeal pain was present only in sitting and worsened if she slouched. Standing eased her pain almost immediately. Her pain was unaltered by sitting on a hard surface, defecation, or squatting.

Signs

The patient's sitting posture was poor, and passive overpressure to the slouched sitting posture reproduced her coccygeal pain. The addition of cervical flexion and knee extension did not alter her pain. Also, the addition of posteroanterior pressure to the coccyx (flexion of the sacrococcygeal joint) did not alter her pain, although the coccyx was very tender.

Lumbar movements were full and pain free to overpressure; however, there was a loss of intersegmental mobility below L3 on both flexion and extension. Testing of intervertebral mobility revealed hypomobility, pain, and spasm on central posteroanterior pressure over L5, but the coccygeal pain was not reproduced. Pain associated with pressure on L5 was unaltered by the addition of posteroanterior pressure on L4. There was no thickening on careful palpation of the sacrococcygeal joint and the ligaments attaching to the coccyx.

Interpretation

Coccygeal pain of musculoskeletal origin can arise from the sacrococcygeal joint or ligamentous attachments to the coccyx, secondary to direct trauma such as sitting heavily on the buttocks, or childbirth, or coccygeal pain can be referred from the low lumbar spine. In this case, the lack of coccygeal trauma, pain on passive movements of the coccyx, and thickening of the sacrococcygeal joint or coccygeal ligamentous attachments negated a local source of pain. Local joint signs at L5-S1 incriminated this joint as the source of symptoms. This could be verified by treating the L5-S1 joint and reassessing symptom production by sitting.

Management

Day 1 (Treatment 1).   The explanation was given that the likely source of symptoms was the lumbar spine and that treatment would entail correction of sitting posture and restoration of low lumbar joint mobility. Large-amplitude accessory posteroanterior mobilization was applied for 60 seconds to L5 to restore normal pain-free mobility. This effected an immediate lessening of the degree of pain on retesting of overpressure to slouched sitting. The technique was repeated with further improvement. The session ended with postural correction of the patient's sitting posture, and she was asked to set up a protocol by which she could monitor her sitting posture at work.

Day 4 (Treatment 2).   The patient reported increased pain associated with sitting, for 2 days following her examination and first treatment; since then her symptoms had greatly improved. On questioning, she reported that she monitored her posture at the completion of each customer transaction. On reassessment, slouched sitting with overpressure was symptom free but her L5-S1 joint remained hypomobile and painful to posteroanterior pressure testing. Day 1 treatment was repeated.

Day 7 (Treatment 3).   The patient reported that she was symptom free. Since her second treatment she had experienced coccygeal aching only twice, associated with periods of prolonged sitting. Posture correction immediately abolished the aching. The L5-S1 joint was firmly mobilized, and the importance of correct sitting posture was emphasized.

Spinal Stenosis

History

A 60-year-old retired nurse complained of a 20-year history of low back pain for which she had never sought treatment. In the last 6 months she had experienced vague aching in both lower limbs, which had become progressively worse to the point at which it now severely interfered with walking.

She found that she could still ride her bicycle without pain. Having been a nurse she suspected peripheral vascular disease, possibly secondary to diabetes mellitus. Tests for these were negative. Plain radiographs of her lumbar spine showed narrowing of the L4-L5 disc space and marked bilateral osteoarthrosis of the zygapophyseal joints at L4-L5 and L5-S1. No spondylolisthesis was present.

Symptoms

Symptoms included deep aching and pain in both calves and the dorsal and lateral aspects of both feet, although worse on the left side. Symptoms were provoked by standing for more than 15 minutes or walking for more than 3 to 4 minutes. They were eased only by sitting.

Signs

Signs included excessive lumbar lordotic curve with adaptive shortening of erector spinae muscles. Extension of the lumbar spine reproduced low back pain, and if the extension was sustained with passive overpressure for 20 seconds, bilateral calf aching developed. Other lumbar movements were hypomobile below L3, but pain free. SLR was equal on both sides, but there was an increased feeling of posterior thigh tightness on the left. There was no neurologic deficit, and peripheral pulses were normal. Deep palpation (through the erector spinae) revealed bilateral thickening, hypomobility, local spasm, and tenderness over the L4-L5 and L5-S1 zygapophyseal joints. Firm pressure did not reproduce referred leg symptoms.

Interpretation

Gradual onset of bilateral extrasegmental lower extremity pain associated with walking suggested vascular or neurogenic (cauda equina) etiology. A neurogenic source for the pain was supported by the easing of symptoms with sitting, which widens the spinal canal, and by reproduction of both back and bilateral leg pain with lumbar extension. A vascular source was unlikely because leg symptoms were not eased by standing still and the patient's peripheral pulses were normal.

In consultation with her medical practitioner, a computed tomography (CT) scan of her low lumbar spine was taken. This confirmed the presence of spinal canal stenosis at L5-S1, with indentation of the thecal sac.

Management

Day 1 (Treatment 1). Management consisted of an explanation to the patient of the likely etiology of her symptoms and the need to widen her spinal canal by flattening her lumbar lordosis. Passive mobilization of her lower lumbar zygapophyseal joints would help to ease her back symptoms, possibly by lessening joint effusion.

In crook lying the patient was unable to actively flatten her lumbar curve; therefore, the tight erector spinae were lengthened using a combination of reciprocal relaxation and passive stretching techniques performed at the limit of lumbar flexion in the sitting posture. This resulted in the patient being able to achieve some flattening of her lumbar spine, and she was instructed to repeat this 10 times at home, four times daily.

Day 3 (Treatment 2). Symptoms were unchanged. Review of active posterior pelvic tilting revealed an improved range of lumbar flexion but poor movement below L3. Lengthening techniques for erector spinae were repeated, but this effected no real improvement in low lumbar flexion. In crook lying, with the abdominal wall relaxed, anteroposterior mobilization was applied by slowly depressing the abdomen with the thumb pads until the anterior aspect of the vertebral bodies was palpated. Following this, there was improvement in the passive range of low lumbar flexion. This was followed by refining the active posterior tilting exercise to encourage recruitment of the low abdominals. The patient was then asked to gently (submaximal effort) flatten her lumbar spine by hollowing her abdomen.[33] The same regimen of home exercises was prescribed.

Day 5 (Treatment 3). Symptoms were unchanged. Treatment 2 was repeated, with emphasis on re-education of low abdominal control of low lumbar/pelvic flexion. This included being able to hold the flattened lumbar position while flexing alternate hips.

Day 8 (Treatment 4). Symptoms were unchanged, and lumbar extension was the same as on day 1. Treatment 2 was repeated, with the addition of unilateral posteroanterior mobilization performed bilaterally L3 to L5. Lumbar extension caused less back pain and, after a second application, extension had to be sustained for 5 seconds before producing back pain. Abdominal hollowing progressed to standing and maintenance during walking.

Day 14 (Treatment 5). The patient was now able to stand for 20 minutes before leg symptoms developed, and walking was unaltered. The improvement gained in lumbar extension from unilateral posteroanterior mobilization had been maintained, so this was repeated. Following this only a vague ache was experienced in the calves after sustaining full extension for 40 seconds. The avoidance of lumbar lordosis when walking was emphasized.

Day 21 (Treatment 6). The patient was now able to walk for 6 minutes before needing to sit to relieve her leg symptoms. Treatment 5 was repeated, with most time spent on maintenance of a flattened lumbar spine during walking and climbing stairs.

Day 28 (Treatment 7). The patient was able to walk 10 to 15 minutes before needing to sit. Treatment 6 was repeated.

Day 56 (Treatment 8). When reviewed 1 month later the patient reported that she could walk for 20 minutes and that standing to do household duties was symptom free as long as she remembered to maintain her slightly flexed lumbar posture. Her lumbar extension and passive intersegmental mobility L3 to L5 were reassessed and found to have been maintained. The need for ongoing abdominal exercises and lumbar posture correction was emphasized.

Sacroiliac Joint Arthropathy

The authors wish to acknowledge Anthony Hogan, Manipulative Physiotherapist, who supplied this case history.

History

A 38-year-old woman walking downstairs missed a step and landed heavily on her right foot with an extended leg. She felt a jarring sensation and immediate sharp pain in the right low back/buttock and was unable to weightbear through her right leg without reproducing the sharp pain. Within an hour she had developed a nasty ache in her buttock. She presented for treatment the next morning unable to weightbear through her right leg. She had no previous history of low back pain but had experienced a less severe low lumbar/buttock ache in the third trimester of her pregnancy that resolved within days of delivery 12 weeks ago.

Symptoms

The sharp pain was localized to the right sacroiliac joint and there was a constant dull ache in the right buttock. Lying down partially relieved the ache, but movements whilst in bed caused the same sharp pain and subsequent increase in dull ache. There was pain on coughing and sneezing; there had been no referral into the lower leg or altered sensation.

Signs

Physical examination of the lumbopelvic region was limited by the inability of the patient to weightbear through the right leg. The low lumbar motion segments were excluded as the primary source of pain by deep soft tissue palpation and passive accessory movement examination. SLR was restricted to 40 degrees on the right and 60 degrees on the left, both producing pain localized to the right sacroiliac region.

Examination of the pelvis, including positional assessment, palpation, and sacroiliac articular movement and stability tests revealed a blocked right sacroiliac joint.

Interpretation

The history, localized area of pain, and lack of findings in the right low lumbar motion segments suggested that the right sacroiliac joint had sustained a traumatic mechanical dysfunction. The physical examination of the pelvis demonstrated a posteriorly rotated upslip of the right innominate, which would be consistent with a vertical force sustained anterior to the axis of sacroiliac joint motion. Given the limited nature of the physical examination in standing it was reasonable to base treatment on findings from accessory movement testing of the lumbar spine and sacroiliac joints.

Management

Day 1 (Treatment 1). The treatment of choice was a manipulative technique to reduce the posteriorly rotated upslip and to regain normal mobility in the right sacroiliac joint.

The patient was positioned supine, and the therapist grasped the right lower leg firmly (above the ankle joint). While palpating the sacral sulcus, the therapist flexed the extended right leg at the hip joint until the posterior rotation limit was felt by the therapist. The position of the leg was finely adjusted with hip abduction and medial rotation until the line of the femur corresponded with the degree of posterior rotation of the innominate. The motion barrier was felt by applying a longitudinal pull through the leg. A high-velocity, small-amplitude tug was applied through the right leg to manipulate the sacroiliac joint.

On reassessment the patient was able to weightbear without the sharp pain, but the buttock ache was unchanged. Articular movement tests for the sacroiliac joint revealed that the manipulation had successfully unblocked the right sacroiliac joint (and the lumbar spine was unchanged). Articular mobility tests revealed excessive superior glide of the innominate on the sacrum compared with the left side. There was inadequate muscle control of this movement on articular stability testing.

Interpretation

Excessive superior glide of the innominate on the sacrum coupled with inadequate muscle stabilization of the joint will leave the joint vulnerable to a recurrence of pain and/or locking. The inadequate muscular stabilization was not evident on initial assessment because the sacroiliac joint was blocked, but it cannot be overlooked at the first treatment session.

Treatment (Continued)

A sacroiliac belt was fitted just above the great trochanter, and the patient was instructed to wear the belt while weightbearing. She was also given advice regarding relative rest from aggravating activities, and a plan was discussed to commence retraining of the muscles required to stabilize the sacroiliac joint once symptoms had subsided. She was instructed to go home and rest as much as possible.

Day 3 (Treatment 2).   The patient reported that the sharp pain on weightbearing through her right leg was much improved and that her main problem was the continuous dull ache in the right buttock, which was quickly aggravated by short periods of walking.

Physical examination revealed almost symmetric movement of the sacroiliac joints; however, the excessive superior glide of the right innominate was still present and could not to be stabilized by muscular contraction.

Interpretation

The presentation indicated that the pain was arising from a traumatized joint. Choices of treatment include manual therapy techniques to relieve pain, strict nonweightbearing on the right leg by use of crutches to further unload the joint, and other anti-inflammatory modalities, excluding anti-inflammatory medication because the patient was breastfeeding.

Treatment

In supine crook lying the sacroiliac joint was treated as an irritable joint. Assessment of anteroposterior and superoinferior gliding of the right sacroiliac joint did not reveal a movement that eased the constant ache, so the movement with the largest amplitude available before an increase in ache was chosen. A small-amplitude anteroposterior movement of the ilia was performed, and care was taken to not increase the ache. After two repetitions the constant ache had subsided considerably, and on reassessment in standing (with sacroiliac belt on) there was a much-reduced constant ache. This treatment was repeated twice, and on reassessment the patient was able to stand with minimal ache localized to the right sacroiliac region and no buttock ache.

Day 5 (Treatment 3).   The patient reported that she was walking pain free for periods of 5 minutes after which the ache, localized to the right sacroiliac region, recurred and the buttock ache recurred after walking for 20 minutes but this settled after lying for 30 minutes. Treatment continued using the anteroposterior and superior accessory movements of the sacroiliac joint by increasing the amplitude to the onset of local ache but care was taken to not reproduce the buttock ache. Treatment using accessory movements was progressed to include posterior rotation of the innominate with the same treatment goals described above. Basic retraining of the stabilizing muscles was commenced in a painfree and unloaded position of the sacroiliac joint (supine crook lying).

Days 8, 10 and 12 (Treatments 4, 5 and 6).   Subsequent passive mobilization treatments were performed to regain full, pain-free range of the sacroiliac joint in all directions of anteroposterior and inferosuperior glides, and both anterior and posterior rotations. On the sixth visit the patient reported being symptom free, and the physical examination revealed pain-free and symmetric movements of the innominate in relation to the sacrum. Although improved, the muscular stabilizers were still not able to fully control the superior glide of the innominate on the sacrum, and for this reason the patient was instructed to continue use of the sacroiliac belt to prevent recurrence until full muscle control of this movement was achieved.

The patient was discharged with a plan to review her exercise program in 3 months. An explanation was offered that the problem may have been influenced by hormonal changes associated with pregnancy. Such hormonal changes may take up to 12 months to resolve, and care to keep adequate strength in the stabilizers of the sacroiliac joint would be required for this time.

CONCLUSIONS

The decision to apply manipulative therapy must be based on a thorough examination and identification of the predominant pain mechanisms in operation. Peripheral nociception, arising from tissue injury to the lumbar joints, ligaments, muscles, and nerve roots, responds well to treatment aimed at the source of the symptoms. Attention must also be directed toward the contributing factors relating to the development and maintenance of the current problem. These include ergonomic factors, past physical and mental traumas, and the patient's physical and mental ability to cope.

Most dysfunctions resulting from peripheral nociception have a mechanical component that responds well to carefully applied manipulative physical therapy. This form of therapy is safe, effective, and an important part of the overall management of patients with these conditions. It is important to select the appropriate technique and to repeatedly reassess the effects of these techniques if optimal results are to be achieved.

REFERENCES

1. Siddall PJ, Cousins MJ: Spine update. Spinal pain mechanisms. Spine 22:1:98, 1997
2. Gifford LS, Butler DS: The integration of pain sciences into clinical practice. J Hand Therapy 10:86, 1997
3. Higgs J, Jones MA: Clinical Reasoning in the Health Professions. Butterworth-Heinnemann, London, 1995
4. Zochodne DW: Epineural peptides: a role in neuropathic pain? Can J Neurol Sci 29:69, 1993
5. Woolf CJ, Doubell TP: The pathophysiology of chronic pain: increased sensitivity to low threshold Aβ-Fibre inputs. Curr Opin Neurobiol 4:525, 1994
6. Shortland P, Woolf CJ: Chronic peripheral nerve section results in a rearrangement of the central axonal arborizations of axotomised A beta primary afferent neurons in the rat spinal cord. J Comp Neurol 330:65, 1993

7. Dubner R, Basbaum A: Spinal dorsal horn plasticity following tissue or nerve injury. In Wall PD, Melzack R (Eds.): Textbook of Pain (3rd Ed.). Churchill Livingstone, Edinburgh, 1994
8. Basbaum AI, Fields HL: Endogenous pain control mechanisms. Ann Neurol 4:451, 1978
9. Fields HL, Basbaum AI: Central nervous system mechanisms of pain control. In Wall PD, Melzack R (Eds.): Textbook of Pain (3rd Ed.). Churchill Livingstone, Edinburgh, 1994
10. Bradley LA: Cognitive-behavioural therapy for chronic pain. In Gatchel RJ, Turk DC (Eds.): Psychological Approaches to Pain Management. The Guildford Press, New York, 1996
11. Turk DC, Meichenbaum D, Genest M: Pain and Behavioural Medicine. A Cognitive-Behavioural Perspective. The Guildford Press, New York, 1983
12. Bogduk N, Tynan W, Wilson AS: The nerve supply to the human lumbar intervertebral discs. J Anat 132:39, 1981
13. Bogduk N: The innervation of the lumbar spine. Spine 8:286, 1983
14. Cyriax J: Dural pain. Lancet 1:919, 1978
15. Wyke B: Neurological aspects of low back pain. In Jayson MIV (Ed.): The Lumbar Spine and Back Pain. Sector, New York, 1976
16. Kimmel D: Innervation of the spinal dural mater and dura mater of the posterior cranial fossa. Neurology 10:800, 1961
17. El Mahdi MA, Latif FYA, Janko M: The spinal nerve root innervation and a new concept of the clinicopathological interrelations in back pain and sciatica. Neurochirurgia 24:137, 1981
18. Pedersen HE, Blunck CFJ, Gardner E: The anatomy of lumbo-sacral posterior rami and meningeal branches of spinal nerves (sinu-vertebral nerves). J Bone Joint Surg 38A:377, 1956
19. Simmons FH, Segil CM: An evaluation of discography in the localization of symptomatic levels in discogenic disease of the spine. Clin Orthop 108:57, 1975
20. Grieve GP: Common Vertebral Joint Problems (2nd Ed.). Churchill Livingstone, London, 1981
21. Maitland GD: Vertebral Manipulation (5th Ed.). Butterworths, London, 1986
22. Mooney V, Robertson J: The facet syndrome. Clin Orthop 115:149, 1976
23. McCall IW, Park WM, O'Brien JP: Induced pain referral from posterior lumbar elements in normal subjects. Spine 4:441, 1979
24. Edgar MA, Nundy S: Innervation of the spinal dura mater. J Neurol Neurosurg Psychiatry 29:530, 1966
25. Edgar MA, Park WM: Induced pain patterns on passive straight-leg-raising in lower lumbar disc protrusion. J Bone Joint Surg 56B:658, 1974
26. Austen R: The distribution and characteristics of lumbar-lower limb symptoms in subjects with and without a neurological deficit. In Proceedings 7th Biennial Conference, Manipulative Physiotherapists Association of Australia, North Fitzroy, Australia, 1991
27. Cyriax J: Textbook of Orthopaedic Medicine (7th Ed.). Vol 1. Baillière Tindall, London, 1978
28. Butler DS: Mobilisation of the Nervous System. Churchill Livingstone, Melbourne, 1991
29. McKenzie RA: The Lumbar Spine. Mechanical Diagnosis and Therapy. Spinal Publications, Waikanae, New Zealand, 1981
30. Kos J, Wolf J: Les menisques intervertebraux et leur role possible dans les blocages vertebraux. Ann Med Phys 15:203, 1972

31. Bogduk N, Jull G: The theoretical pathology of acute locked back: a basis for manipulative therapy. Man Med 1:78, 1985

32. Bodguk N, Twomey LT: Clinical anatomy of the lumbar spine (2nd Ed.). Churchill Livingstone, Melbourne, 1991

33. Richardson C, Jull G, Toppenburg R, Comerford M: Technique for active lumbar stabilisation for spinal protection: a pilot study. Aust J Physiotherapy 38:105, 1992

7

Lumbar Segmental Instability: Pathology, Diagnosis, and Conservative Management

James R. Taylor
Peter O'Sullivan

Part 1 of this chapter describes the pathology and pathomechanics of common forms of instability, based principally on the observations of Taylor and research colleagues Dr. C.C. McCormick, Professor K. McFadden, and Dr. Nils Schönström (as cited in the text). Part 2 outlines the neuromuscular control of lumbar motion segments, then describes the clinical diagnosis of segmental instability and a conservative management program that has been successfully tested in two groups of patients with different forms of instability. This is based on the doctoral research and clinical experience of Dr. Peter O'Sullivan.

PART 1: PATHOLOGY AND PATHOMECHANICS OF INSTABILITY

Lumbar segmental instability develops when the structure of the intervertebral disc, zygapophyseal joints, and their ligaments is damaged and there is loss of segmental neuromuscular control. This is associated with abnormal segmental movement and recurrent episodes of back pain. In patients with chronic or recurrent back pain, the presence of lumbar segmental instability is often missed or only diagnosed after many other causes for the back pain have been proposed and a variety of treatments have been tried with no lasting response. Despite this poor level of recognition, lumbar instability is said to be responsible for 20% to 30% of chronic low back pain.[1,2,3,4] In some patients, instability may resolve spontaneously with the passage of time.[5,6]

This chapter does not present a comprehensive account of all forms of instability but instead an account of common forms of segmental instability associated with spondylolysis and with degenerative segmental changes associated with injury to the joints and ligaments of the segment.

Definitions

Segmental instability remains a controversial topic despite many years of debate. Early pathologic studies referred to it simply as a "loose motion segment."[7,8] More sophisticated biomechanical analysis of the abnormal movement in an unstable segment focused on loss of the normal "passive" restraints to motion, with loss of "active" neuromuscular control giving an abnormal center of motion or "enlarged neutral zone."[9–11] The emphasis is on the abnormality of the movement rather than on hypermobility, which may exist in normal individuals.[2,5,12,13,14]

Panjabi[15] defined spinal instability in terms of a region of laxity around the neutral resting position of a spinal segment, called the "neutral zone." This neutral zone is shown to increase with intersegmental injury and intervertebral disc degeneration[16–18] and to decrease with simulated muscle forces across a motion segment[16,18–20] and with spinal fixation.[14] In this way the size of the neutral zone is considered to be an important measure of spinal stability. It is influenced by the interaction between what Panjabi[15] described as the passive, active, and neural control systems.

Passive, Active, and Neural Segmental Controls

The passive system constitutes the vertebrae, intervertebral discs, zygapophyseal joints, and ligaments. The active system constitutes the muscles surrounding and acting on the motion segment. The neural system comprises the relevant parts of the central and peripheral nervous systems that direct and control the muscles in providing dynamic stability of the segment.[15] In this light Panjabi[15] defined spinal instability as a significant decrease in the capacity of the stabilizing systems of the spine to maintain intervertebral neutral zones within physiologic limits, so there is not necessarily any major deformity, neurologic deficit, or incapacitating pain.

One of the limitations in the clinical diagnosis of lumbar instability lies in the difficulty to accurately detect abnormal or excessive intersegmental motion because conventional radiologic testing is often insensitive and unreliable.[21] Traditionally the radiologic diagnosis of spondylolisthesis, in patients with chronic low back pain attributable to these findings, has been considered to be one of the most obvious manifestations of lumbar instability,[22] with a number of studies reporting increased translational and rotational motion occurring segmentally in the presence of this condition and also with spondylolysis.[23–26]

Clinical Instability

Clinicians are more concerned with the symptoms that may arise from an unstable segment than with the pathology of the segment involved. They coined the term *clinical instability* to describe the syndrome in which the abnormal segment is the source of chronic or recurrent pain.[4,14,27]

Clinical instability is characterized by a syndrome of recurrent painful episodes brought on by minimal trauma or by a sudden, unguarded or unexpected movement. Affected individuals usually show a "catch in the back" during examination of lumbar spinal movements or a painful arc in semi-flexion, or, when returning erect from flexion, when they often push themselves erect with their hands on their thighs. Some may be aware of a clunk or a feeling that something "gives way" with a sharp pain in the back during a particular movement.

Anatomy and Pathology of Segmental Instability

Instability results from damage to the passive restraints of normal motion, with loss of the normal stiffness in these structures. From the radiologic or pathologic perspective, different varieties of instability may be recognized. Radiologic examination may diagnose instability associated with fractures, fracture dislocations, or spondylolisthesis but it is unreliable in diagnosing the lesser forms of instability associated with injuries to the intervertebral joints with subsequent degenerative disease or loosening of these joints. Instability associated with acute unstable fractures is not considered here, but "degenerative" forms of instability from injuries to the intervertebral joints, spondylolytic spondylolisthesis, and pseudolisthetic instability (degenerative spondylolisthesis) will be considered. We accept the views of Farfan and Kirkaldy-Willis that rotational strains are responsible for the most common injuries to intervertebral joints leading to instability.[5, 28]

Studies of Fresh, Unfixed Lumbar Spines at Autopsy

Studies of large series of fresh, unfixed spines at postmortem include descriptions of what Schmorl called the "loose motion segment."[8, 29, 30, 31] In the normal lumbar spine there is resistance to bending moments in the sagittal and coronal planes, with an elastic recoil on releasing the bending force. Application of torque forces to normal lumbar motion segments shows them to be very stiff in attempted axial rotation, with an elastic resistance to twisting and no perceptible, true axial rotation in the horizontal plane, but when torque is applied to the unrestrained complete lumbar spine there is some apparent axial rotation, which accompanies coupled sagittal and coronal plane movements.[32] By contrast, unstable segments reveal abnormal "loose" movements, with no real resistance and loss of the normal elastic recoil. This contrast between normal and unstable segments is most obvious on twisting the spine by applying torque forces. This is because it is easier to perceive the presence of an unphysiologic axial rotary movement than to judge when there is hypermobility in the sagittal or coronal plane. Grossly unstable segments also show abnormal translation with loss of the normal elastic recoil. These abnormal movements may be associated with spondylolisthesis, whether spondylolytic or degenerative (pseudolisthesis), or with rotational strains involving damage to the disc and zygapophyseal joint capsule and ligaments.

Spondylolytic Instability

The best-known type of instability is associated with bilateral spondylolysis, with pseudarthroses giving abnormal movement at the fracture sites in the partes interarticulares. This is often accompanied by marked deformity of the affected laminae, and it is seen most frequently in the laminae of L5. There may be excessive angular and translatory movement of L5, or there may be a semipermanent forward slip or listhesis of L5 on S1 (Fig. 7-1). There is loss of the normal restraint to movement offered by the zygapophyseal joint facets of L5, which hook down behind the superior sacral facets at S1. This essential stabilizing factor no longer operates, and the defects in the partes interarticulares act like false joints, with increases in the ranges of motion and increased shearing forces in the L5-S1 disc. Spondylolysis is found in about 5% of adults[7]; it is relatively rare in children and unknown in fetuses and newborn infants.[7] Affected individuals are frequently asymptomatic because the pars defects are often present without painful instability, but there is an increased risk of developing clinical instability because the disc is subject to injury and accelerated degeneration when it is deprived of the normal protection afforded by the facets. Internal disc disruption is more likely than in a normal lumbar motion segment due to the increased shearing, which produces tears or fissures in the annulus of the unprotected disc. When spondylolysis occurs as a stress fracture in athletes, the segment is acutely painful, and this injury results in recurrent pain related to physical activity. In other patients with spondylolysis that may have been present and unrecognized since puberty and who have remained asymptomatic for many years, the segment may become symptomatic after an injury, such as a severe lifting strain or a significant motor vehicle accident. There may at this stage be movement at the pseudarthroses with a tear in the unprotected annulus of the disc. When the affected segment becomes unstable, flexion extension radiographs show excessive translation or angular movement.[12] An unstable bilateral spondylolysis is liable to slip into spondylolisthesis, with increased deformity of the laminae or separation of the inferior articular processes from the remainder of the vertebra at the fracture sites, leading to progressive disc degeneration with a risk of neural impingement and radicular symptoms.

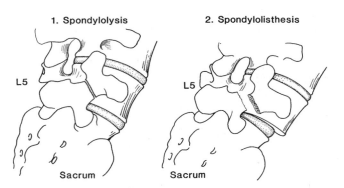

Fig. 7-1   Diagram of posterior oblique views of the lumbosacral spine showing (1) spondylolysis (fracture of neck of "Scotty dog") and (2) spondylolisthesis.

Degenerative Spondylolisthesis

The zygapophyseal facets and the disc are equally important in ensuring segmental stability. Wear-and-tear damage to the facets, or developmentally sagittally oriented facets, can reduce their capacity to provide segmental stability and lead to degenerative disc changes with instability. Primary disc degeneration with gross loss of disc height and fissuring of the annulus can also lead to instability. So-called pseudolisthesis was first described by Schmorl in 1932. He described 14 cases of anterolisthesis and 9 cases of retrolisthesis in an series of 600 autopsy spines.[8] These did not have spondylolytic defects in the neural arches but each segmental instability was associated with disc degeneration and facet remodeling. This represented about 5% of an unselected autopsy series, but Morgan and King[8] gave radiographic evidence of listhesis varying in the range from 3 mm to 17 mm in 28.6% of a consecutive series of 500 patients who presented with low back pain, although none of them showed spondylolysis. The higher incidence in Morgan and King's series[8] suggests a strong association of degenerative spondylolisthesis with low back pain. The degenerative form occurs in elderly patients, in whom the facets degenerate and become more sagittally oriented so that they are no longer competent to restrain forward translation of the upper vertebra, causing degeneration and failure of the intervertebral disc. Some cases of instability are post-surgical. Before the essential function of the facets in ensuring stability was realized, surgical decompression for stenosis often included removal of the facets, leading to instability.[33] Even after microdiscectomy there is an increased incidence of instability.[34] Sagittal plane instability correlates well with disc degeneration.[35]

Rotational Strain Instability

A less-well known but possibly more common and often unrecognized form of segmental instability probably results from a rotational strain. This is most likely to occur when the lumbar spine is loaded in flexion because in that posture the zygapophyseal facets are less congruous and less able to prevent overstretch of the spiral fibers of the annulus of the disc. In axial rotation there is also a risk of stretching or tearing the capsular structures of one or both zygapophyseal joints.[5,28,29,36] As this common form of instability is not well known it will be described in more detail, with some of the secondary segmental changes observed in our own research in low back pain patients.

In studies of lumbar movements in cadavers and living subjects, Taylor and Twomey[32] showed that torque could produce axial rotation as a coupled movement in the whole lumbar spine. This contrasted with the observation that when twisting individual segments, the lumbar facet orientation blocked true axial rotation.[36,37] While studying the coupled nature of axial rotation in fresh, unfixed, cadaver lumbar spines, from which the muscles had been removed, McFadden and Taylor[38] identified lumbar motion segments that showed abnormal movement with hypermobility. On manual

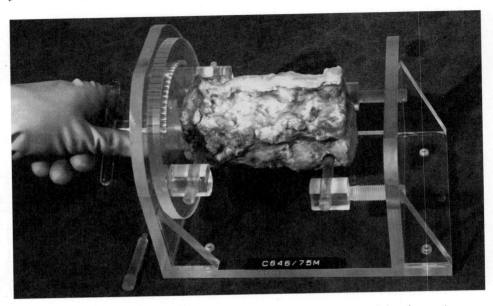

Fig. 7-2 The "torque apparatus" with a (three-motion segment) lumbar spine mounted between two Perspex rods. Torque is applied to the specimen by turning the handle on the left. The specimen can be held in a twisted position in the apparatus for CT scanning.

twisting of the lumbar spines, normal motion segments had a stiff, elastic feel. On testing the same specimens in a "torque apparatus" (Fig. 7-2)—which fixed one end of the lumbar spine with a Perspex rod through the sacrum and applied torque to the opposite end through a short lever, operating a Perspex rod inserted through the vertebral body of L2—the small amount of rotary movement achieved in normal segments was accompanied by coupled coronal plane and sagittal plane movements.

Manual attempts to twist the normal lumbar spine did not achieve any significant segmental movement—only a slight elastic "give" with a stiff feeling and an immediate elastic recoil as soon as the force was released. By contrast, abnormal segments showed immediate, clearly palpable and visible movement on application of torque with a slack feeling and an absence of the normal elastic recoil on releasing the torque force. Such segments were found in 2.5% of 150 motion segments tested, all in subjects in the age range 36 to 80 years except for a 14-year-old subject killed in a motor vehicle accident, who proved to have a fracture of the lumbar pedicles. The abnormal movements were found in L4-5, L5-S1, or L3-4 in that order of frequency.

Five of the columns showing such abnormal segmental movement were submitted to CT scanning with a constant torque applied to the spine in the radiolucent torque apparatus. The abnormal segments showed separation of the facets, on one side, some with vacuum phenomenon (air) in the loose joints (Fig. 7-3). By contrast, the adjacent segments in these lumbar spines, when submitted to the same force, did not show any increase in the space between the facets.

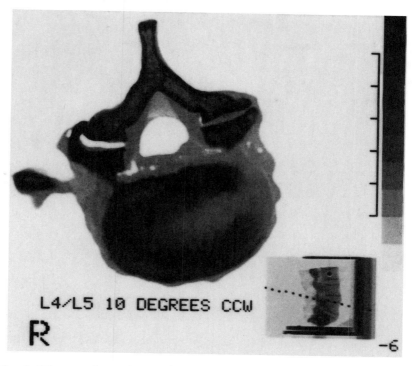

Fig. 7-3 A CT scan of a cadaver L4-5 motion segment from a 57-year-old man showing "gapping" or facet separation with air in the joint. The loose joint shows evidence of previous injury in the form of a large marginal osteophyte on the superior articular process. This segment showed abnormal movement compared with adjacent segments on manual testing.

Subsequent transverse serial sectioning of the abnormal segments showed internal disc disruption, varying from a single radial annular fissure in younger subjects to severe disc degeneration with extensive fissuring and loss of disc height in elderly subjects. The zygapophyseal joints showed capsular laxity or tears, usually on one side only, with signs of osteoarthrosis in the more stable contralateral zygapophyseal joint. Some segments showed abnormally enlarged fat pads within the loose zygapophyseal joint (Fig. 7-4), extending through the joint from the upper polar recess to the inferior polar recess, with increased fat in the extracapsular recesses. Large fat pads extending through the midjoint level probably indicate a "loose" segment.[39] Unstable motion segments showed increased ranges of axial rotation compared with normal segments,[38] with irregular movement observed in the unstable segments and abnormal motion around variable, eccentric centers of motion.

Schönström and Taylor,[40] in a study of movements in response to torque forces in fresh unfixed cadaver spines using three-plane photography to measure the movements, found abnormal movement patterns in lumbar motion segments that showed disc and unilateral facet laxity when they were transversely sectioned after testing. These segments had eccentric centers of axial rotation situated unilaterally in or near the more stable zygapophyseal

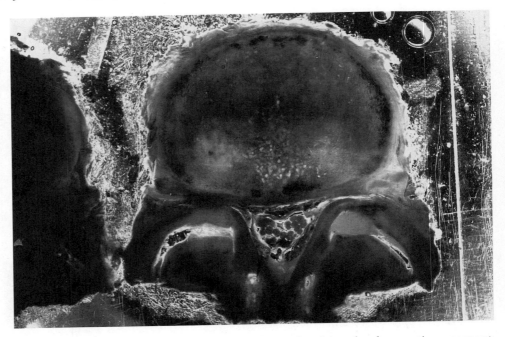

Fig. 7-4   A grossly enlarged fat pad at mid-joint level in a lumbar motion segment from a 43-year-old man. This segment, in contrast with adjacent segments, showed abnormal movement on manual testing. The contralateral joint shows cartilage damage and osteoarthrosis (dark ground illumination of a 2 mm thick transverse section).

joint, which often showed evidence of osteoarthrosis. Mimura[24] showed that axial rotational instability correlated with translational instability and a changed center of rotation.

Signs Indicating Possible Instability in CT Scans of Back Pain Patients

In addition to these functional studies in cadavers, we have identified changes suggestive of instability in zygapophyseal joints viewed in axial computed tomography (CT) scans of back pain patients and controls. We have also identified similar appearances in transverse sections of postmortem zygapophyseal joints. Some of the changes we shall describe in CT scans of the zygapophyseal joints of back pain patients may be remodeling changes secondary to established segmental instability. Their presence may aid in identifying a suspect unstable segment. Comparison of the CT scans from these living patients with transverse sections of postmortem zygapophyseal joints adds further information on the nature of the pathologic changes observed in the CT scans.

CT and anatomic studies of the L3-L4, L4-L5, and L5-S1 motion segments suggested that Z-joint subluxation may be a feature of rotary instability.[41,42] In unilateral subluxations (Fig. 7-5), the zygapophyseal joint articular sur-

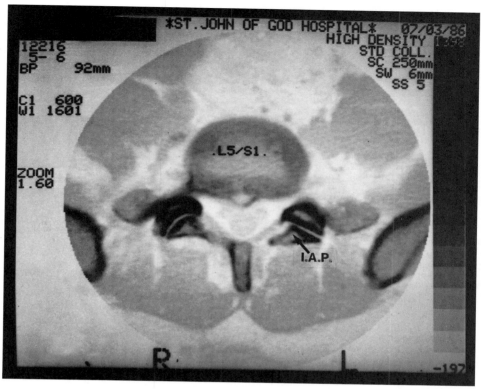

Fig. 7-5   A print from a CT scan of a 38-year-old man with back pain showing retrolisthesis or subluxation of the left inferior articular process (IAP). The facets of the subluxed joint are flat compared with the contralateral facets, and the superior articular process shows a small marginal osteophyte in its ligamentum flavum attachment. There are increased fat planes posterior to the laminae of this L5-S1 segment, which may represent either fatty replacement of the deep fibers of multifidus or possibly accumulation of excess fat around a hypermobile segment.

faces no longer fitted close together, and remodeling changes had appeared in the subluxed facets. There was retrolisthesis of the inferior articular process (IAP) from the superior articular process (SAP) so that the articular surface of the IAP did not fit within the articular margins of the SAP. By contrast, normal facets showed congruent articular surfaces, the convex IAPs fitting closely within the concave SAPs.

Accurate measurements in CT scans from 191 low back pain patients showed IAP retrolisthesis in 40 motion segments.[41,42] First, three independent observers classified the facets of the L3-L4, L4-L5, and L5-S1 segments as normal, subluxed, or severely subluxed on visual inspection; then the degree of subluxation from a congruent position was measured and corrected for magnification error. Joints were defined as subluxed when they showed IAP retrolisthesis of more than 1 mm from a congruent position on the SAP (Fig. 7-6). Structural changes in subluxed joints were studied by comparing them with matched congruent joints of the same segmental level, sex, and age.

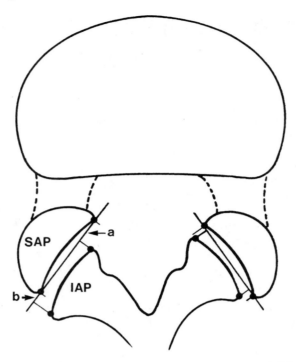

Fig. 7-6   A diagram showing how retrolisthesis was measured. The average of **a** and **b,** corrected for magnification error, was taken as the measured retrolisthesis. This was arbitrarily regarded as significant if it exceeded 1 mm.

Joint parameters recorded in mid-joint scans included:

1.   Marginal osteophytes (see Fig. 7-5)
2.   Widening of the joint space
3.   Smooth rounding of the posterior margin of the subluxed IAP (Fig. 7-7)
4.   Flat facets in the subluxed joint (see Fig. 7-5).

In the 191 patients with back pain, 573 motion segments were examined. IAP retrolisthesis was found in 40 motion segments, and IAP anterolisthesis was found in 3 motion segments (Table 7-1). The IAP retrolisthesis was unilateral in 33 of the 40 cases. One or more example of facet subluxation was found in 22% of the back pain patients. The L5-S1 segment was involved in 62% of all examples, most frequently in young adult males; the other subluxed joints were evenly distributed between L4-L5 and L3-L4 segments; most L3-L4 subluxations were seen in the oldest age groups. The average subluxation was 1.8 mm ± 0.62 mm.

Structural Changes Associated With Facet Subluxation

The most frequent accompaniments of facet subluxation were changes in the joint capsule at the articular margins and structural changes in the subluxed facet compared with the contralateral congruent facet. The most com-

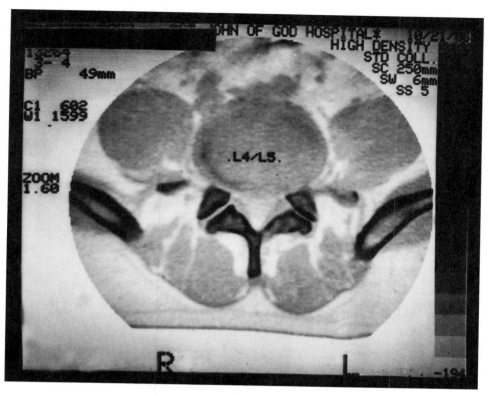

Fig. 7-7   This CT scan of an L4-L5 segment from a 49-year-old man with back pain shows rounding of the posterior margins of both inferior articular processes (IAP). Both show retrolisthesis from their superior articular facets, with remodeling of the facets. The retrolisthesis is more marked on the left, where there is a triangular thickening of the ligamentum flavum projecting into the "deficit" due to the posterior slip of the IAP. The fat planes behind the laminae are increased compared with normal. This may represent wasting of the deep fibers of multifidus.

mon structural association was the presence of flat articular surfaces on the subluxed facets compared with reciprocally concave and convex articular surfaces in the congruent contralateral facets. With posterior subluxation of the IAP, the "space" at the anterior joint margin was filled by an angular thickening of the ligamentum flavum, which projected into the joint along its anterior margin (Fig. 7-7). The posterior margin of the backward prolapsing IAP developed a "wrap-around-bumper," with extension of the articular cartilage onto the area resting on the posterior capsule.

The presence of flat facets was ten times more common in the subluxed facets than in the congruent joints; all the other features listed for three age groups in Table 7-2 were much more common in subluxed facets than in congruent facets.

The back pain patients collected in the study showed a skew in the age distribution of patients when comparing males and females. This reflects the observation of Borenstein[43] that back pain is equally common in males and females but occurs earlier in males.

Table 7-1 Age and Gender Distribution of Patients With Back Pain and Incidence of Subluxed Joints in CT Scans

Age Range	Males			Females			Totals		
(Years)	T	S	%	T	S	%	T	S	%
20–34	50	11	22%	17	3	18%	67	14	21%
35–49	50	11	22%	30	4	13%	80	15	19%
50–78	19	8	42%	25	4	16%	44	12	27%
Totals	119	30	25%	72	11	15%	191	41	22%

T = total numbers of back pain patients; S = number of patients with subluxed joints.

Measurements of the joint angle between the joint line of each SAP and the median plane, recorded in this same group of back pain patients[44] using the method of Kenesi and Lesur[45] showed a marked and progressive increase in zygapophyseal joint angle asymmetry with age in motion segments with subluxed joints. There was no increase of joint angle asymmetry with age in congruent joint pairs. This age-related increase in angular asymmetry (tropism), only in subluxed motion segments, suggests an age-related bone remodeling influence in the incongruent joints.

For comparison, we also collected 70 sets of CT scans from patients with no history of back pain over the preceeding 3 years. Zygapophyseal joint subluxation was also found in this control series, mostly in the older sub-

Table 7-2 Changes Associated With Subluxation: A Comparison of Congruent and Subluxed Joints

Age Group (Years)	No. of Joints		Flat Facets	Capsule Changes	Inclusions	"Wrap-around Bumpers"
20–34	S	14	11	12	4	3
	C	14	1	5	1	0
35–49	S	15	10	15	6	4
	C	15	1	6	0	0
50–80	S	14	8	9	3	1
	C	14	1	5	1	0
Totals: (S)		43	29	36	13	8
(C)		43	3	16	2	0

Key: S = subluxed joints; C = congruent joints

Capsule changes: include marginal osteophytes and calcification in the ligamentum flavum. Inclusions: includes marginal "capsular" inclusions and enlarged intra-articular fat pads. "Wrap around bumper" = extension of the articular surface onto the posterior surface of the IAP.

jects, but in the patients younger than 50 years of age, subluxation was twice as frequent in the back pain patients as in the asymptomatic patients. In older patients (over 50 years) the frequency of joint subluxation was just as common in asymptomatic controls as in back pain patients.

We concluded that zygapophyseal joints do not "sublux" in healthy young motion segments and that subluxation probably indicates a loosening of the motion segment due to injury or degeneration in the passive restraints of the joints with weakness in the muscles.

Anatomic Study

In studies of age changes in lumbar zygapophyseal joints[46] and subsequent additional autopsy studies,[47,48] similar findings of facet subluxations were found in association with capsular laxity and other joint changes (Figs. 7-8 and 7-9). Eighty-three spines were transversely sectioned through each complete zygapophyseal joint and the posterior third of the corresponding intervertebral disc and adjacent vertebral bodies. Subluxed facets with retrolisthesis of the IAP were identified and found to be associated with capsular tears, capsular laxity, the presence of enlarged intra-articular fat pads, and facet remodeling changes.[42] IAP retrolisthesis was often associated with partial detachment of the ligamentum flavum from the anterior

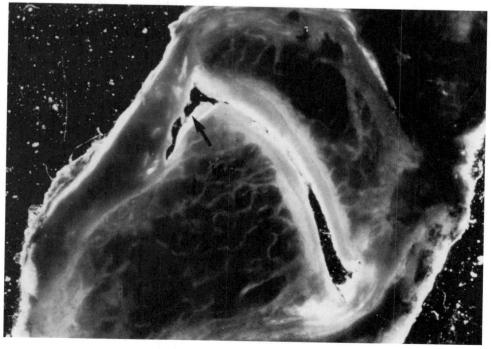

Fig. 7-8 A transverse section of a lower lumbar zygapophyseal joint showing capsular laxity with partial tear or detachment of the ligamentum flavum away from the anterior surface of the inferior articular process (arrowed). There is retrolisthesis of the inferior articular process.

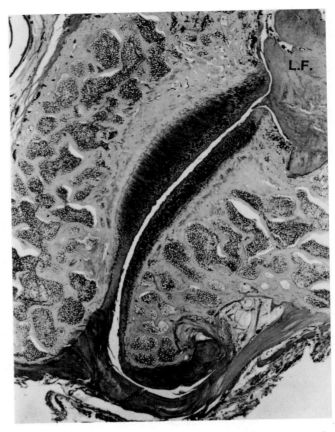

Fig. 7-9   A stained 100 μm transverse section of an L3-L4 zygapophyseal joint from a 73-year-old man shows a "wrap-around bumper" extension of articular cartilage around the posterior surface of the inferior articular process and projection of a small triangular portion of the ligamentum flavum *(LF)* into the anterior joint.

surface of the IAP. In some joints, the ligamentum flavum had expanded into the anterior gap in the joint as a triangular projection to fill the space left by retrolisthesis of the IAP. The posterior margin of the subluxed IAP was often rounded, with metaplastic extension of the articular surface around the posterior aspect of the IAP where it rubbed on a thickened, fibrous capsule. This rounded articular extension resembled the "wrap-around bumper" of a car (see Fig. 7-9). Enlarged fat pads often extended right through the joint from the polar recesses. The fat pads are normally present in the superior and inferior joint recesses and only extend to midjoint level if they are grossly enlarged, as when they act like "space-fillers" in a "loose joint."[39]

In summary, lumbar motion segment instability is a common degenerative phenomenon related to injury and aging.[5,7] We support the suggestion of Farfan[28] and Liu et al[36] that damage to the motion segment may result from torsional strain. The obliquely oriented fibers of the annulus fibrosus are vulnerable to overstretch in combined torsion and flexion, when the articular surfaces of the zygapophyseal joints are no longer congruent. Since

CT demonstrates the structure of the osseous Z joints better than the soft tissues of the disc, a loosening of the motion segment may be suspected from the changes we have described in these joints. The structural changes accompanying subluxation are not unique to instability but are strongly associated with it.

Clinical Studies

Dynamic radiologic investigations may aid in the diagnosis of instability by revealing abnormally increased translatory or rotational movements, as in flexion-extension views or dynamic CT scans ("twist CT scans"). These tests are at present insufficient to be diagnostic of instability, because of the variety of views as to what constitutes the limits of normal rotation and translation.[2, 12, 24] More time-consuming analysis of movement may provide more valuable confirmation of a clinical diagnosis by demonstrating an abnormally enlarged or abnormally situated centroid in movements of the suspect segment. This abnormal movement is more relevant to the diagnosis of segmental instability than hypermobility.

In patients referred to a pain clinic with chronic or recurrent low back pain, who were diagnosed as having clinical instability with clinical hypermobility at a painful motion segment, two types of pathologic processes were found. One group showed spondylolysis, usually with grade 1 listhesis, and flexion-extension radiographs confirmed excessive translation or angular movement. In the other group, a twist CT scan was performed (Fig. 7-10), as advocated by Kirkaldy-Willis[5]; an axial scan across the middle of the Z-joints in supine posture, with flexed hips and knees, was supplemented by mid-joint scans with the pelvis in left and right rotation, with maintenance of hip and knee flexion, by inserting a wedge cushion under each side of the pelvis in turn. A skilled radiographer can obtain comparable mid-joint views without repeated exposure to x-rays, though there may be a tendency toward coupled side flexion on full twisting.

Separation of the facets by more than 1 mm in the suspect, symptomatic segment, usually unilateral, without separation of facets in adjacent asymptomatic segments, was viewed as supporting the clinical diagnosis. It should be noted that the amount of gapping or facet diastasis probably depends on the force applied and any pain-related resistance to twisting by the patient. When Schönström and Taylor[40] examined 28 fresh unfixed cadaver lumbar spines from which all muscle had been removed, using a 35 cm lever inserted through the vertebral body, with bilateral weight a pulley circuits producing 7 Nm of torque, they deduced from external photographic measurements that 1 mm of gapping could occur in normal joints. By contrast, in loose degenerate segments, with this fairly large force and without any muscle resistance, 2.5 mm or more of gapping or facet separation was measured. It is suggested on the basis of our observations in patients, that the much smaller range of 1 mm of gapping in a twist CT scan in living patients with intact muscles may correspond approximately to the much wider gapping obtained by Schönström and Taylor[40] in the cadaver spines.

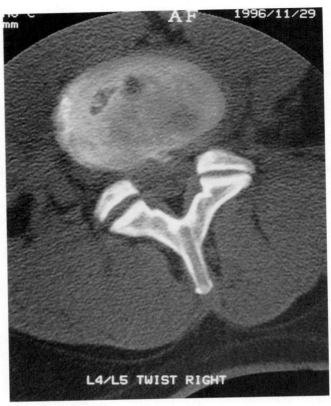

Fig. 7-10 A "twist CT scan" of the L4-L5 segment from a young man with recurrent low back pain who showed signs of clinical instability at L4-L5. Note the vacuum phenomenon in the disc, indicating disc damage.

PART 2: CONSERVATIVE MANAGEMENT OF INSTABILITY

The Role of the Neuromuscular System

A wide range of conservative interventions has been advocated for the treatment of instability. These include orthotic bracing, flexion exercises, abdominal trunk curls, hamstring stretching, pelvic tilt exercises, and general aerobic exercises such as swimming and walking.[22,49–54] However, few clinical trials have evaluated the effectiveness of these different conservative measures for this clinical problem, which often results in surgical fusion after failure of conservative management.[51,52,54]

There is growing evidence to indicate that the neuromuscular system employs complex and varying strategies of cocontraction of the trunk muscles to provide stiffness and stability to the lumbar spine during functional movement.[55–59] It is thought that the central nervous system adopts patterns of cocontraction for two main reasons. First, to stiffen the moving joint so as to minimize the effect of potential internal and external disturbances on posture, and second to equilibrate moments at other joints and regulate loads at the moving joint.[59] The concept of different trunk muscles playing differing roles in the provision of dynamic stability to the spine was proposed by Bergmark.[60] He hypothesised the presence of two muscle systems in the maintenance of spinal stability.

1. The "global muscle system" consisting of large, torque-producing muscles that act on the trunk and spine without directly attaching to it. These muscles include rectus abdominis, external oblique, and the thoracic part of lumbar iliocostalis and provide general trunk stabilization, but are not capable of having a direct segmental influence on the spine.
2. The local muscle system, consisting of muscles that directly attach to the lumbar vertebrae, which are responsible for providing segmental stability and directly controlling the lumbar segments. By definition lumbar multifidus, psoas major, quadratus lumborum, the lumbar parts of the lumbar iliocostalis and longissimus, transversus abdominis, the diaphragm, and the posterior fibers of internal oblique all form part of this local muscle system, as do smaller muscles such as interspinalis and intertransversarii.

Increasing evidence supports the hypothesis by Bergmark[60] that the local system muscles function differently than global system muscles. Furthermore, the relationship between the two muscle systems alters, depending on the loading conditions placed on the spine. This evidence is apparent in biomechanical studies investigating the capacity of individual muscles and their actions on the spine and in electromyographic studies, which investigate the patterns of activation of different muscles during different activities and under different loading conditions.[61]

Cholewicke and McGill[62] reported that the lumbar spine is more vulnerable to instability in its neutral zone and at low load when the muscle forces are low. They confirmed that under these conditions lumbar stability is maintained in vivo by increasing the activity (stiffness) of the lumbar segmental muscles (local muscle system). Furthermore, they highlighted the importance of motor control to coordinate muscle recruitment between large trunk muscles (the global muscle system) and small intrinsic muscles (the local muscle system) during functional activities to ensure that mechanical stability is maintained. Under such conditions they suggest that intersegmental muscle forces as low as 1% to 3% maximal voluntary contraction may be sufficient to ensure dynamic stability. Although the global muscle system provides most of the stiffness to the spinal column, the activity of the local muscle system is considered necessary to maintain the mechanical stability of the whole spine. In situations where the passive stiffness of a motion segment is reduced, the vulnerability of the spine instability is increased.[62]

Coordinated patterns of muscle recruitment are essential between the global and local system muscles of the trunk in order to compensate for the changing demands of daily life and ensure that the dynamic stability of the spine is preserved.[62,63] To accomplish this the neuromuscular system must provide the necessary compressive forces along the spine to ensure stability, while controlling its curvature at a segmental level.[64] In this way the muscle forces act to maintain and stabilize the arch-like structure of the lumbar spine. The activation of the erector spinae and psoas major, known to significantly increase the compressive loading to the lumbar spine when active,[65,66] enhance the segmental stiffness and therefore the stability of the spine. The segmental stabilizing role of muscles such as lumbar multifidus, with separate segmental innervation, acts to maintain the lumbar lordosis and ensure control of individual vertebral segments, particularly within the neutral zone.[15,16,19,20,67] The deep abdominals on the other hand, while applying some compressive forces to the spine,[35] are primarily active in providing rotational and lateral stability to the spine via the thoracolumbar fascia, while maintaining levels of intra-abdominal pressure.[69,70] As well as the provision of coronal spinal stability, the thoraco-lumbar fascia is considered to enhance the efficiency of the lumbar erector spinae muscles in controlling the lumbar spine. This action is dependent on the co-activation of the transversus abdominis and lateral fibers of internal oblique and the production of intra-abdominal pressure. The intra-abdominal pressure mechanism, primarily controlled by the diaphragm, transversus abdominis, and pelvic diaphragm, also provides an important stabilizing role in the lumbar spine.[64]

During static postures and dynamic movements of the spine, local system muscles such as transversus abdominis and lumbar multifidus display tonic muscle activation[71] that occurs throughout all ranges of motion irrespective of direction of movement, suggesting a stabilizing function. On the other hand, global system muscles, such as external oblique, rectus abdominis, and the erector spinae display activity consistent with torque production and movement initiation, and therefore their function is more direction specific.[72,73] With higher loading conditions significant co-activation of both the local and global system muscles occurs to meet the increased demands for spinal stability.[74] During rapid movement initiation or sudden loading of the spine the neuromuscular system utilizes strategies of pre-activation of muscles such as transversus abdominis and the diaphragm, in conjunction with increases in intra-abdominal pressure, to provide a stable base on which other torque-producing trunk muscles can safely move.[69,72,75] Inappropriate timing or altered control of these complex patterns of muscle co-contraction could result in tissue damage rather than stability to the motion segment.[63,76]

Dysfunction of the Neuromuscular System in the Presence of Low Back Pain

The literature reports varying disruptions in the activity of the trunk muscles in low back pain patients, both at rest and during movement. Often these disruptions relate to disruptions in the patterns of recruitment and cocontraction within and between different muscle synergies.[77] There is growing evidence that the muscles particularly vulnerable to these changes are those known to provide stability in the lumbar spine, such as the deep abdominals and lumbar multifidus. Segmental changes have been well documented with particular reference to lumbar multifidus, but it appears that the manner of the dysfunction may vary with different lumbar segments.[78,79] There is also evidence to suggest that the presence of chronic low back pain often results in a general loss of function and deconditioning as well as changes to the neural control system, affecting timing of patterns of cocontraction, balance, reflex, and righting responses.[77]

There is some evidence that these changes in neuromuscular system may predispose to the onset of low back pain. There is certainly evidence to suggest that many of the changes in the neuromuscular system occur as a result of a painful condition in the lumbar spine.[44] Generalized changes to the trunk musculature, such as a loss of strength and endurance and muscle atrophy, are believed to result from disuse and inactivity in this population. The more specific and segmental changes are considered to result from either motor or sensory nerve damage, or altered habitual movement patterns of activity, and reflex excitation or inhibition of the muscles proximal to the site of the injury.[79,80] The altered mechanoceptive and proprioceptive afferent input into the neural system is likely to result in further disruption to patterns of muscle activation, leaving the patient biomechanically vulnerable to further injury or increased chronicity.

There is growing evidence that the deep abdominals and lumbar multifidus muscles are preferentially adversely affected in the presence of chronic low back pain[58,75,45,81,82,83] and lumbar instability.[84,85,86,87] Similarly, there have been reports that in the presence of local muscle system dysfunction there is a compensatory substitution of global system muscles. This appears to be the neural control system's attempt to maintain the stability demands of the spine.[85,88]

On the basis of this growing body of knowledge a recent focus in the physiotherapy management of chronic low back pain patients has been the identification of specific motor control deficits and the specific training of those muscles affecting the spine whose primary role is considered to be the provision of dynamic stability and segmental control to the spine, i.e., transversus abdominis and lumbar multifidus.[61,89,90] This focus is based on a motor control model whereby the faulty movement pattern or patterns are identified and the components of the movement are isolated and retrained into functional tasks specific to the patient's needs.[61]

Clinical Diagnosis of Lumbar Segmental Instability

One of the inherent problems regarding the accurate diagnosis of lumbar segmental instability is that the condition has been separately defined from patho-anatomic, radiologic, and clinical points of view, all of which, when viewed alone, have inherent limitations. For example, patho-anatomic abnormalities are commonly observed in people without low back pain,[91] and researchers have reported the presence of increased intersegmental spinal motion in asymptomatic individuals.[84,92,93] Furthermore, the sensitivity, specificity, and predictive value of clinical examination findings for the diagnosis of these conditions have not been fully established.[54,94] This has led to situations in which the radiologic finding of increased intersegmental motion has been viewed without in-depth consideration of the clinical presentation, nor the recognition of the powerful influence that the neuromuscular system has on the control of intersegmental spinal motion.

Because of these limitations, the clinical diagnosis of lumbar segmental instability requires the presence of a concurrent number of "diagnostic" criteria. Kirkaldy-Willis[5] outlined a typical clinical presentation of lumbar segmental instability. He described patients with this condition as presenting with a history of recurrent dysfunction or repetitive painful traumatic incidents. After each incident the degree of disability becomes more pronounced. The patient commonly complains that the back feels weak or is going to give way or that certain movements, such as returning to an upright position from flexion, produce a catch of pain in the back (commonly known as the "instability catch"). It is a condition where a minor provocation can change the patient from being mildly symptomatic to suffering disabling pain.[29] Other symptoms suggestive of instability are reported to be the onset of sharp pain with sudden or unexpected movement or during twisting motions of the trunk. An inability to sustain loaded positions, such as sitting or standing, due to increased low back pain have also been reported[95,96] although these symptoms are common to many low back conditions.

Kirkaldy-Willis[5] reported that with active movement, the presence of a "catch," sway, or shift at one level may be observed as the patient returns to the standing position from forward bending. The patient usually assists this movement by placing both hands on the knees or thighs. Signs of abnormal increased movement between one vertebra and the next can be detected by inspection and palpation. Confirmation that the abnormally mobile segment detected is in fact symptomatic and reproductive of the patient's symptoms is essential.[97] The predictive value of these signs is largely unproved,[94] but recent research indicates that skilled manipulative physiotherapists can distinguish patients with symptomatic spondylolysis from low back pain patients without spondylolysis based on the finding of increased intersegmental motion at the involved level.[23,98] Clinical examination by skilled manipulative physiotherapists was able to identify a symptomatic spinal level accurately, as compared with a positive facet joint block procedure, and of 60 patients with low back pain, 6 patients were also accurately identified as having a spondylolisthesis based on the finding of increased intersegmental motion at the corresponding level.[98]

Trial Data

Questionnaire data completed by patients diagnosed with lumbar segmental instability involved in recent clinical trials revealed that half of them developed their back pain condition secondary to a single-event injury and the other half developed their back pain gradually in relation to multiple minor traumatic incidents.[99] The patients' main complaint was of chronic and recurrent low back pain with increasing levels of functional disability over time. They controlled their symptoms by reducing their levels of activity. Patients also reported a poor conservative treatment response with either aggravation from spinal manipulation and mobilization or only short-term relief from this form of therapy, which did not alter the natural history of the condition.

The back pain was most commonly described as recurrent (70%), constant (55%), "catching" (45%), "locking" (20%), "giving way" (20%), or accompanied by a feeling of "instability" (35%). The most frequently reported aggravating postures were sustained sitting (85%), prolonged standing (70%), and semiflexed postures (70%). The most common aggravating movements were forward bending (75%), sudden unexpected movements (75%), returning to an upright position from forward bending (65%), lifting (65%), and sneezing (60%).[68] These symptoms and signs are commonly reported as consistent with the presence of segmental instability.[5,54,95]

On physical examination, active spinal movement commonly revealed good ranges of spinal mobility, with the presence of "through range" pain or a painful arc rather than end-of-range pain, and the inability to return to erect standing from forward bending without the use of the hands to aid this motion. Segmental shifts or hinging were commonly associated with the painful movement. Another common feature was the reported abolition or significant reduction of pain with deep abdominal muscle activation during the provocative movement. Also noted in the physical examination was the absence of abnormal neurologic examination findings in all the patients. Similarly, neural tissue provocation tests such as straight leg raise, slump, and prone knee bend were generally normal.[99] These physical examination findings have also been reported by other authors as indicative of a lumbar segmental instability condition.[5,54,95] These findings support the theory that there is a complex of symptoms and signs suggestive of the diagnosis of lumbar segmental instability that may have predictive value for patients with this condition.

Palpatory Examination

Passive physiologic motion segment testing was used to detect increased segmental motion. Flexion/extension and rotation were reported to be the most sensitive movement tests to detect excessive intersegmental motion. For spondylolisthesis and spondylolysis the excessive segmental motion was detected at the level above the pars defects. Palpatory techniques then were employed to determine if the mobile segment was in fact symptomatic.[99]

Neuromuscular Examination

The model used employs two forms of examination of the neuromuscular system. The first employs movement tests and movement analysis, and the second involves specific muscle testing. The first is a qualitative form of examination and demands a high level of therapist skill for accurate detection and interpretation. Some aspects of this form of examination have been previously described by Sahrmann.[100] The critical aspects of this part of the examination are first to analyse the strategy of dynamic stabilization that the patient has adopted; second to identify whether there is a directional basis to the instability problem or whether it is a multidirectional problem; and third to determine whether the patient's subjective complaint corresponds to the level of pathology detected on the physical examination.

Specific muscle testing forms the second part of the neuromuscular examination. This seeks to specifically examine the patient's ability to consciously isolate the activation of the local muscle system without dominant activation of the global muscle system. More specifically it tests the ability of the patient to cocontract the transversus abdominis with segmental multifidus in a neutral lordotic posture while controlling respiration. This aspect of the examination seeks to identify the presence of local muscle system dysfunction and faulty patterns of global muscle substitution. This form of examination has been previously described in detail.[90, 101]

Aims of the Neuromuscular Examination

1. To determine the neuromuscular system's strategy of dynamic stabilization
2. To observe any loss of dynamic trunk stabilization with limb loading (movement faults)
3. To observe patterns of muscle recruitment
4. To determine the relationship between symptoms and neuromuscular system control
5. To observe segmental hinging (relative flexibility)
6. To identify direction specificity of the "instability" problem
7. To identify local muscle system dysfunction
8. To identify faulty patterns of global muscle system substitution

Directional Patterns of Lumbar Segmental Instability

The clinical experience of O'Sullivan has revealed four common but distinctly different patterns of clinical presentation observed in patients with lumbar segmental instability. It is important to note that these are observations and are not based on scientific research. Furthermore, they do not represent the only clinical presentations to be seen with patients with an instability problem. They are presented to illustrate the four most common patterns observed by the author and help the reader to identify these patients in a clinical situation.

Flexion Pattern.   This appears to be the most common pattern. Patients who predominantly report control problems in spinal flexion commonly relate their injury to either a single flexion/rotation injury or to repetitive strains involving flexion/rotational activities. These patients' prime complaint is of an inability to perform or sustain flexion and in particular semiflexed postures. These patients usually present with a loss of segmental lumbar lordosis at the level of the "unstable motion segment." This is particularly noticeable in standing and sitting postures, with an associated tendency to hold the pelvis in a degree of posterior pelvic tilt. This loss of seg mental lordosis is accentuated in flexed postures and is usually associated with increased tone in the upper lumbar and lower thoracic erector spinae muscles and an associated increase in lordosis present in the thoraco-lumbar region (Figs. 7-11 and 7-12). Movements into forward bending are commonly associated with a tendency to flex more at the symptomatic level than at the adjacent levels and to hold the upper lumbar spine in lordosis. This movement is usually associated with an arc of pain into flexion and an inability to return from flexion to neutral without use of the hands to assist the movement. In extension one observes a tendency to preferentially extend above the symptomatic segment, with an associated loss of extension at the affected segment and absence of anterior pelvic tilt. On specific movement testing there is an inability to differentiate anterior pelvic tilt and low lumbar spine extension independent of upper lumbar and thoracic spine extension. Also commonly noted is the inability to control the lumbar lordosis in forward-loaded postures. The quality of the movement during attempts to initiate segmental lordosis and independent anterior pelvic tilt motion from the upper lumbar and thoracic spine is usually associated with "jerky" and "staccato" movements rather than with smooth, controlled movement. This is most pronounced on the eccentric phase of these movement tests. Movement tests such as squatting, sitting with knee extension, and hip flexion, and "sit to stand" tests usually reveal an inability to control segmental lordosis and an anterior pelvic tilt position, with a tendency to segmentally flex at the unstable motion segment and posteriorly tilt the pelvis.

Specific muscle tests reveal an inability to activate lumbar multifidus in cocontraction with the deep abdominal muscles at the "unstable" motion segment. Many patients are unable to assume the start position of a neutral lordotic lumbar spine, particularly in four-point kneeling and sitting, due to

Fig. 7-11 Flexion pattern: patient who sustained a flexion injury complains of flexion-related pain. Note in sitting position the posterior tilt of the pelvis and a segmental loss of lower lumbar lordosis with upper lumbar and lower thoracic compensatory lordosis.

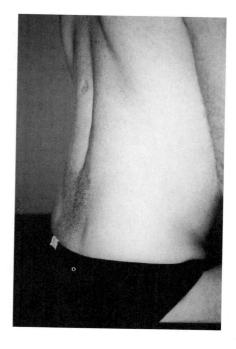

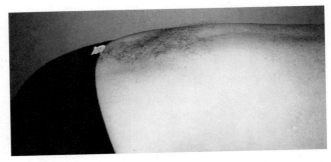

Fig. 7-12   Flexion pattern: patient four-point kneeling in his neutral resting position with posterior tilt of the pelvis and a segmental loss of lower lumbar lordosis with upper lumbar compensatory lordosis.

an inability to initiate anterior pelvic tilt and lordose the lower lumbar spine (see Fig. 7-12). These patients' attempts to activate these muscles are commonly associated with a Valsalva maneuver and bracing of the abdominal muscles with a loss of breathing control and excessive coactivation of the thoracolumbar erector spinae muscles. Attempts to specifically activate the deep abdominal muscles usually result in excessive recruitment of external oblique and rectus abdominis, a loss of breathing control, and a further flattening of the segmental lordosis, often resulting in pain. Indeed, a common observation is an inability to breathe using the diaphragm, with an apical respiration pattern being assumed. It appears that the diaphragm becomes dysfunctional at the same time as the deep abdominal and segmental multifidus muscles, with patients unable to initiate deep abdominal muscle activation and control respiration at the same time.

Palpatory examination reveals a segmental increase in flexion mobility at the symptomatic motion segment, and extension may appear to be stiff. Palpatory examination may reveal a decrease in posteroanterior accessory motion at the "unstable" motion segment.

These patients present with segmental dysfunction of the lumbar multifidus, psoas major, deep abdominal muscles, and diaphragm. Their strategy for dynamically stabilizing the lumbar spine appears to be the excessive activation of the thoracolumbar erector spinae and external oblique muscles and bracing with the diaphragm. In this case the dominant activation of the thoracolumbar erector spinae and superficial abdominal muscles appears to stabilize the motion segment by "locking" it into an end-of-range flexion position rather than providing stabilization to the motion segment within the neutral zone. Sacroiliac joint dysfunction is also noted to be common in this patient group, and this appears to be closely related to dysfunction of the lumbar multifidus and deep abdominal muscles and associated loss of pelvic control and force closure mechanisms.

Extension Pattern.   A second group of patients predominantly report extension movement–related control problems resulting in pain during standing, forward bending postures, walking, and carrying out overhead activities and usually associated with an inability to walk fast, run, and swim

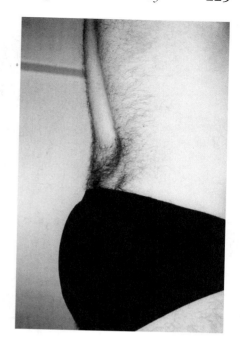

Fig. 7-13 Extension pattern: patient with L5-S1 grade 1 spondylolisthesis complaining of extension-related pain and presenting with an anterior pelvic tilt and increased lower lumbar lordosis with associated hyperactivity of the lumbar erector spinae and lumbar multifidus muscles and an inability to activate the deep abdominal muscles.

These patients commonly recount their injury as relating to an extension/rotation incident or repetitive trauma frequently associated with sporting activities involving extension. In the standing position they commonly exhibit an increase in segmental lordosis at the unstable motion segment, often with an increased level of segmental muscle activity at this level, and the pelvis is often positioned in anterior pelvic tilt (Fig. 7-13). Extension activities usually reveal segmental hinging at the affected segment, with a loss of segmental lordosis above this level and associated "sway" posture (Figs. 7-14 and 7-15). Similarly, hip extension and knee flexion movement tests in a prone position reveal a loss of cocontraction of the deep abdominal muscles and dominant patterns of activation of the lumbar erector spinae, resulting in excessive segmental lumbar spine extension at the unstable level (Fig. 7-16). Forward bending movements commonly reveal a tendency to hold the lumbar spine in lordosis (particularly at the level of the unstable motion segment) with a sudden loss of lordosis at mid-range flexion commonly associated with an arc of pain. Return to neutral again reveals a tendency to hyperlordose the spine segmentally before the upright posture is achieved, with pain on returning to the erect posture and the need to aid the movement with the hands. Specific movement tests reveal an inability to initiate posterior pelvic tilt independent of hip flexion and activation of the gluteals, rectus abdominis, and external obliques.

Specific muscle tests reveal an inability to cocontract segmental lumbar multifidus with the deep abdominal muscles in a neutral lumbar posture—with a tendency to lock the lumbar spine into extension. This may represent an attempt of the neuromuscular system to stabilize the motion segment outside the neutral zone in an extension posture. Attempts to isolate the deep abdominal muscle activation is commonly associated with excessive activa-

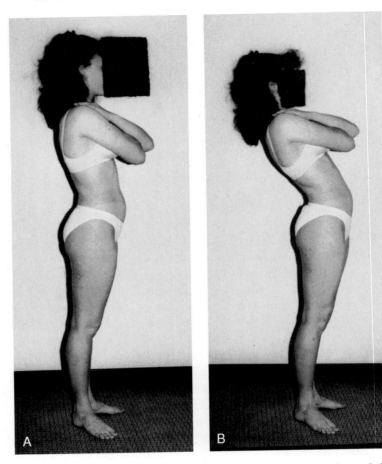

Fig. 7-14   A, Extension pattern: patient with a lumbar segmental instability condition complaining of extension-related pain. The patient's natural standing posture holds the low lumbar spine in lordosis with associated anterior tilt of the pelvis and associated upper lumbar and thoracic spine kyphosis. **B,** Extension pattern: patient during backward bending. Note the segmental extension at the lower lumbar spine and the lack of associated posterior pelvic rotation and upper lumbar and thoracic spine extension.

tion of the lumbar erector spinae, external oblique, and rectus abdominis, and an inability to control diaphragmatic breathing.

Palpatory passive movement testing reveals a segmental increase in extension mobility at the symptomatic motion segment. Flexion may feel stiff. Palpatory examination in a prone position reveals an increased posteroanterior accessory motion at the "unstable" motion segment.

These patients present with a loss of cocontraction of the lumbar multifidus and deep abdominal muscles. Their attempts to dynamically stabilize the lumbar spine appear to be carried out by excessive activation of the lumbar erector spinae and in some cases the superficial fibers of lumbar multifidus and associated bracing with the diaphragm and abdominal muscles. In this case lumbar multifidus and the lumbar erector spinae (with the absence of cocontraction with the deep abdominal muscles) stabilize the mo-

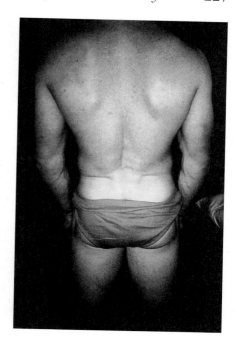

Fig. 7-15 Extension pattern: patient with L5-S1 grade 1 spondylolisthesis complaining of extension-related pain and presenting with a segmental hinging pattern with backward bending.

tion segment by "locking" it into an end-of-range extension position rather than providing stabilization to the motion segment within the neutral zone.

Lateral Shift Pattern. A third presentation is the recurrent lateral shift, where with minimal precipitation the patient's spine locks into a lateral shift position in flexion. This is usually unidirectional, but in some cases it is bidirectional. These patients commonly relate a vulnerability to reaching or rotating in one direction. They present in standing with a loss of lumbar segmental lordosis at the affected level (similar to the patient presentation in the flexion pattern), usually with an associated lateral shift in the lower lumbar spine. Palpation of the lumbar multifidus muscles in standing commonly reveals resting muscle tone on the side ipsilateral to the shift, but atrophy and

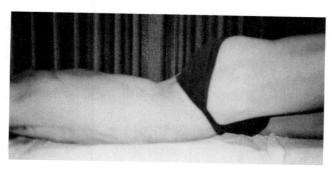

Fig. 7-16 Extension pattern: patient with L4-L5 grade 1 spondylolisthesis complaining of extension-related pain and presenting with a segmental hinging pattern during active hip extension in prone position. Also noted is the associated lack of extension movement at the hip joint.

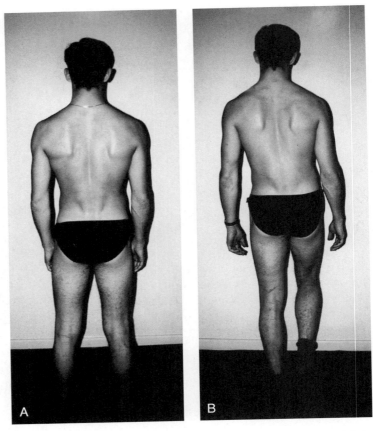

Fig. 7-17 Lateral shifting pattern: patient with L5-S1 grade 1 spondylolisthesis complaining of flexion/rotation–related pain and presenting with a left lateral shifting pattern standing (**A**) exacerbated when single leg standing on the left foot (**B**).

the absence of resting tone on the contralateral side. The lateral shift is accentuated when standing on the foot ipsilateral to the shift, and during gait as a tendency to transfer weight through the trunk and upper body rather than through the pelvis (Fig. 7-17). Spinal sagittal movements reveal a tendency to shift further laterally at mid-range flexion, and this is commonly associated with an arc of pain. Side bending in the direction of the shift commonly reveals a lateral translatory motion rather than a side-bending motion at the "unstable" level. Movement tests reveal dominant activation of the thoracolumbar erector spinae and lumbar multifidus on the ipsilateral side of the shift and a loss of rotary and lateral trunk control in the direction of the shift. This can be observed in supine postures with a lateral leg lowering and in four point kneeling when flexing one arm. Sitting to standing and squatting usually reveals a tendency toward lateral trunk shift during the movement, with increased weightbearing on the lower limb on the side of the shift.

Specific muscle testing reveals an inability to bilaterally activate segmental lumbar multifidus in cocontraction with the deep abdominal muscles with an inability to activate the muscles on the side contralateral to the shift.

Palpation reveals a unidirectional increase in intersegmental motion at the symptomatic level on rotation and side bending in the direction of the shift.

These patients present with a loss of cocontraction of the lumbar multifidus and deep abdominal muscles on the side contralateral to the segmental lateral shift. Attempts at dynamically stabilizing the lumbar spine appear to be carried out by dominant activation of the lumbar erector spinae, and in some cases the lumbar multifidus, on the ipsilateral side to the shift and associated bracing with the diaphragm and abdominal muscles. This appears to represent the tendency in these patients to stabilize the motion segment by "holding" it into a lateral shifted position rather than providing stabilization to the motion segment within the neutral zone.

Multidirectional Pattern. This is the most serious and debilitating of the clinical presentations and is usually associated with a severe traumatic injury. Patients complain of extreme pain and functional disability. They describe their provocative movements as being multidirectional. All weight-bearing postures are painful, and difficulty is reported in obtaining relieving positions during weightbearing. Locking of the spine is commonly reported following sustained flexion and extension postures. These patients may assume a flexed, extended, or laterally shifted spinal posture. Excessive segmental shifting and hinging patterns may be observed in all movement directions, with associated "jerky" movement patterns and reports of "jabbing" pain on movement in all directions. There is associated lumbar erector spinae muscle spasm. These patients have great difficulty assuming neutral lordotic spinal positions, and attempts to facilitate lumbar multifidus and transversus abdominis cocontraction (especially during weightbearing positions) are usually associated with a tendency to flex, extend, or laterally shift the spine segmentally, with associated global muscle substitution, bracing of the diaphragm, and pain. These patients have the poorest prognosis for conservative exercise management.

A common observation with all the patients with lumbar segmental instability is the tendency to hold the lumbar spine out of the neutral zone (as in flexion, extension, or a lateral shifted position), although they may describe this resting position as their normal neutral posture. This loss of position sense and segmental control is greatest within the neutral zone. It appears that the neuromuscular system strategy in these patients is to stabilize the motion segment out of the neutral position (in either flexion, extension, or a lateral shifted posture) in an attempt to maintain stability.

Management of Lumbar Segmental Instability

The specific exercise intervention as described in this chapter has been shown to be effective in reducing pain and functional disability in patients with chronic low back pain and a clinical and radiologic diagnosis of lumbar segmental instability.[89,99] A brief description of the methods and results of the two randomized controlled clinical trials that tested the efficacy of this specific exercise approach is described in greater detail later in the chapter.

Before entering the clinical trials, the majority of the patients had undergone various forms of conservative treatment approaches in an attempt to manage their pain condition. Many patients reported significant aggravation of pain from previous resistance-based exercise programs and general rehabilitation and aerobic exercise approaches. Although there is evidence supporting the benefits of general exercise training for the management of chronic low back pain, nonspecific exercise approaches do not appear to address the specific motor control faults we have observed in these patients. The approach presented in this chapter does not propose to replace general exercise training but rather to "re-program" the patient so that, at a later date, they can carry out a general exercise with pain control.

Motor Control Model

The findings of the physical examination dictate the treatment approach to be taken. As stated, the aim of the examination is to identify the movement faults present, the neuromuscular control strategy utilized by the patient to stabilize his or her spine, the presence of dysfunction in the local muscle system, and faulty substitution patterns of the global muscle system. Once this has been achieved, the specific exercise intervention aims to retrain appropriate motor control strategies and integrate this in a functional manner. This specific exercise intervention represents, in its simplest form, the process of motor learning described by Fitts and Posner[102] who reported three stages in learning a new motor skill (Figs. 7-18 and 7-19).

First Stage of Training

The first stage is the cognitive stage or early training period, during which a high level of awareness is demanded of patients so that they isolate the co-contraction of the local muscle system without global muscle substitution. This can be facilitated by the use of auditory, visual, palpatory, and pressure

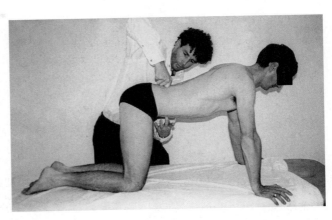

Fig. 7-18   Patient in four point kneeling with neutral lumbar lordosis being instructed to activate the transversus abdominis muscle with controlled breathing.

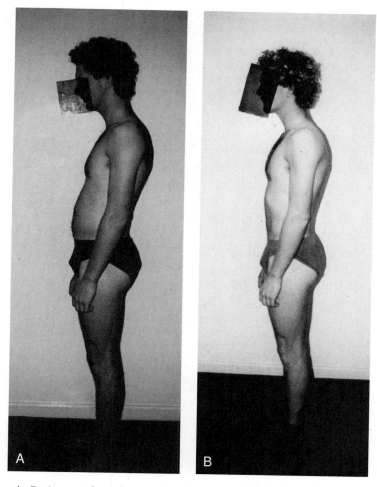

Fig. 7-19 **A,** Patient with a chronic low back pain condition associated with an unstable spondylolisthesis at L5-S1 prior to specific exercise intervention. **B,** Patient with a chronic low back pain condition associated with an unstable spondylolisthesis at L5-S1 following the specific exercise intervention.

biofeedback and, in some cases, EMG biofeedback. The aim in the early stages is to train the specific isometric cocontraction of the deep abdominal muscles with lumbar multifidus at low levels of maximal voluntary contraction and with controlled respiration. No focus is usually placed on the lumbar multifidus contraction at this early stage until a deep abdominal muscle contraction is isolated, apart from stressing the importance of maintaining the lumbar spine in a **neutral lordotic posture.** If the focus is placed on training the lumbar multifidus muscles before the patient isolates a deep abdominal contraction, then attempts to activate the lumbar multifidus frequently result in inappropriate patterns of cocontraction, with an associated loss of the neutral lordosis, abdominal bracing patterns and impaired breathing control and resultant exacerbation of pain. The start position selected by the therapist to facilitate the activation of the deep abdominal muscles is based on that which best isolates the activation of these muscles in a neutral lordotic posture, as identified in the physical examination. The optimal positions are usually supine crook lying (with hips and knees flexed), four-point kneeling, prone lying, or sitting. Many patients with profound local muscle system dysfunction will be unable initially to assume a neutral lordotic posture (especially in four-point kneeling or sitting), and the first training session for these patients will need to focus on training pelvis control independent of the thoracic spine and hips so that they can assume this position.

For patients with flexion, lateral shift, or multidirectional patterns of instability, training is usually needed to facilitate anterior pelvic tilt and low lumbar spine lordosis independent from the upper lumbar and thoracic spine extension. This is because the habitual postures that these patients assume hold the pelvis in posterior tilt with associated loss of low lumbar lordosis (see Figs. 7-11 and 7-12). This control is best taught in four-point kneeling and sitting, which then becomes the start position for the deep abdominal muscle facilitation with a neutral lordosis. For patients with extension patterns of instability where there is a tendency toward increased segmental lordosis, initial training is needed to facilitate posterior pelvic tilt and posture the lumbar spine out of a hyperlordosis and toward a more pelvic position and neutral lordosis. This is best facilitated in four-point kneeling, sitting, prone lying, or crook lying.

Once the ideal starting position has been achieved, the key focus in this early stage is to isolate the activation of the deep abdominal muscles (transversus abdominis) with minimal coactivation of global system muscles (such as the rectus abdominis, external oblique, and erector spinae muscles) and with controlled diaphragm breathing (Fig. 7-20). The majority of patients with significant local muscle system dysfunction will be unable to perform this pattern of muscle activation due to an inability to control breathing and the dominant substitution of global system muscles such as external oblique and rectus abdominis. In these cases, initial training of diaphragm breathing is required before facilitation of the deep abdominal muscles (it may take a week or two for the patient to learn this pattern). Indeed, apical patterns of respiration are commonly noted with these patients, who appear frequently unable even to initiate diaphragm breathing. These patients are capable of using the diaphragm to dynamically "brace" the spine by increasing intra-abdominal pressure while breathing apically or performing a Valsalva maneuver, but are unable to isolate a low-level activation of the transversus abdominis while maintaining normal respiratory patterns. This appears to reflect a dysfunction in the dual respiratory and stabilizing roles of the diaphragm with the deep abdominal muscles.

Once diaphragm breathing has been taught, the other difficulty at this early stage is usually a dominance of activation of global system muscles such as the rectus abdominis, external oblique, and erector spinae muscles. If dominant muscle substitution of rectus abdominis and/or external oblique is encountered during attempts to isolate transversus abdominis, it is useful for the therapist to place the focus of the muscle contraction away from the abdominal muscles and toward the pelvic floor, and also to focus on lateral costal diaphragm breathing because this action is antagonistic to that of ex-

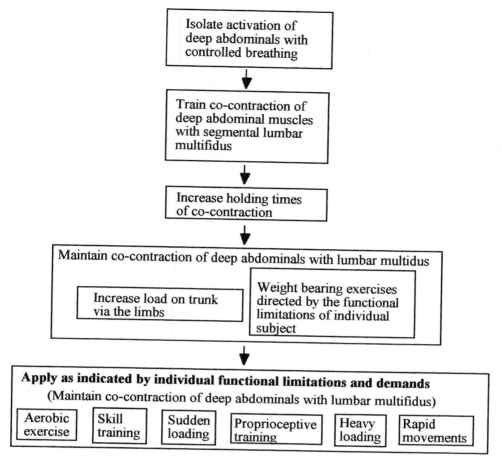

Fig. 7-20 Specific exercise training progression.

ternal oblique. A focus on maintaining an ideal starting position is always essential—deviation away from the neutral lordotic posture during muscle activation is an indication of substitution of global muscle systems.

It is important to note that the activation of low and middle fibers of transversus abdominis that attach to the pelvic rim and the thoracolumbar fascia is a focused contraction of the muscles of the lower and middle abdomen (below the level of the lateral rib cage). No dominant abdominal muscle activation is encouraged above a level of about midway between the umbilicus and the xiphisternum. If abdominal muscle activation occurs above this level, it will restrict movement of the rib cage, limit respiration, and inhibit the desired pattern of muscle activation. The pattern of muscle activation focuses on a "drawing up and in" of the pelvic floor and lower and midbelly toward the spine while controlling breathing and maintaining a neutral lordotic posture. In weightbearing positions such as sitting and standing there is a greater vertical loading of the abdominal contents on the pelvic floor and lower abdomen, so the focus is more of a "lifting" contraction with the "drawing in" contraction. If it is noted that the neutral lumbar lordosis is lost, controlled lateral costal diaphragm breathing ceases, and there is a narrowing of the sternal angle or flexion of the thorax, then the patient is instructed to stop the contraction.

These cocontractions involve a high level of specificity, good patient compliance, and low levels of voluntary contraction. It is important to educate the patient that the exercises are more "brain" exercises than "muscle" exercises in the early stages of training and the focus is on control. Some patients take up to 4 or 5 weeks of specific training before an accurate pattern of cocontraction can be achieved in weightbearing postures. The greater the effort or higher the level of voluntary contraction to the motor task, the more likely subjects are to substitute with other synergistic muscles such as rectus abdominis and external oblique.

In the early stages the patient is not given set holding times. Rather, the instruction is to hold the contraction only until global muscle substitution occurs, breathing control is lost, or muscle fatigue occurs. This training must be performed in a quiet environment without interruption over a period of 10 to 15 minutes because a high level of concentration is required. Training should be carried out at least once a day. Once this pattern of muscle activation has been isolated, then the contractions must be performed in sitting and standing and the holding contraction increased from 10 to 60 seconds before its integration into functional tasks and aerobic activities such as walking.

Once the isolated deep abdominal muscle activation has been achieved in the optimal position, with good breathing control and without global muscle substitution, the patient will usually describe a deeply situated muscle "fatigue" over the lumbar multifidus muscle lateral to the spinous process at the level of the unstable spinal segment. Palpatory examination just lateral to the spinous process will confirm this. At this stage the focus is on reinforcing the cocontraction of the lumbar multifidus segmentally with the deep abdominal contraction. It should also be noted that in the case of lumbar segmental instability in the absence of pars defects, the cocontraction of lumbar multifidus is at the level of the "unstable" motion segment, whereas in the case of isthmic spondylolysis and spondylolisthesis the focus is the level above the pars defects.

Throughout this muscle training period there should be no increase or aggravation of back pain at any time because the pattern of muscle activation occurs within the neutral zone and therefore does not stress the motion segment at the end of range.

This early form of training is consistent with assertions that motor learning and control are not simply a process of strength training, but depend on patterning and inhibition of inappropriately active motor neurons. The acquisition of skills occurs through selective inhibition of unnecessary muscular activity as well as the activation and synchronization of additional motor units.[88, 103] This stage of training may take between 3 and 6 weeks.

As soon as a controlled cocontraction of the deep abdominal muscles with lumbar multifidus has been achieved in upright postures such as sitting and standing, a degree of pain control is expected in these postures. This provides a powerful biofeedback for the patient.

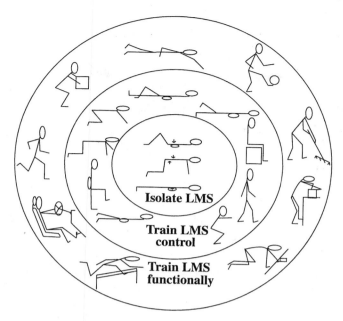

Fig. 7-21 Stages of rehabilitation.

Summary of First Stage of Training. The steps involved in the first stage of training are as follows.

1. Teach start position—neutral lumbar lordosis. Training the independence of the lumbar spine and pelvis to the thoracic spine and hips
2. Teach diaphragm breathing—central and lateral costal breathing
3. Teach isolated contraction of transversus abdominis with controlled diaphragm breathing and without substitution of the external oblique, rectus abdominis, and erector spinae within a neutral lumbar lordosis
4. Focus on cocontraction of transversus abdominis with lumbar multifidus within a neutral lordosis (pain free position), again with controlled diaphragm breathing and without substitution of the external oblique, rectus abdominis, and erector spinae
5. Train pattern of cocontraction in weightbearing postures such as sitting and standing with postural correction (Fig. 7-21)

Second Stage of Training

The second phase of motor learning is the associative stage, where the focus is on refining a particular movement pattern. Once the pattern of cocontraction is achieved it is immediately incorporated into dynamic tasks or static holding postures as determined by the patient's individual complaint. This is based on the patient's individual presentation and primary movement faults detected in the clinical examination. The pain-provocative faulty movement pattern is identified and broken down into simple steps. The patient is taken through these steps while isolating the cocontraction of the local muscle system. This is carried out first while maintaining the spine in a neutral lordotic posture and finally with normal spinal movement. Segmental control and pain control must be ensured at all times.

For example, if the patient complains of pain when transferring from sitting to standing, then the components of the movement are isolated and trained. Initially, the patient is taught to hold the cocontraction within a neutral spine position in sitting and then to move the weight forward maintaining the same spinal position while flexing at the hips, and then during weight transference from sitting to standing. At all times the cocontraction pattern is maintained because neutral zone control is imperative. If the patient loses segmental control—either with a loss or increase of segmental lordosis or a lateral shifting pattern—then the movement is ceased, and retraining to this point is repeated until it can be performed with normal, segmental, pain-free movement. Once normal movement has been achieved this becomes the training exercise. When it can be carried out with relative ease, the patient is trained to flex the spine, beginning with the cervical spine, then the thoracic spine, and finally the lumbar spine, and then flexing at the hips while maintaining the pattern of cocontraction in a pain-free manner. In this manner neutral zone control is established with normal movement patterns rather than a rigid movement pattern of "fixing" the spine in a neutral position. For patients with a flexion pattern the tendency is to lose low lumbar lordosis and anterior pelvic tilt control with an accentuated increased lordosis in the upper lumbar spine. Patients with a lateral shifting pattern usually have a similar tendency, and during weight transference will shift their weight laterally and lose symmetry of weightbearing in the sagittal plane. For patients with extension patterns, the tendency will be to increase the segmental lordosis during load transfer and lose the deep abdominal muscle contraction. This must be carefully monitored and corrected by the therapist.

The aim of the therapist is to identify two or three faulty and pain-provocative movement patterns and break them down into component movements with high repetitions (i.e., 50 to 60). This breakdown of movement components for retraining motor control strategies can be performed for walking, lifting, bending, twisting, etc. The patients carry out the movement components at home on a daily basis with pain control and gradually increase the speed and complexity of the movement pattern until they can move in a smooth, free, and controlled manner without pain. Patients are also encouraged to carry out regular aerobic exercise such as walking while maintaining a low-level cocontraction of the local muscle system. Therefore, if the patient goes for a 30-minute walk, they have performed a 30-minute low-level contraction of the muscles. This helps to increase the tone within the muscles and aids the automaticity of the pattern. Focus must be placed on correct postural alignment, low-level local muscle system cocontraction, and controlled respiration.

Patients are also encouraged to perform the cocontractions many times throughout the day, particularly in situations where they experience or anticipate pain or feel "unstable." This is essential so that the patterns of cocontraction eventually occur automatically without need for conscious control during activities and habitual postures of daily living. Interestingly, only once this pattern of muscle cocontraction is isolated do patients report a reduction in symptoms when integrating this control into static postures (such as sitting, standing, and sustained flexion), functional activities (such as bending, twisting, and lifting), and aerobic activities (such as walking, swimming, or running). This ability to control pain, reported by many patients when performing the muscle cocontraction, appears to act as a powerful biofeedback to reinforce the integration of this muscle control into functional tasks. This stage can last between weeks to months depending on the performer, the degree and nature of the pathologic process, and the intensity of practice before the motor pattern is learned and becomes automatic. It is at this stage that patients commonly report an ability to carry out (with minimal discomfort) the regular aerobic, general exercise, or loaded physical or recreational activities that previously aggravated their condition. It is at this stage that patients are able to cease the formal specific exercise program. They are instructed to maintain local muscle system control functionally with postural awareness while maintaining regular levels of general exercise.

Third Stage of Training

The third stage of training is the autonomous stage, where a low degree of attention is required for the correct performance of the motor task.[102] The third stage was indeed the aim of the specific exercise intervention, whereby subjects can dynamically stabilize their spines in an automatic manner during the functional demands of daily living (see Fig. 7-21, *B*). Evidence that this automatic change was achieved in the trial groups lies in the results of the surface EMG data and in the long-term outcome in patients who had undergone this treatment intervention. This will be discussed in detail in the following section.

The design of examination-based specific exercise programs addresses the specific motor dysfunction of each patient in a functional manner, while taking into account the level at which they experience pain or sense "instability." However, this treatment approach requires a high degree of skill and expertise on the part of the treating physiotherapist, first to train the cocontraction of local system muscles without the dominant substitution of global system muscles and then to integrate this new motor skill into the previously painful postures and activities that were a part of the patient's normal lifestyle. This approach also depends on a high level of patient motivation, understanding, and compliance. A possible reason for the high levels of compliance and motivation observed in patients with this exercise approach may be the knowledge that this approach allows the exercises to be performed during normal daily activities and that it focuses on the patient's ability to control his or her own symptoms.

Requirements for Success of this Treatment Approach.
Accuracy of examination and diagnosis
Specificity of exercise training
Proprioceptive awareness of patient
High level of patient compliance

Factors Contributing to Failure of this Treatment Approach.

Severe pathology (multidirectional instability)
Constant unremitting pain (neuropathic pain disorder)
Radicular pain
Psychologic factors such as depression
Compensation (patients seeking financial compensation for their condition)
Lack of proprioceptive awareness
Poor patient compliance

Clinical Research Results

Two randomized controlled clinical trials were performed to establish the efficacy to this specific exercise approach for the management of lumbar segmental instability in two specific patient groups. The full, detailed results of the trials have been reported previously.[89,99]

Trial One

The aim of this study was to evaluate the efficacy of this specific exercise intervention in a group of patients with chronic low back pain whose symptoms were considered to be attributable to the radiologic diagnosis of spondylolysis or spondylolisthesis.[89,99]

The study design used was a randomized controlled trial–test/retest design, with a postal questionnaire follow-up at 3, 6, and 30 months. Forty-four patients with chronic low back pain diagnosed with this condition entered the study. Their average duration of symptoms was 2½ years. Before intervention, testing was carried out on all patients by an independent investigator to establish baseline data for each subject. The measures used were previously validated and shown to be reliable and sufficiently sensitive to detect changes over time in a chronic low back pain population. These measures were:

1. the short-form McGill Pain questionnaire—used to measure average pain intensity levels.[104]

2. The Oswestry functional disability questionnaire—used to measure functional disability levels.[105]

3. A Cybex electronic inclinometer—used to measure sagittal range of movement of the lumbar spine and hips in standing.[106]

4. Surface electromyography—employed to measure abdominal muscle recruitment patterns from internal oblique and rectus abdominis during the abdominal drawing in maneuver.[108] This maneuver was chosen because in the normal situation it has been shown to result in preferential activation of the deep abdominal muscles relative to rectus abdominis.[107–109] However, in the chronic low back pain population this pattern has been reported to be disrupted.[108]

The subjects were then randomly assigned to two treatment groups. The first group underwent a 10-week treatment program directed on a weekly basis by a manipulative physiotherapist. This involved the specific training of the deep abdominal muscles in cocontraction with lumbar multifidus muscles proximal to the pars defect. The activation of these muscles was incorporated into static postures and functional tasks, to provide a dynamic corset to the lumbar spine during activities of daily living.

The second group underwent treatment over the same period, as directed by their treating practitioner. This predominantly involved regular general aerobic exercise and "sit-up" exercises.

On completion of the treatment period both groups were again retested by the same independent investigator, who was blind to group allocation. Forty-two patients completed the trial. At 30-month follow-up two patients were lost from the specific exercise group and five were lost from the control group (one was excluded from the analysis and underwent the specific exercise intervention after the 6-month follow-up).

Results. There were no statistically significant differences between the two groups before the intervention. Statistical analysis of the data following intervention revealed significant changes in the specific exercise group with:

- A reduction in pain intensity levels ($F (1,20) = 75.5$, $p < 0.0001$) (Fig. 7-22)
- A reduction in pain descriptor scores ($F (1,20) = 35.8$, $p < 0.0001$)
- An decrease in functional disability levels ($F (1,20) = 49.1$, $p < 0.0001$) (Fig. 7-23)
- An increase in the range of hip flexion mobility in standing ($F (1,20) = 6.2$, $p = 0.0215$)
- An increase in the activation of the internal oblique abdominal muscles relative to rectus abdominis ($F (1,20) = 5.53$, $p = 0.029$)

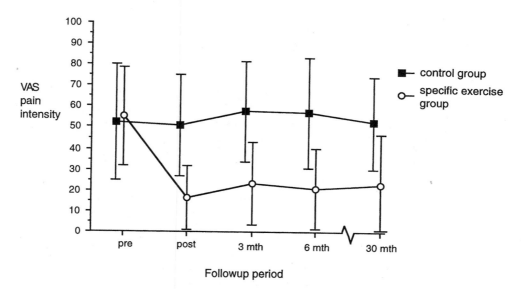

Fig. 7-22 Pain intensity scores for the specific exercise and control groups following the intervention period and at 3, 6 and 30-month follow up.

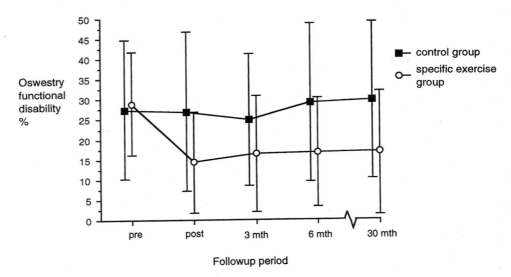

Fig. 7-23   Functional disability scores for the specific exercise and control groups following the intervention period and at 3, 6 and 30-month follow up.

There was no significant change in the lumbar spine range of motion in either group. The control group showed no significant change based on these parameters. These differences were significant between the groups based on change scores.

At 3-, 6-, and 30-month follow-up, the improvement in the specific exercise group was maintained on the basis of the level of pain intensity (F $(1,32) = 14.4, p = 0.0006$) (see Fig. 7-22); pain descriptor scores ($F (1,32) = 6.1, p = 0.0187$); and functional disability ($F (1,32) = 4.2 \, p = 0.0481$) (see Fig. 7-23), with an interaction effect occurring. The second group again showed no statistically significant change (Figs. 7-22 and 7-23). At 30-month follow-up the specific exercise group reported a reduced need for medication intake and ongoing treatment as compared with the control group.

Summary.   These findings support the view that a functionally integrated specific exercise approach to treatment, directed at training the deep abdominal muscles in cocontraction with lumbar multifidus proximal to the pars defect, is effective in reducing pain and functional disability levels in patients with chronically symptomatic spondylolysis or spondylolisthesis. Furthermore, the results of this study indicate that a "specific exercise" treatment approach directed at these muscles is more effective than other conservative treatment interventions commonly prescribed for patients with this condition, and the benefits of this intervention were still maintained at 30-month follow-up. Accordingly, where the stability of the basic morphology of the lumbar spine is compromised (such as with symptomatic spondylolysis or spondylolisthesis), specific training of these muscles may act to provide dynamic stability to the spine during activities of daily living. This intervention may provide a significant alternative treatment approach in a patient population where such pathology is commonly treated with surgical fusion. This treatment approach may also have implications for the wider low back pain population where "instability" of the lumbar spine is suspected.

Trial 2

The aim of this study was to (1) evaluate the efficacy of this intervention in patients with chronic low back pain who had a clinical presentation of a lumbar segmental instability problem, confirmed by motion radiology, in the absence of spondylolysis and spondylolisthesis; and (2) determine whether the intervention results in a change in the motor control strategy by which the lumbar spine is stabilized.[85,99]

Methods. Twenty subjects were selected for entry to this trial on the basis that they had:

- A chronic low back pain condition and a clinical presentation consistent with a lumbar segmental instability problem
- Clinically detected symptomatic hypermobility at a lumbar segment detected by a skilled manipulative physiotherapist
- Radiologic finding of increased segmental motion at the same level using the twist-test CT scan or flexion-extension x-rays.

Subjects were assessed by an independent examiner before and after treatment intervention to establish the:

- Pain intensity and functional disability levels
- Sagittal range of motion of the lumbar spine and hips in standing
- Ratio of activation of internal oblique, external oblique, rectus abdominis, and diaphragm during the abdominal drawing in maneuver
- Time to onset of the diaphragm, internal oblique, external oblique, rectus abdominis, and lumbar multifidus, relative to anterior deltoid during rapid upper limb flexion, using surface electromyography

Subjects were randomly assigned to two treatment groups. The first group underwent a 10-week treatment program directed on a weekly basis by a manipulative physiotherapist. This involved the specific training of the deep abdominal muscles in cocontraction with lumbar multifidus at the level of the symptomatic hypermobile segment. The activation of these muscles was incorporated into static postures and functional tasks during activities of daily living. The second group underwent conservative treatment, as directed by their treating practitioner.

Results. On completion of the treatment period, the specific exercise group showed the following statistically significant results:

- Reduction in pain intensity and functional disability levels compared with the control group

- Increase in the ratio of activation of internal oblique relative to rectus abdominis during the abdominal drawing in maneuver
- Increase in the speed to onset of activation of the diaphragm and internal oblique relative to anterior deltoid during rapid upper limb flexion

These changes were significant between the groups. No significant changes were observed in the ratio or muscle onset data in the control group following the intervention period.

Discussion.   These findings indicate that a "specific stabilizing exercise" treatment approach when integrated functionally is effective in reducing pain and functional disability levels in patients with chronic low back pain where lumbar segmental instability is detected. The findings also provide evidence that patients can be trained to isolate the contraction of the deep abdominal muscles relative to rectus abdominis and external oblique. More importantly the findings indicate that the "specific stabilizing exercise" intervention resulted in a change in the automatic motor control strategy within the trunk muscles, during self-imposed trunk loading.[99, 108] It is hypothesized that these findings represent an enhanced ability of the neuromuscular system to dynamically stabilize the lumbar spine during functional tasks.

REFERENCES

1. Lehmann TR, Braun, RA: Instability of the lower lumbar spine. Orthop Trans 7:97, 1983
2. Friberg O: Lumbar instability: a dynamic approach by traction compression radiology. Spine 12:119–129, 1987
3. Paajanen H et al: Disc degeneration and lumbar instability: MR examination of 16 patients. Acta Orthop Scand 60:375–378, 1989
4. Phuc V, Macmillan M: The aging spine: clinical instability. M South Med J 87:S26–S35, 1994
5. Kirkaldy-Willis WH: Managing Low Back Pain. Churchill Livingstone, New York, 1983
6. Sato H, Kikuchi S: The natural history of radiographic instability of the lumbar spine. Spine 18:2075–2079, 1993
7. Schmorl G, Junghanns H: The Human Spine in Health and Disease (2nd Ed.). Grune & Stratton, New York, 1971
8. Morgan FP, King T: Primary instability of lumbar vertebrae as a common cause of low back pain. J Bone Joint Surgery 39B:6–22, 1957
9. Wilder D, Seligson D, Frymoyer J, et al: Objective measurement of L4-5 instability. Spine 5:56, 1980
10. Pope M, Panjabi M: Biomechanical definitions of instability. Spine 10:255, 1985
11. Gertzbein S: Segmental instability of the lumbar spine. Semin Spinal Surgery 3:130, 1991
12. Dupuis PR, Yong-Hing K, Cassidy D, et al: Radiological diagnosis of lumbar instability. Spine 10:262, 1985
13. Kalebo P: Compression traction radiography in the diagnosis of lumbar segmental instability. Spine 15:351, 1990

14. Panjabi M, Lydon C, Vasavada A, et al: On the understanding of clinical insta-blity. Spine 19:2642, 1994

15. Panjabi M: The stabilizing system of the spine. Part 2. Neutral zone and insta-bility hypothesis. Spinal Disord 5(4):390, 1992

16. Kaigle A, Holm S, Hansson T: Experimental instability in the lumbar spine. Spine 20(4):421, 1995

17. Mimura M, Panjabi M, Oxland T, et al: Disc degeneration affects the multidi-rectional flexibility of the lumbar spine. Spine 19(12):1371, 1994

18. Panjabi M, Abumi K, Duranceau J, Oxland T: Spinal stability and interseg-mental muscle forces. A biomechanical model. Spine 14(2):194, 1989

19. Goel V, Kong W, Han J, et al: A combined finite element and optimisation in-vestigation of lumbar spine mechanics with and without muscles. Spine 18(11):1531, 1993

20. Wilke H, Wolf S, Claes L, et al: Stability increase of the lumbar spine with dif-ferent muscle groups. Spine 20(2):192, 1995

21. Dvorak J, Panjabi M, Novotny J, et al: Clinical validation of functional flexion-extension roentgenograms of the lumbar spine. Spine 16(8):943, 1991

22. Frymoyer J, Selby D: Segmental instability. Spine 10(3):280, 1985

23. Avery A: The reliability of manual physiotherapy palpation techniques in the diagnosis of bilateral pars defects in subjects with chronic low back pain. Master of Science Thesis, Curtin University of Technology, Western Australia, 1996

24. Mimura M: Rotational instability of the lumbar spine—a three dimensional motion study using bi-plane x-ray analysis system. Nippon Seikeigeka Gakkai Zasshi 64(7):546, 1990

25. Montgomery D, Fischgrund J: Passive reduction of spondylolisthesis on the operating room table: A prospective study. J Spinal Disord 7(2):167, 1994

26. Wood K, Popp C, Transfeldt E , et al: Radiographic evaluation of instability in spondylolisthesis. Spine 19(15):1697, 1994

27. Dunsker, SB: The Unstable Spine. Grune & Stratton, New York, 1986

28. Farfan HF: Mechanical Disorders of the Low Back, Lea & Febiger, Philadel-phia, 1973

29. Kirkaldy-Willis WH, Farfan HF: Instability of the lumbar spine. Clin Orthop 165:110, 1982

30. Taylor JR, Corker M: Age-related responses to stress in the vertebral column. In Schmitt LH, Freedman L, Bruce NW (Eds.): The Growing Scope of Human Biology. The Centre for Human Biology, University of Western Australia, Perth, Australia.

31. Twomey L: Age changes in the human lumbar vertebral column. PhD thesis. University of Western Australia, Perth, Australia, 1981.

32. Taylor J, Twomey L: Sagittal and horizontal plane movements of the lumbar vertebral column in cadavers and in the living. Rheumatol Rehab 19:223, 1980

33. Hopp E, Tsou PM: Post decompression lumbar instability. Clin Orthop 227:143, 1988

34. Katilainen E, Valtonen S: Clinical instability after microdiscectomy. Acta Neu-rosurg 125:120, 1993

35. Weiler PJ, King GJ, Gertzbein SD: Analysis of sagittal plane instability of the lumbar spine in vivo. Spine 15:1300, 1990

36. Liu YK, Goel VK, Dejong A, et al: Torsional fatigue of the lumbar interverte-bral joints. Spine 10:894, 1985

37. Ahmed A, Duncan N, Burke D: The effect of facet geometry on the axial torque-rotation response of lumbar motion segments. Spine 15:391, 1990

38. McFadden K, Taylor J: Axial rotation in the lumbar spine and gaping of the zygapophyseal joints Spine 15:295, 1990

39. Taylor JR, McCormick CC: Lumbar facet joint fat pads: their normal anatomy and their appearance when enlarged. Neuroradiology 33:38, 1990

40. Schönström N, Taylor J: A three plane photographic and measurement analysis of normal and abnormal axial rotary movememts of lumbar motion segments in response to torque. 1992 (unpublished)

41. Taylor JR, McCormick CC, Willen, J: Lumbar zygapophyseal incongruity as a sign of lumbar motion segmental instability. J Anat 165:299, 1989

42. Taylor MM, Taylor JR, McCormick CC: Features associated with subluxation in lumbar facet joints: Anatomical and radiological comparisons. Proc Australasian Soc Human Biol 5:359, 1992

43. Borenstein D: Low back pain. Curr Opin Rheumatol 2:233, 1990

44. Taylor JR, McCormick CC: Variation and asymmetry in lower lumbar zygapophyseal joint angles. Proceedings of the Australian Association of Orthopaedic Surgeons, Perth, Australia, 1987

45. Kenesi C, Lesur L: Orientation of the articular processes at L4, L5 and S1: Possible role in the pathology of the intervertebral disc. Anatomia Clinica 7:43, 1985

46. Taylor JR, Twomey LT: Age changes in lumbar zygapophyseal joints: Observations on structure and function. Spine 7:739–745, 1986

47. Taylor JR, Twomey LT: Structure and function of lumbar zygapophyseal joints. In Boyling J, Palastanga N: Manual Therapy of the Vertebral Column. (2nd Ed.). Churchill Livingstone, Edinburgh, 1992

48. Taylor JR, Twomey LT: Structure and function of lumbar zygapophyseal joints. J Orthop Med 14:71, 1992

49. Bell D, Ehrlich M, Zaleske D: Brace treatment for symptomatic spondylolisthesis. Clin Orthop Related Research, 236:192, 1988

50. Blanda J, Bethem D, Moats W, et al: Defects of the pars interarticularis in athletes: A protocol for non-operative treatment. J Spinal Disord 6(5):406, 1993

51. Hardcastle P: Repair of spondylolysis in young fast bowlers. J Bone Joint Surg 75B(3):398, 1993

52. Hensinger R, Michigan A: Spondylolysis and spondylolisthesis in children and adolescents. J Bone Joint Surg 71A(7):1098, 1989

53. Lettin A: Diagnosis and treatment of lumbar instability. J Bone Joint Surg 49B(3):520, 1967

54. Nachemson A: Lumbar spine instability. Spine 10(3):290, 1985

55. Lavender S, Marras W, Miller R: The development of response strategies in preparation for sudden loading to the torso. Spine 18(14):2097, 1993

56. Lavender S, Tsuang Y, Andersson G: Trunk muscle activation and co-contraction while resisting applied moments in a twisted posture. Ergonomics 36(10):1145, 1993

57. Pope M, Anderson G, Broman H, et al: Electromyographic studies of the lumbar trunk musculature during development of axial torques. J Orthop Research 4(3):288, 1986

58. Roy S, Deluca C, Casavant D: Lumbar muscle fatigue and chronic low back pain. Spine 14:992, 1989

59. Thelen D, Schultz A, Ashton-Miller J: Co-contraction of lumbar muscles during development of time-varying triaxial moments. J Orthop Research 13(3):390, 1995

60. Bergmark A: Stability of the lumbar spine. A study in mechanical engineering. Acta Orthop Scand Suppl 230(60):20, 1989

61. O'Sullivan P, Twomey L, Allison G: Dynamic stabilisation of the lumbar spine. Crit Rev Physical Rehab Med 9:315, 1997a

62. Cholewicke J, McGill S: Mechanical stability of the in vivo lumbar spine: implications for injury and chronic low back pain. Clin Biomechan 11(1):1, 1996

63. Gardener-Morse M, Stokes I, Laible J: Role of muscles in lumbar spine stability in maximum extension efforts. J Orthop Res 13(5):802, 1995

64. Aspden R: Review of functional anatomy of the spinal ligaments and the lumbar erector spinae muscles. Clin Anat 5:372, 1992

65. Bogduk, N: Anatomy and biomechanics of psoas major. Clin Biomechan 7:109, 1992

66. Bogduk N, Macintosh J, Pearcy M: A universal model of the lumbar back muscles in the upright position. Spine 17(8):897, 1992

67. Steffen R, Nolte L, Pingel T: Importance of the back muscles in rehabilitation of postoperative segmental lumbar instability—a biomechanical analysis. Rehab Stuttgart, 33(August 3):164, 1994

68. McGill S, Norman R: Reassessment of the role of intra-abdominal pressure in spinal compression. Ergonomics 30(11):1565, 1987

69. Cresswell A, Oddsson L, Thorstenson A: The influence of sudden perturbations on trunk muscle activity and intra-abdominal pressure while standing. Exper Brain Res 98:336, 1994

70. McGill S: Electromyographic activity of the abdominal and low back musculature during the generation of isometric and dynamic axial trunk torque: Implications for lumbar mechanics. J Orthop Res 9:91, 1991

71. Cresswell A, Grundstrom H, Thorstensson A: Observations on intra-abdominal pressure and patterns of abdominal intra-muscular activity in man. Acta Physiol Scand 144:409, 1992

72. Hodges P, Richardson C: Feedforward contraction of transversus abdominus is not influenced by the direction of arm movement. Exper Brain Res 114:362–370, 1997

73. Valencia F, Munro R: An electromyographical study of the lumbar multifidus in man. Electromyograph Clin Neurophysiol 25:205, 1985

74. McGill S: A myoelectrically based dynamic three-dimensional model to predict loads on lumbar spine tissues during lateral bending. J Biomechan 25(4):395, 1992

75. Hodges P, Richardson C: Dysfunction of transversus abdominus associated with chronic low back pain. In Manipulative Physiotherapy Association of Australia Ninth Biennial Conference. Gold Coast, Queensland, Australia, 1995

76. McGill S, Hoodless K: Measured and modelled static and dynamic axial trunk torsion during twisting in males and females. J Biomed Engineer 12:403, 1990

77. O'Sullivan P, Twomey L, Allison G: Dysfunction of the neuro-muscular system in the presence of low back pain—implications for physical therapy management. J Manual Manip Therapy 5(1):20, 1997b

78. Hides J, Stokes M, Saide M, et al: Evidence of lumbar multifidus muscle wasting ipsilateral to symptoms in patients with acute/subacute low back pain. Spine 19(2):165, 1994

79. Stokes M, Cooper R, Jayson M: Selective changes in multifidus dimensions in patients with chronic low back pain. Euro Spine J 1:38, 1992

80. Grabiner M, Koh T, Ghazawi AE: Decoupling of bilateral paraspinal excitation in subjects with low back pain. Spine 17(10):1219, 1992

81. Hides J, Richardson C: Multifidus inhibition in acute low back pain: recovery is not spontaneous. In Manipulative Physiotherapist Association of Australia Ninth Biennial Conference. Gold Coast, Queensland, Australia, 1995

82. Biedermann HJ, Shanks GL, Forrest WJ, et al: Power spectrum analysis of electromyographic activity. Spine 16(10):1179, 1991

83. Jull G, Richardson C, Hamilton C, et al: Toward the validation of a clinical test for the deep abdominal muscles in back pain patients. In Manipulative Physiotherapists Association of Australia Ninth Biennial Conference, Gold Coast, Queensland, Australia, 1995

84. Lindgren K, Sihvonen T, Leino E, et al: Exercise therapy effects on functional radiographic findings and segmental electromyographic activity in lumbar spine instability. Arch Phy Med Rehab 74:933, 1993

85. O'Sullivan P, Twomey L, Taylor, J: Specific stabilising exercise in the treatment of chronic low back pain with a clinical and radiological diagnosis of lumbar segmental "instability." In Manipulative Physiotherapists Association of Australia Tenth Biennial Conference, Melbourne, Australia, 1997

86. Sihvonen T, Partanen J: Segmental hypermobility in lumbar spine and entrapment of dorsal rami. Electromyograph Clin Neurophysiol 30:175, 1990

87. Sihvonen T, Partanen J, Hanninen O, et al: Electric behaviour of low back muscles during lumbar pelvic rhythm in low back pain patients and healthy controls. Arch Phys Med Rehab 72:1080, 1991

88. Edgerton V, Wolf S, Levendowski D, et al: Theoretical basis for patterning EMG amplitudes to assess muscle dysfunction. Med Sci Sports Exercise 28(6):744, 1996

89. O'Sullivan P, Twomey L, Allison G: Evaluation of specific stabilising exercise in the treatment of chronic low back pain with radiological diagnosis of spondylolysis and spondylolisthesis. Spine (Volvo specialty issue) 24:2959, 1997e

90. Richardson CA, Jull, GA: Muscle control—pain control. What exercises would you prescribe? Man Therapy 1(1):2, 1995

91. Tulder M, Assendelft W, Koes B, et al: Spinal radiological findings and non-specific low back pain. Spine 22(4):427, 1997

92. Boden S, Wiesel S: Lumbosacral segmental motion in normal individuals. Have we been measuring instability properly? Spine 15:571, 1990

93. Hayes M, Howard T, Gruel C, et al: Roentgenographic evaluation of lumbar spine flexion-extension in asymptomatic individuals. Spine 14:327, 1989

94. Nachemson A: Instability of the lumbar spine. Neurosurg Clin North Am 2(4):785, 1991

95. Paris S: Physical signs of instability. Spine 10(3):277, 1985

96. Tokuhashi Y, Matsuzaki H, Sano S: Evaluation of clinical lumbar instability using the treadmill. Spine 18(15):2321, 1993

97. Stokes I, Frymoyer J: Segmental motion and instability. Spine 12:688, 1987

98. Phillips D: A comparison of manual diagnosis with a diagnosis established by a uni-level spinal block procedure. Master of Science Thesis, Curtin University of Technology, Perth, Western Australia, 1994

99. O'Sullivan P: The efficacy of specific stabilising exercise in the management of chronic low back pain with radiological diagnosis of lumbar segmental instability. PhD Thesis, Curtin University of Technology, Perth, Western Australia, 1997

100. Sahrmann S: Diagnosis and treatment of muscle imbalances associated with regional pain syndromes. In Singer K (Ed.): Manipulative Physiotherapists As-

sociation of Australia—Eighth Biennial Conference—post conference workshop, Perth, Western Australia, 1993

101.   Richardson C, Jull G, Hodges P, et al: Therapeutic exercise for the spinal segmental stabilisation in low back pain: Scientific basis and clinical approach. Churchill Livingstone, Edinburgh, 1999

102.   Shumway-Cook A, Woollacott M: Motor control: Theory and practical applications. Williams & Wilkins, Baltimore, 1995

103.   Basmajian J: Motor learning and control: A working hypothesis. Arch Phys Med Rehab 58:38, 1977

104.   Melzack R: The short form McGill Pain Questionnaire. Pain 30:191, 1987

105.   Fairbank J, Couper J, Davies J, et al: The Oswestry low back pain questionnaire. Physiotherapy 66(8):271, 1980

106.   Saur P, Ensink F, Frese K, et al: Lumbar range of motion: reliability and validity of the inclinometer technique in the clinical measurement of trunk flexibility. Spine 21(11):1332, 1996

107.   Richardson CA, Jull GA, Toppenberg RM, et al: Techniques for active lumbar stabilisation for spinal protection: A pilot study. Austral J Physiother 38(2):105, 1992

108.   O'Sullivan P, Twomey L, Allison G, et al: Altered patterns of abdominal muscle activation in patients with chronic back pain. Austral J Physiother 43(2):91, 1997

109.   Strohl K, Mead J, Banzett R, et al: Regional differences in abdominal muscle activity during various maneuvers in humans. J Appl Physiol 51(6):1471, 1981

8

A New Clinical Model of the Muscle Dysfunction Linked to the Disturbance of Spinal Stability: Implications for Treatment of Low Back Pain

Carolyn A. Richardson
Gwendolen A. Jull
Julie A. Hides

Historically, therapeutic exercise has always played an essential role in the management of low back pain with aims to alleviate pain and prevent recurrent episode, as well as being a primary prevention strategy. Research to understand the muscle problems present in low back pain sufferers is being undertaken worldwide in an effort to help clinicians understand the mechanisms through which therapeutic exercises exert their seemingly beneficial effect. Nevertheless, it is difficult to decide on the most effective exercise program for a particular low back pain patient. A review of the international literature reveals many different exercise protocols, all of which either have some proven value or purport to be of value to the low back pain sufferer. They encompass a diversity of approaches, including a variety of strengthening programs,[1] functional capacity training,[2] walking and aerobic fitness programs,[3,4] stabilization programs focusing on trunk cocontraction exercises,[5,6,7] "ball" programs,[8] programs addressing "muscle imbalances,"[9,10] programs that address a variety of trunk muscles with the focus of minimizing loading of the spine,[11] or programs that encourage the patient to merely stay active.[12] Although it is well recognized that a "one size fits all" approach to the treatment of any condition is irrational, the diversity in the current methods of exercise for the low back pain patient suggest that we have not yet developed a logical approach to therapeutic exercise for these patients.

This chapter presents a new clinical model to describe the nature of muscle dysfunction in low back pain, leading to different directions for management. It is a developing model, but its purpose is to assist clinicians and researchers to look afresh at muscle dysfunction in low back pain. The clinical model is based on the muscle system's function to provide support and control or active stabilization to the lumbar spine. It is based on our current research and the discovery of problems in motor control, which present in the deep muscles of the back and trunk in low back pain patients. These muscles have a primary function for spinal segmental stabilization. This model also considers how other muscles might react and presents hypotheses to link the nature and extent of motor control problems to the magnitude of the back pain problem. The model emphasizes the need for a problem-solving approach for the individual back pain patient in the assessment and management of muscle dysfunction and the need for new measures to depict and define problems in motor control. The model also presents proposals to guide decisions regarding the precision and extent of therapeutic exercise that may be required in the individual back pain sufferer.

CLINICAL AND RESEARCH BACKGROUND

All the muscles of the lumbopelvic region are capable of providing some support for the lumbar vertebral joints as well as the sacroiliac joints. The muscles of this region generally fall into one of two categories in terms of their stabilization role. Bergmark[13] has described the two muscle systems linked to stabilization of the lumbar spine as the local muscle system and the global muscle system. The muscles of the local system are closely related anatomically to the individual vertebrae and are capable of increasing spinal segmental stiffness and providing segmental support.[14, 15] Transversus abdominis and multifidus would fall into this category. The global muscle system comprises the larger torque-producing muscles, which are anatomically more remote from the joint. They function to control spinal orientation and to balance the external load demands placed on the spine. Rectus abdominis and the external oblique muscles belong to this category. Other authors have put forward similar concepts in relation to the categorization of muscles used to stabilize a joint. In the context of muscles that stabilize the shoulder, Wilk et al[16] describe the rotator cuff as primary stabilizers of the joint and the larger superficial muscles (such as latissimus dorsi) as the secondary stabilizers of the joint. These categories would be in line with local and global muscles respectively.

In line with the ideas of Bergmark[13] and Wilk et al,[16] our clinical and research experience with the muscle system of the spine would suggest that local muscles should be described functionally as the primary continuous stabilizers of the spine, affecting the stability of the joints in all functional movements and postures. Global muscles functionally could be described as the secondary demand stabilizers of the spine. The functional role of global muscles is readily understood because these muscles are used to balance external loads and generally contract to counteract the biomechanical loading of the spine. The function of the local muscles as primary continuous stabilizers of the spine has only recently been investigated through several neurophysiologic studies.

A series of studies aimed at investigating the stability role of transversus abdominis and multifidus have highlighted the important role of the local muscle system in spinal stability. Cresswell et al[17] discovered that the transversus abdominis contracted continuously during flexion-extension movements of the trunk while the muscles of the global system (e.g., rectus abdominis and external oblique) turned off and on in line with the forces required to balance the trunk during the flexion-extension movements. In contrast to the transversus abdominis, where activity was relatively consistent, the global muscles increased their activity in line with the biomechanical requirements of the trunk movement. Studies undertaken by Hodges and Richardson[18, 19] have revealed how the central nervous system prepares and modulates the activity of the transversus abdominis to support the lumbar spine and its segments for functional activities and load. Of particular interest has been the discovery that the muscle demonstrates an ability to function independently of the other trunk muscles.[19]

The lumbar multifidus (especially the deep fibers) has also been highlighted in both biomechanical[20, 21, 22, 23] and physiologic research[24–28] as a local muscle that is capable of providing direct support to the spine through its ability to provide control of individual lumbar vertebral segments. The role of the local muscle system in the stabilization of the spine has also been highlighted by Cholewicki et al.[29] In their in vivo biomechanical model these researchers estimated that the spine was completely unstable if the global muscles were controlling spinal movement without any contribution of the local muscles. A contraction of the local muscles (e.g., multifidus) of only 3% of maximal voluntary contraction (MVC) was enough to re-establish spinal stability.

Besides studies highlighting the importance of the local muscles transversus abdominis and multifidus in spinal stability, research on back pain patients has demonstrated that these particular muscles are impaired and do not function adequately in this patient group. It could be argued that such deficits, if not addressed in management, would directly affect spinal support and leave the spine vulnerable to reinjury and thus vulnerable to recurrences of low back pain. The deficits found in the local muscles relate to their coordination and control rather than their ability to generate force (strength).[30, 31] These deficits include:

Loss of anticipatory function[30, 32]
Loss of ability to function independently of the other trunk muscles[30, 32]
Delays in activation and thus a loss of preprogrammed function for support[30, 32]
Asymmetric timing between the two sides of transversus abdominis, lessening its mechanical mechanism for support[33]
Lumbar multifidus inhibition in an acute episode of low back pain[31, 34]
Phasic activity rather than a tonic supporting contraction[30]

While scientific laboratory studies have gradually shed light on the problems in the local system, this knowledge has also been used by physiotherapists to gradually improve the conservative management of low back pain patients. Over several years exercise techniques evolved in which the transversus abdominis and multifidus were contracted together isometrically by instructing patients to slowly draw in the abdominal wall without moving the spine.[35] This new treatment approach was accepted by many research groups,[36,37] and evidence that this new exercise strategy was successful in decreasing pain and disability emerged through the clinical trial of O'Sullivan et al.[36] Hides et al[31] demonstrated that the treatment approach was linked to an improvement in muscle impairment in multifidus.

Clinical tests of deep muscle impairment were derived by analysis of the muscles' anatomical action. In the clinical situation, the motor skill aligned to a normal pattern of transversus abdominis muscle activation is an action of drawing in the abdominal wall.[7,38] When performed with a normal motor pattern, this should activate the horizontal fibers of transversus abdominis in its deep muscle corset action. It has also been found that when this action is performed correctly, it results in a simultaneous contraction of the deep fibers of lumbar multifidus, which can be palpated in the test.[35] Some indirect quantification of the transversus abdominis contraction, and the patient's ability to contract this muscle relatively independently of the other muscles of the abdominal wall, has been achieved in a prone test with the use of a pressure biofeedback unit.[35,39] The air-filled bag of the feedback device is placed under the patient's abdomen (Fig. 8-1). The patient, after appropriate instruction,[39] is asked to very slowly draw in his or her abdominal wall without moving the spine. The pressure should gradually decrease if the patient is able to move the abdominal wall inward without spinal or

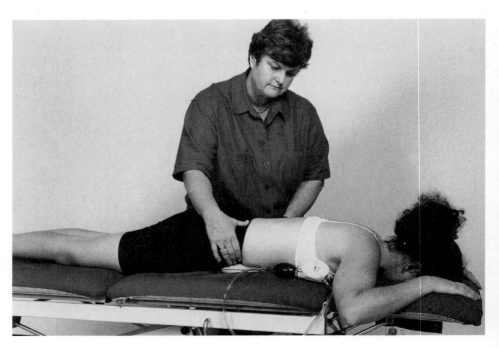

Fig. 8-1 The air-filled back of the pressure biofeedback device is placed under the patient's abdomen. (With permission from Richardson C, Jull H, Hodges P, Hides J: Therapeutic Exercise for Spinal Segmental Stabilisation in Low Back Pain: Scientific Basis and Clinical Approach. Churchill Livingstone, Edinburgh, 1999.)

rib cage movement, as well as maintaining normal breathing. The basis of this test for transversus abdominis is that this muscle is the predominant one in the abdominal group capable of drawing the weight of the abdominal contents off the sensor and creating a concavity in the abdominal wall, causing the decrease in pressure in the sensor. The majority of fibers of the other abdominals, the rectus abdominis and the external and internal obliques, are oriented either vertically or obliquely. When these muscles contract, they may flatten the abdominal wall but cannot draw in the waist and abdomen beyond this. The test identifies predominance of external oblique and rectus abdominis, or impairment of transversus abdominis, when there is no change in pressure, or an increase in pressure, as when the subject is unable to perform the test without moving the spine. In summary the clinical test performed in the prone position simply reflected the ability of patients to draw in the abdominal wall in an action similar to the exercise. Back pain patients found this action very difficult to perform.

In preliminary validation studies the clinical test, performed in prone posture, was found to be related to the motor control problem detected by Hodges et al[40] through the use of fine-wire electromyography (EMG) inserted into the transversus abdominis. Importantly, the action of drawing in the abdominal wall was used in the clinical trials on treatment of specific groups of chronic low back pain patients undertaken by O'Sullivan et al[36] and was found to be the measure that changed in line with their decreasing pain and disability. In addition, in an earlier randomized clinical trial involving acute low back pain sufferers, Hides et al[31] found that an improvement in this clinical measure was linked to a restoration of multifidus size at the symptomatic level.

Efforts had to be made to further investigate the muscle test action to understand the muscle patterns observed in subjects without low back pain. Reasons had to be found why low back pain patients could not draw in their abdominal wall while keeping their spine in a steady position, and why they used different compensation strategies in an attempt to achieve the drawing-in action. Clinical observations of back pain patients over many years indicated that it was not only the local system that was dysfunctional in low back pain patients. Unsuitable control strategies could also develop in the global muscle system to compensate for local muscle impairment. This became another key element in the new model of therapeutic exercise.

THE CLINICAL MODEL: A BASIS FOR THERAPEUTIC EXERCISE FOR ACTIVE STABILIZATION

The creation of models provides hypotheses and directions for research. Low back pain is multifactorial, and different models have been created to study the many factors involved. Biomechanical models have progressed knowledge and understanding of the factors that may be involved in the breakdown and development of pathology in the osseo-articular structures of the lumbar motion segment. The potential adverse effects of, for example, repetitive cyclic loading, static loading, and vibration have received considerable attention. The repetitive microtrauma to either the anterior or posterior elements of the motion segment that may result from such conditions have revealed a potential for gradual loss of passive structural integrity ultimately resulting in the disturbance or irritation of pain-sensitive structures. Interestingly, a lack of trunk muscle strength and endurance is often considered to contribute to the mechanical overload or acute traumatic episode, and preventive exercise programs have had a measure of success.[3,4]

Panjabi[41,42] presented a more expansive model to explain the development of low back pain, and this model centers around the concept of clinical instability. He presents spinal stability as being accomplished through the coordinated function of three subsystems, the passive subsystem (the osseoarticular structures), the active subsystem (the spinal muscles), and the neural subsystem (the control of the muscle system by the central and peripheral nervous systems). These three systems cannot act independently of each other and are considered part of a unique entity of spinal stabilization (Fig. 8-2). The role of muscles in the stabilization of the spine and their links to the passive system have been clearly highlighted in this model. Although the interaction of these three subsystems is extremely complex, and to a large extent ill defined in scientific studies, this simple model helps clinicians to understand Panjabi's concept of the development of low back pain.

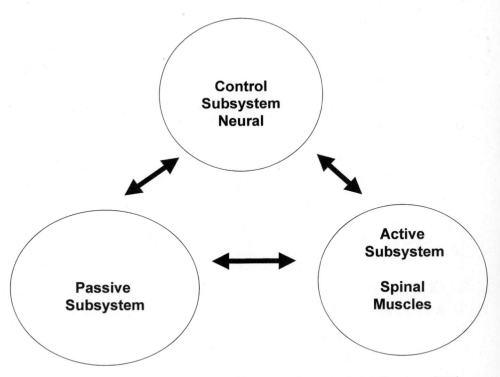

Fig. 8-2 The three systems that contribute to active spinal stabilization. (With permission from Panjabi MM: The stabilising system of the spine. Part I. Function, dysfunction, adaptation and enhancement. Part II. Neutral zone and stability hypothesis. 5:383–397, 1992.)

In this model, a disturbance in one subsystem can be compensated by the other subsystems in an attempt to maintain spinal stability and a pain-free functioning status. A point can be reached where the compensation is not sufficient, resulting in clinical instability and the onset of low back pain. Similarly, injury to the spine may lead to deficits in one system with resultant compensation in the other systems. Panjabi[41] has defined clinical instability as "a significant decrease in the capacity of the stabilising system of the spine to maintain the intervertebral neutral zones within physiologic limits, which results in pain and disability." Panjabi's model and concepts of instability have influenced the way in which the contribution of the muscle system can be viewed in relation to the development of low back pain. These concepts also provide a reasonable explanation as to why, in conditions where the passive system may be compromised, exercises designed to improve the functional supporting role of the muscle system may be useful in increasing spinal stability and in preventing the development of recurrent episodes or persistent low back pain.

Our clinical model for the development of the muscle dysfunction linked to the disturbance of spinal stability has evolved from that of Panjabi.[41,42] It is based on our research and clinical findings and describes how the relationship between the neural (control) and active (muscles) subsystems in particular might be disturbed. The model expands on the detail of the type of impairments that might be found in the muscle system. The model is presented schematically in Fig. 8-3.

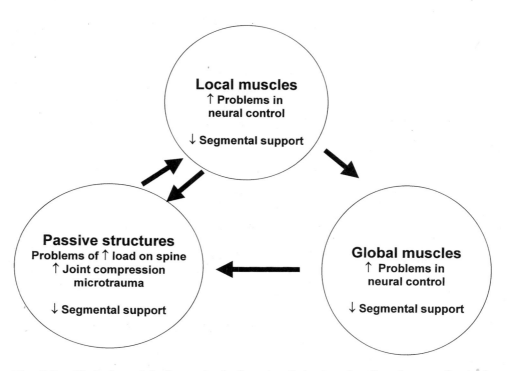

Fig. 8-3 Clinical model of muscle dysfunction linked to the disturbance of spinal segmental stability.

Decrease in Support of the Passive System

The passive system can suffer loss of support due to both direct and indirect influences. Considerable research has been conducted on the biomechanics of the lumbar spine motion segments, including the disc, vertebral body, ligaments, and zygapophyseal joints. Abnormal mechanics of the lumbar motion segment may result in inflammation, biomechanical, and/or nutritional changes that adversely affect nociceptive sensors.[43] In vitro studies have been conducted on cadaveric specimens where sequential lesioning of support structures has been performed to simulate injury conditions. Resultant increases in displacement and translations of the motion segment have been measured, allowing the effects of the muscles on the biomechanics of the spine to be assessed.[14, 21]

The passive system can also be exposed to a decrease in support indirectly due to a secondary response to injury. Joint or ligament injury can lead to pain and reflex inhibition. Reflex inhibition is elicited by abnormal afferent information from a damaged joint, resulting in decreased motor drive to muscle groups acting across the joint.[44, 45, 46] The joint involved is then predisposed to further injury. Research has also demonstrated a clear link between passive joint structures and the support and control of the surrounding muscles. A link has been found between ligament damage and fusimotor support to the surrounding muscles.[47, 48, 49]

The Problem in Neural Control of the Local Muscles

The control of the muscles that support the spine comes to a large extent from the motor programs emanating from the central nervous system. As described earlier, an impairment in this system has been found in low back pain patients.[30] Research studies,[30, 31] as well as clinical data gathered through the use of real-time ultrasound imaging,[39] have highlighted the problems in neural control in the local muscles of the spine (transversus abdominis and the deep fibers of multifidus) found in low back pain patients. It is conceivable that a problem in control in the local muscle system would result in a decreasing contribution of the neural system to overall spinal stability, as indicated in the model (Fig. 8-3). At this stage, even with a normal global system, a cycle of progressive loss of spinal segmental stability could occur, with decreased support of the local muscle system adversely affecting the passive structures, which then lead to more problems in the local muscle system and so on.

An Increasing Contribution by the Global System

Weakness and loss of endurance in the whole muscle system are commonly aligned to the condition of low back pain. In contrast, in our clinical model of active stabilization, the contractile elements of the muscle system demonstrate a range of responses to low back pain. Some can show an increase in their activity with time. This is quite a new concept and has important implications for management. The model predicts an increasing contribution of the global muscles, the muscles that have been described as the demand stabilizers or force generators in the stability system. Alteration in function ranges from a mild abnormality of the pattern of compensation to marked over-activation of the global muscles even at rest. Their contraction is in excess of their normal functional demand and thus seems to indicate a compensation mechanism for the decreasing contributions of the passive system and neural control of the local system. This compensation is more obvious in low-load activities, where normally minimal global muscle activity is required to maintain spinal stabilization. In its worst form, the increased activity of the global muscles above demand (especially in everyday activities) could lead to increased forces on the spine for longer periods, causing unnecessary heightened tissue loading and fatigue. Because the global demand stabilizers of the spine have no direct effect on segmental support, the consequences of their increased activity may be further damage to passive structures such as the disc, zygapophyseal joints, and spinal ligaments. The damage, pain, and progressive pathology in passive structures would in turn further reinforce and increase the problems in the local muscle system. The cycle is perpetuated, with gradually increasing compensations in the global system (see Fig. 8-3).

Some recent studies on muscle dysfunction associated with low back pain are producing findings that, we believe, support this model of increasing global muscle activity above demand in the low back pain sufferers. Cholewicki et al[50] postulated that patients with a lack of passive support may achieve sufficient stability by increasing cocontraction of their trunk muscles. Gardiner-Morse et al[51] agree that higher values of coactivation are required when normal joint stiffness is reduced. In their EMG study involving low back pain patients and matched controls, Peach and McGill[52] found increased levels in external oblique activity in some trunk movements in the low back pain population. This activity was above levels required for the same movement in the matched controls. In further support of the model, Joseph Ng (personal communication) has found a trend, although not significant, toward less fatigability in the oblique abdominals in low back pain patients when compared to asymptomatic control subjects. This current research is important because most clinicians would imagine that these muscles would be more fatigable in the low back pain population.

QUANTIFYING THE CHANGES IN MUSCLE FUNCTION

Relevant measures are required to test the hypotheses put forward in any new model. This clinical model for active segmental stabilization presents significant challenges, especially in the clinical situation. Many of the key muscles of interest are deep and not readily accessible. The measures required are ones that can reflect properties of motor control, not of the conventional parameters of muscle strength, endurance, or extensibility. Our research objective is to develop appropriate measures that are able to be used in the clinical situation. In line with our clinical model, our direction has been to develop assessments that will provide information on the local and global systems separately as well as their relationship to each other.

In this era of evidence-based medicine, relevant measures of the physical impairments linked to low back pain are also vital for the conduct of future clinical trials. Methods must be available to permit applicable measurement of any changes occurring in motor control in the low back pain patient as a result of exercise. Evidence is needed to evaluate whether such changes proceed in parallel with decreasing pain and disability.

Measurement of Problems in Local Muscles

Fine-wire EMG, as described in the experiments of Hodges and Richardson,[30] is used to measure the motor control problem in the deep, local muscles of the trunk. Although a good and exacting measurement technique, this method has disadvantages. It is invasive, with a minimal risk of infection. The method can be uncomfortable for many people because the hypodermic needles used for the fine-wire insertion, in the case of transversus abdominis, need to pass through three thick fascial layers of the abdominal wall. In addition, a high level of skill and training is required to complete the insertion and obtain high-quality signals. However, the method is not suitable for the clinical setting or even for use in large-scale treatment or back pain prevention trials to test the effect of exercises. Noninvasive measurements of the motor control deficits are required, and this is the continuing challenge in our laboratory and back pain clinics.

The prone test with pressure biofeedback has been a basic clinical test. It has several drawbacks that make it unsuitable for the rigors of a research setting. It requires operator skill in instruction and in monitoring the correct performance of the test. For example, false-positive reductions in pressure may occur if undetected subtle flexion of the spine occurs with the action of the external oblique muscle and the trunk is merely lifted off the sensor. Nevertheless, initial research into aspects of validity of the test with back pain patients and asymptomatic control subjects did demonstrate a link between performance in the prone test and the presence or absence of timing deficits in transversus abdominis.[40] In addition, the clinical philosophy behind this approach of testing the independent function of transversus abdominis is based on laboratory findings of the way the central nervous system seems to recruit the transversus abdominis. Hodges and Richardson,[19] in their trunk perturbation studies, demonstrated that the activation of transversus abdominis was functionally independent of the other abdominal muscles in its stabilization role. The contraction of lumbar multifidus in the prone test also appears to be independent of the thoracic and thoracolumbar portions of erector spinae, although more research is required into this aspect.

Further dimensions need to be added to the prone test of drawing in the abdominal wall to gain better direct quantification of the independent action of transversus abdominis and more information on the patient's control of

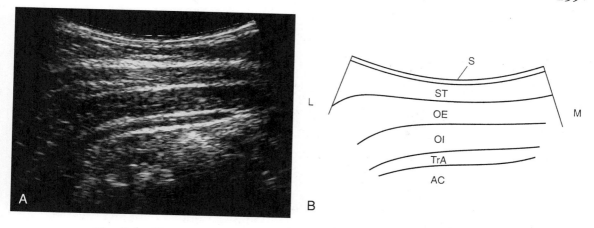

Fig. 8-4   Ultrasound images of the abdominal wall in transverse section (transducer placed anterolaterally) with relaxed abdominal wall. Note the curved skin *(S)* is due to the convex shape of the transducer. *ST* = subcutaneous tissue; *OE* = obliquus externus abdominis; *OI* = obliquus internus abdominis; *TrA* = transversus abdominis; *AC* = abdominal contents; *M* = medial; *L* = lateral. (With permission from Richardson C, Jull H, Hodges P, Hides J: Therapeutic Exercise for Spinal Segmental Stabilisation in Low Back Pain: Scientific Basis and Clinical Approach. Churchill Livingstone, Edinburgh, 1999.)

the muscle. Real time ultrasound imaging is adding another dimension to the test. It allows direct visualization of the contraction of the deep muscles, both of the abdominal wall (Fig. 8-4) and of the fascicles of the segmental multifidus (Fig. 8-5) during attempts at the motor skill of drawing in the abdominal wall.[53] In the development of noninvasive measures depicting con-

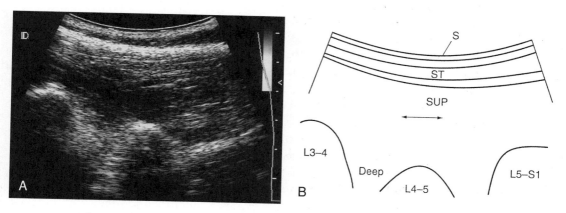

Fig. 8-5   **A,** Ultrasound image of the multifidus in longitudunal section. **B,** Superiorly are the skin *(S)* and subcutaneous tissue *(ST)*. The multifidus fibers run in the direction of the arrow (↔). Inferiorly are the zygapophyseal joints L3-L4, L4-L5, and L5-S1. The deep fibers of the multifidus are seen surrounding the zygapophyseal joints. *Deep,* deep multifidus fibers; *SUP,* superficial fibers. (With permission from Richardson C, Jull G, Hodges P, Hides J: Therapeutic Exercise for Spinal Segmental Stabilisation in Low Back Pain: Scientific Basis and Clinical Approach. Churchill Livingstone, Edinburgh, 1999.)

trol, factors such as the speed of contraction of the local muscles and their loss of independent function from muscles of the global system are now being investigated with the goal of quantification through the use of imaging. In all assessments, laboratory and clinical studies on low back pain patients have reinforced the need for separate measurements of both sides of the transversus abdominis muscle[33,54] and each side of the five lumbar levels of multifidus.[34] Problems in motor control of transversus abdominis can present on one side alone or bilaterally and at one segment of the lumbar multifidus and not the adjacent levels.

The prone test of the motor skill of drawing in the abdominal wall, like all muscle tests, is a cognitive or volitional test of muscle function. This again is an inherent drawback in the test. The possibility of a noninvasive test of automatic deep muscle function is currently being investigated.

Measurement of Developing Problems in the Global System

Quantification of the activation levels of the global muscles is not as difficult a task as that posed by the local muscle system. Surface EMG can be applied to most trunk muscles. In the context of the clinical model of detecting overdemand in the global muscle system as a compensation for impairments in the deep muscle system, the best order in which to monitor muscles in the abdominal group appears to be the external oblique, the internal oblique, and the rectus abdominis. In the back muscles, the erector spinae in the low thoracic, thoraco-lumbar region need to be monitored for overdemand activity. Through our use of many different testing conditions, it has been found that the detection of any unwanted heightened or compensatory activity in muscles of the global system is easier to depict in conditions of low load or gradually increasing loads with the trunk in a static position. Conditions requiring no trunk movement with low load should not demand substantial activity in the global muscles, and thus excessive activity beyond demand can be more easily recognized. The prone test of the abdominal drawing-in action is one of the tests employed for the assessment of overactivity in the global muscles. Currently, low-level leg loading tests are being investigated toward the development of a noninvasive test of automatic motor control of the trunk muscles.

Various types of data can be gathered to obtain information on the global muscles to help detect whether their activity is a reflection of overdemand and impaired motor control strategies. These include the following:

1. Level of contribution (percentage) to a standard test. We have chosen to use a maximum expiratory effort to provide the standard maneuver to allow the EMG data to be normalized during the selected movements or tests. This method of standardization was chosen in preference to the more usual method of using EMG levels during force generation, for several reasons. First, it is difficult to achieve a maximal contraction for the trunk muscles when dealing with people in pain and with compromised passive sup-

port systems. In addition a maximal expiratory effort allows all trunk muscles to be normalized in one automatic maneuver. This maneuver can be checked to be repeatable and reliable through the use of a vitalograph.[55]

2. Degree of cocontraction in a standard test. Clinical evidence of the poor global muscle patterns is often reflected in an increased cocontraction of the trunk flexor and extensor muscle groups beyond demand. That is, an increased level of co-contraction, similar to the bracing action of the trunk muscles required in heavy loaded efforts (e.g., lifting) is often detected in low back pain patients during an activity normally requiring low levels of effort.

3. Temporal pattern of the global muscles in a standard test. Problems in motor control may be detected by findings that muscles of the global system are recruited earlier than required or do not "turn off" in an appropriate time period following cessation of the test.

IMPLICATIONS OF THE CLINICAL MODEL FOR PRESCRIPTION OF EXERCISE

As a result of the model, the exercise approach of drawing in the abdominal wall has been refined and made more efficient. In essence, the exercise approach is concerned, in the first instance, with activation of the local muscles as a functional entity, viewing this action as a separate motor skill that has to be learned. The exercise therefore involves a motor learning approach. In the motor learning exercise protocol the local muscles (primarily the transversus abdominis and the deep fibers of the lumbar multifidus) are activated and repeatedly contracted independently of the global muscle system to restore their stabilization role. This approach is based on known methods of retraining a specific motor skill. An essential part of such an exercise is performing a vast number of repetitions of the skill in order to change the motor programs.[56] In facilitating this cocontraction, the clinician makes a conscious effort to choose a technique that will minimize the contraction of global muscles such as the rectus abdominis, the external oblique, and the long thoracolumbar erector spinae. Details of the facilitation techniques are described elsewhere.[39] This approach, which we have named segmental stabilization training, is in direct contrast to all other exercise programs designed for the low back pain populations. In these, global muscle activation is an essential element. For example, in general stability programs, exercises are employed that train both local and global muscles simultaneously without any differentiation between the systems.

The proposal in this new clinical model that global muscle activity could be "above demand" in many low back pain sufferers presents some interesting questions in light of many traditional views on the treatment of low back pain. Regimens of exercise for low back pain patients that revolve around strength and endurance training of global muscles would operate on the assumption of the presence of "underdemand" levels of the global muscles for spinal support. The apparent disparate assumptions between this new model and the traditional model of muscle dysfunction in low back pain may not be as vast as first assumed if the (1) back pain patient's muscle problem is viewed individually with a problem solving approach to analysis; (2) the "one size fits all" approach to treatment is abandoned; and (3) problems in the muscle system of low back pain patients are primarily considered as problems of motor control.

In studying both low back pain patients and patients without low back pain in our clinic, the futility of regarding low back pain patients as a homogeneous population with respect to the prescription of therapeutic exercise has become clearly evident. The clinical examination of very large numbers of back pain patients has led us to develop an hypothesis regarding the motor control problems in low back pain patients. This hypothesis may provide a more rational basis for the prescription of therapeutic exercise. It may also be of value in formulating future research questions. Our hypothesis is that muscle and motor control problems in the context of the model should be viewed as a continuum (Fig. 8-6). This continuum relates directly to the treatment options that are appropriate for the patient.

At one end of the continuum of motor control are the patients with a minor problem in the local muscles, with minimal compensation in function by the global muscles. At the other extreme are patients with maximal loss of segmental control due to effects on the local muscles, and maximal compensation of the global muscles. This may even occur at rest. Although the relationship between loss of passive joint support and degree of motor control problem may not be a direct one, examples of patients in this latter category may include those with a severely compromised motion segment and more serious problems of recurrent low back pain and disability. The reason for this extreme compensation of the global muscles may be linked to a gen-

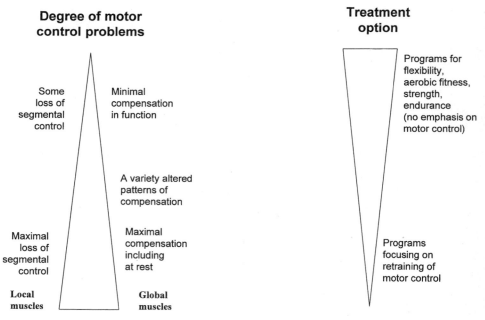

Fig. 8-6 Treatment options in relation to the continuum of motor control deficits.

eral response of the body to protect the segment from further damage. The irony is that the compensatory strategy is not the most efficient or effective one with respect to the motion segment and probably holds the trunk as a whole in a semirigid state. In line with the proposal of the continuum and the relations between motor control problems and the severity of the back condition, Cholewicki et al[50] have suggested that "the increased levels of muscle coactivation may constitute an objective indicator of the dysfunction in the passive stabilizing system of the lumbar spine."

In between the two extremes of the continuum are the majority of the low back pain population. While decreased support of segmental control provided by the local muscles is evident, a variety of altered patterns of compensation in the global system may present. In other words, the global muscle system may not show increased activation at rest, but when segmental control is challenged, the global muscles may either overrespond or respond at inappropriate times.

The application of the model to the prescription of therapeutic exercise may provide more rational guidelines to the exercise approach for the individual back pain sufferer. Patients with minor problems in the local muscles with minimal or no compensatory changes in the global muscles may do well with general stabilization training and gym work. Such training should emphasize drawing in the abdominal wall to ensure that the local muscle system is activated appropriately for any of the strength, flexibility, or fitness work. As patient's problems are assessed to be located further up the continuum, so the relative emphasis on specific training of the local system or training the interaction between local and global muscle systems is adjusted. Once patients demonstrate a loss of control of the deep muscles, which is associated with increasing levels of global muscle activity, very specific training of the local system is required to re-establish the supporting role of the local muscle system. This necessitates an exercise technique where the compensation pattern of the global muscles is minimized until the spinal supporting role of the local muscle system is re-established. This is the basis of segmental stabilization training.[39] In the context of the clinical model, it is worth reflecting on patients with severe muscle coordination problems with evidence of marked overactivity in global muscles. It may be that strength and endurance training in the first instance, which focuses on the large global muscles of the trunk (such as the external obliques), may be harmful to low back pain patients and may even cause their motor control problems and low back condition to worsen.

THE FUTURE

Initial randomized controlled clinical trials have demonstrated the beneficial effect of exercises that focus on transversus abdominis and multifidus in decreasing pain and disability in chronic low back pain patients with radiologic evidence of spondylolysis and spondylolithesis and patients diagnosed with clinical instability[36,57] as well as influencing return of multifidus size after an initial acute episode.[31] Although the benefit of these exercise techniques has been established, there have not been any further randomized controlled trials to determine whether a more efficient exercise technique has been devised.

It is hoped that in the near future the measurements developed from the new clinical model will allow changes in the motor control problems in low back pain patients to be reliably determined with noninvasive techniques. This would facilitate clinical research to investigate if the changes occurring with a particular treatment or exercise regimen are related to both changes in motor control and decreasing pain and disability in the low back pain patient. Databases for the noninvasive assessments of deep muscles and the compensatory activation of the global muscles representing the continuum of muscle problems, from mild to severe, are required. The degree of muscle problems may give a guide to the overall patient management and could help direct the most efficient treatment for low back pain patients. This would be a significant step forward in decision making for exercise treatment options and would ensure best practice exercise regimens for the back pain patient. It may bring us closer to meeting the yet unconquered challenge of the prevention of recurrent and persistent back pain

CONCLUSION

It is generally recognized that there are many treatments, especially different types of exercises, that seem to benefit low back pain sufferers. The difficulty has been in deciding which treatment would most likely benefit the individual patient. The ideas presented in this chapter are based on research and a new clinical model. They suggest that treatment must be individualized and based on a clinical problem-solving approach. New, noninvasive measures of the coordinated control of the spine, assessed by analyzing the functional integration of the local and global muscles, may hold the key to these future treatment decisions.

REFERENCES

1. Mooney V, Andersson GBJ: Controversies—trunk strength testing in patient evaluation and treatment. Spine 19:2483–2485, 1994
2. Torstensen TA: The physical therapy approach. Proceedings from the Third Interdisciplinary World Congress on Low Back Pain and Pelvic Pain. Vienna, Austria, 1998
3. Cady LD, Bischoff DP, O'Connell ER, et al: Strength and fitness and subsequent back injuries in fire fighters. J Occupation Med 3:269–272, 1979
4. Nutter P: Aerobic exercise in the treatment and prevention of low back pain. State Art Rev Occupation Med 3:137–145, 1988
5. Saal JA, Saal JS: Nonoperative treatment of herniated lumbar intervertebral disc with radiculopathy. An outcome study. Spine 14:431–437, 1989
6. Robison R: The new back school prescription: Stabilisation training. Part 1. Occupation Med 7:17–31, 1992
7. Richardson CA, Jull GA: Muscle control—pain control. What exercises would you prescribe? Man Therapy 1:2–10, 1995

8. Klein-Vogelbach S: Therapeutic exercise in functional kinetics. Springer-Verlag, Berlin, 1991

9. Janda V: Evaluation of muscular imbalance. In Liebenson C (Ed.): Rehabilitation of the Spine: a Practitioners Manual. Williams & Wilkins, Philadelphia, 1996

10. Sahrmann SA: Muscle imbalances in the orthopaedic and neurological patient. Proceedings of Tenth International Congress of the World Confederation for Physical Therapy, Sydney, Australia, Book 2:836–841, 1987

11. McGill S: Low back exercises: evidence for improving exercise regimens. Phys Therapy 78:754–765, 1998

12. Indahl A, Velund L, Reikeraas O: Good prognosis for low back pain when left untampered: a randomized clinical trial. Spine 20(4):473–477, 1995

13. Bergmark A: Stability of the lumbar spine. A study in mechanical engineering. Acta Orthop Scand (suppl) 230:20–24, 1989

14. Wilke HJ, Wolf S, Claes LE, et al: Stability increase of the lumbar spine with different muscles groups. A biomechanical in vitro study. Spine 20:192–198, 1995

15. Crisco JJ, Panjabi MM: The intersegmental and multisegmental muscles of the spine: a biomechanical model comparing lateral stabilising potential. Spine 7:793–799, 1994

16. Wilk KE, Arrigo CA, Andrews JR: Current concepts: The stabilising structures of the glenohumeral joint. J Orthop Sports Phy Therapy 25(6):364–379, 1997

17. Cresswell AG, Grundstrom A, Thorstensson A: Observations on intra-abdominal pressure and patterns of abdominal intra-muscular activity in man. Acta Physiol Scand 144:409–418, 1992

18. Hodges PW, Richardson CA: Contraction of the abdominal muscles associated with movement of the lower limb. Phys Therapy 77:132–144, 1997

19. Hodges PW, Richardson CA: Feedforward contraction of transversus abdominis is not influenced by the direction of arm movement. Exper Brain Res 114:62–370, 1997

20. Kaigle AM, Holm SH, Hansson TH: Experimental instability in the lumbar spine. Spine 20:421–430, 1995

21. Panjabi M, Abumi K, Duranceau J, Oxland T: Spinal stability and intersegmental muscle forces. A biomechanical model. Spine 14:194–200, 1989

22. Wilke HJ, Wolf S, Claes LE, et al: Stability increase of the lumbar spine with different muscles groups. A biomechanical in vitro study. Spine 20:192–198, 1995

23. Steffen R, Nolte LP, Pingel TH: Rehabilitation of postoperative segmental lumbar instability. A biomechanical analysis of the rank of the back muscles. Rehabilitation 33:164–170, 1994

24. Macintosh JE, Valencia F, Bogduk N, Munro RR: The morphology of the human lumbar multifidus. Clin Biomechan 1:196–204, 1986

25. Lewin T, Moffett B, Viidik A: The morphology of the lumbar synovial joints. Acta Morpho Neerlando Scand 4:299–319, 1962

26. Donisch EW, Basmajian JV: Electromyography of deep back muscles in man. Am J Anat 133:15–36, 1972

27. Jonsson B: The functions of individual muscles in the lumbar part of the spinae muscle. Electromyography 10:5–21, 1970

28. Valencia FP, Munro RR: An electromyographic study of the lumbar multifidus in man. Electromyo Clin Neurophysiol 25:205–221, 1985

29. Cholewicki J, McGill SM: Mechanical stability of the in vivo lumbar spine: implications for injury and low back pain. Clin Biomechan 11:1–15, 1996

30. Hodges PW, Richardson CA: Inefficient muscular stabilisation of the lumbar spine associated with low back pain: a motor control evaluation of transversus abdominis. Spine 21:2640–2650, 1996

31. Hides JA, Richardson CA, Jull GA: Multifidus muscle recovery is not automatic following resolution of acute first episode low back pain. Spine 21:2763–2769, 1996

32. Hodges PW, Richardson CA: Delayed postural contraction of transversus abdominis in low back pain associated with movement of the lower limbs. J Spinal Disord 11:46–56, 1998

33. Henry SM, Scott Q, Richardson CA: Asymmetric activation of transversus abdominis muscle in subjects with low back pain. North American Spine Society, San Francisco, 1998

34. Hides JA, Stokes MJ, Saide M, et al: Evidence of lumbar multifidus muscle wasting ipsilateral to symptoms in patients with acute/subacute low back pain. Spine 19:165–172, 1994

35. Richardson CA, Jull GA: An historical perspective on the development of clinical techniques to evaluate and treat the active stabilising system of the lumbar spine. Austra J Physiother Mono 1:5–13, 1995

36. O'Sullivan PB, Twomey LT, Allison GT: Evaluation of specific stabilizing exercise in the treatment of chronic low back pain with radiologic diagnosis of spondylolysis or spondylolisthesis. Spine 22:2959–2967, 1997

37. Pool-Goudzwaard AL, Vleeming A, Stoeckart R, et al: Insufficient lumbopelvic stability: a clinical, anatomical and biomechanical approach to 'a-specific' low back pain. Man Therapy 3(1):12–20, 1998

38. Lacote M, Clevalier AM, Mirander A, et al: Clinical Evaluation of Muscle Function. Churchill Livingstone, Edinburgh, 1987

39. Richardson CA, Jull GA, Hodges PW, Hides JA: Therapeutic Exercise for Spinal Segmental Stabilisation in Low Back Pain: Scientific Basis and Clinical Approach. Churchill Livingstone, Edinburgh, 1999

40. Hodges PW, Richardson CA, Jull GA: Evaluation of the relationship between the findings of a laboratory and clinical test of transversus abdominis function. Physiother Res Internat 1:30–40, 1996

41. Panjabi MM: The stabilising system of the spine. Part 1. Function, dysfunction, adaption, and enhancement. J Spinal Disord 5:383–389, 1992

42. Panjabi M: The stabilising system of the spine. Part II. Neutral zone and stability hypothesis. J Spinal Disord 5:390–397.

43. White AA: New Perspectives on Low Back Pain. In Frymoyer JW, Gordon SL (Eds.). American Academy of Orthopaedic Surgeons Symposium, Park Ridge, Illinois, 1988

44. Hurley MV, Newham DJ: The influence of arthrogenous muscle inhibition on quadriceps inhibition on quadriceps rehabilitation of patients with early unilateral osteoarthritic knees. Br J Rheumatol 32:137–131, 1993

45. Stokes M, Young A: The contribution of reflex inhibition to arthrogenous muscle weakness. Clin Sci 67:7–14, 1984

46. Stokes M, Young A: Investigations of quadriceps inhibition: Implications for clinical practice. Physiotherapy 70:425–428, 1984

47. Grigg P, Harrigan EP, Fogarty KE: Segmental reflexes mediated by joint afferent neurons in cat knee. J Neurophysiol 41:9–14, 1978

48. Johansson H, Sjolander P, Sojka P: Receptors in the knee joint ligaments and their role in the biomechanics of the joint. CRC Crit Rev Biomed Engineer 18:341–368, 1991

49. Johansson H, Sjolander P, Sojka P: A sensory role for the cruciate ligaments. Clin Orthop Related Res 268:161–178, 1991

50. Cholewicki J, Panjabi MM, Khachatryan A: Stabilizing function of trunk flexor-extensor muscles around a neutral spine posture. Spine 22:2207–2212, 1997

51. Gardner-Morse M, Stokes IAF, Laible JP: Role of muscles in lumbar spine stability in maximum extension efforts. J Ortho Res 13:802–808, 1995

52. Peach JP, McGill SM: Kinematics and trunk muscle myoelectric activity in the chronic low back pain patient. Submitted to J Phys Therapy, 1997

53. Hides JA, Richardson CA, Jull GA, Davies SE: Ultrasound imaging in rehabilitation. Austral J Physiother 41:187–193, 1996

54. Jull GA, Scott Q, Richardson C, Henry S, et al: New concepts for the control of pain in the lumbopelvic region. Proceedings from the Third Interdisciplinary World Congress on Low Back Pain and Pelvic Pain. Vienna, Austria, 1998

55. Guyton AC: Textbook of Medical Physiology (8th Ed.). W.B. Saunders, Philadelphia, 1991

56. Kottke FJ, Halpern D, Easton JKM, et al: The training of coordination. Arch Phys Med Rehab 59:567–572, 1978

57. O'Sullivan P, Twomey L, Allison G: Altered pattern of abdominal muscle activation in chronic back pain patients. Austral J Physiother 43:91–98, 1997

9

Exercise and Spinal Manipulation in the Treatment and Rehabilitation of Low Back Pain

Lance T. Twomey
James R. Taylor

The widespread and increasing incidence of low back pain (LBP) in western society and the inability of medicine to comprehensively or effectively manage it have created the opportunity for development of a variety of approaches to its treatment. The many "therapies" that have been tried with some success during this century include active exercise regimens and passive (or manual) mobilization and manipulation. The physical/manual therapist is concerned with the application of primary physical modalities incorporating postural assessment and modification, ergonomic advice, exercise, mobilization and manipulation, massage, and traction to musculoskeletal pain and dysfunction problems, including LBP.

Much of the current treatment for LBP remains empirical. This is not surprising in an environment where the current knowledge of the pathogenesis of LBP is incomplete and controversial, and where many of the diagnostic labels attached to patients with LBP are unclear and confusing. However, in recent years biologic and clinical studies have added considerably to the understanding of development, age-changes, pathology, and effects of trauma on spinal structures.[17,18] This chapter considers evidence to support the place of exercise and spinal manipulation and mobilization in the treatment of LBP.

EXERCISE AND BACK PAIN

Bed rest and analgesics remain the treatments prescribed by most physicians in the management of LBP.[18] This is in spite of the lack of evidence that prolonged bed rest or the avoidance of movement and exercise brings about a reduction in back pain. Indeed, current research shows that, apart from a brief period of rest immediately after the onset of acute LBP, bed rest has no effect on the natural history of back pain.[2] Similarly, if the literature on the use of physical activity is considered, it is clear that well designed exercise and movement programs play an important role in the treatment of many musculoskeletal disorders, including most acute and chronic LBP syndromes, and are essential in the restoration of function necessary to maintain the productivity, self-respect and well-being of affected individuals.[8, 16, 18, 20] This view is reinforced by the observation that prolonged rest or the avoidance of exercise are associated with an increase in the duration and the severity of back pain.[3] To be useful, initial bed rest where prescribed for LBP should be of limited duration.

All elements of the musculoskeletal system react adversely to prolonged inactivity (including bed rest), resulting in widespread weakness and loss of tissue. Prolonged inactivity leads to a loss of muscle bulk and reductions in bone density, connective tissue thickness, and extensibility. These changes bring about reductions in joint ranges of motion, muscle strength, and endurance, and a marked decline in physical fitness.[15] This situation is especially problematic for the elderly, and it is clear from current research that the musculoskeletal system (including the vertebral column) demands the loading and stress of exercise and movement at all stages during the life cycle, even into old age, to maintain its function and strength.[16]

Spinal Joints

In the spine the health of the joints is dependent on repeated low stress movements. The intervertebral discs and the zygapophyseal (facet) joints require movement to ensure the proper flow of fluid and nutrients across and through joint surfaces. Although movement and exercise may not reduce the number of episodes of LBP that a person undergoes, it ensures that those affected are better able to manage and live with their problem, to recover from it more quickly, to remain or return to productive work more rapidly, and to have a considerably improved quality of life.[16, 18] Recent evidence for the use of exercise in the treatment of joint and back pain is considered in this chapter.

All of the cartilaginous structures of the body respond adversely to disuse and conditions of sustained loading and respond positively to movement and exercise.[5, 14] Thus in the spine the articular cartilage and ligaments of the facet joints and the fibrocartilage of the intervertebral discs (IVD) are negatively affected by inactivity and especially by prolonged loading in one position. The IVDs are the largest avascular, cartilaginous structures in the body and rely for their nutrition on the diffusion of nutrients, mostly across the vertebral end-plates. Disc nutrition is very dependent on movement, and it is movement in the sagittal plane that brings about the greatest fluid transfer into and out of the lumbar discs. Thus regular, large-range spinal movement is important to ensure adequate disc nutrition. On the other hand, it has been shown that sustained disc loading, especially at or toward the limit of lumbar flexion, is associated with the expression of a considerable quantity of fluid from the IVDs and, if habitual, as in some occupations, is associated with disc degeneration and LBP.[16]

Similarly, the articular cartilage of the facet joints demands regular movement and mechanical loading and unloading to remain healthy. Exercise and joint movement ensure the passage of synovial fluid over the articular cartilage and, together with the alternate compression and relaxation of cartilage that occurs in movement, enable the synovial fluid to be expressed and then "sucked back" into the articular cartilage as the pressure changes over the surface during movement.[14] The regular loading and unloading of joint cartilage that occurs throughout exercise or passive movement facilitates this process.[5] While joint cartilage responds favorably to movement, it (like the IVD) responds poorly to immobilization, especially under conditions of prolonged loading, leading to atrophy and degeneration of articular cartilage and sclerosis of the underlying subchondral bone. Similarly, ligaments, as dynamic collagenous structures, undergo hypertrophy with exercise and atrophy with disuse.[14]

Spinal Bone and Muscle

Both bone and muscle are dynamic tissues that respond positively to exercise and adversely to disuse. A strong inverse relationship exists between muscle mass and osteoporosis wherein a decline in muscle mass is matched by an increasing fragility of bone. There is now compelling evidence demonstrating that much of the reduction in muscle mass and the accompanying decline in strength and endurance that occur with increasing age in western society are due to disuse and can be prevented and reversed by exercise programs.[10, 16] Thus it is now well-established that bone density can be increased by regular physical exercise, even in postmenopausal elderly women. The bone gain after exercise is both site-specific and exercise-specific. To this effect, exercise involving impact and torsion loading of parts of the body has been shown to cause the largest increases in local bone density. Thus bone density of lumbar vertebrae is enhanced by resisted trunk exercise and by exercises involving the impact and shear stresses of walking and running.[16]

Similarly, it is clear that it remains possible to increase muscle strength, endurance, and hypertrophy even in quite elderly people. Thus there is an abundance of evidence on the relationship between exercise and aging to show evidence of considerable increases in muscle size and function in older people, especially when the strengthening programs are individualized and are consistent with personal goals.[15, 16] In recent years the improved understanding of the relationship between back pain, exercise, and the effects of prolonged disuse have resulted in programs of **intensive physical therapy and work "hardening" regimens,** appropriate to the physical condition (as carefully measured) of individuals with chronic LBP.[8] The success of such programs can be evaluated by the marked improvement in physical capacity and function of patients and by the ability of many affected individuals to return to the workplace. It is important to note that at the conclusions of such programs of intensive physical "reconditioning" a significant reduction in subjective pain measures are also consistently reported.[8, 21] Thus McQuade et al[11] have shown that the stronger the individual with chronic LBP, the less that person appears to be limited by the condition, and also that the higher the aerobic work capacity, the more active and flexible is that individual. A considerable number of studies indicate that back pain intensity is not consistently increased by exercise; indeed many subjects report feeling significantly better following vigorous exercise, while those with higher exercise levels are shown to have fewer episodes of back pain and fewer days away from work.[8, 11, 13, 18, 20] There is obviously an important central role for the use of exercise and movement in the management of both acute and chronic LBP, but the experience of pain clinics is that there remains a number of patients with chronic pain who cannot persist with such programs.

Recent studies by physical therapists have improved understanding of the role that spinal muscles play in the control and stability of the lumbar motion segment and the relationship between chronic LBP and a breakdown in neuro-muscular control.[22, 26] Essentially, they indicate a major role played by the segmental muscles that control individual motion segments and look to the ability of patients to gain effective control over their activity. These studies are detailed in Chapters 7 and 8 and are useful indicators of future study and clinical application.

MANIPULATION AND MOBILIZATION

Manipulation and mobilization are passive joint movement procedures in which the operator takes a joint or joint complex through all or part of its range of motion (ROM). Mobilization involves repetitive low-velocity passive movements, usually within or at the limit of ROM, while manipulation involves a small-amplitude, high-velocity thrust at the limit of a patient's joint range so that the joint is briefly taken beyond the restricted ROM. These techniques, aimed at maintaining or restoring a ROM and reducing LBP, are performed by both medical and nonmedical practitioners, involve considerable patient cooperation, and need to be carried out with the patient relaxed so that the practitioner is able to achieve the desired joint range. Manipulation may also be performed under anesthesia, but this controversial procedure is considered to involve greater risk of tissue injury than when performed with the patient awake and cooperative.[1] The terms *manipulative therapy* and *manual therapy* are often used to encompass both mobilization and manipulation as defined above, while *manipulation* describes only the more forceful procedure. Spinal manipulative therapy has become one of the most widely used methods of treating vertebral column pain, and millions of patient treatments are performed each year, mostly in western societies.[4, 7, 25]

Although there has been a considerable growth in the volume of research on the place of manipulation in recent years, most of the research is hindered by inadequate study design and bias and has failed to use the appropriate methodology necessary for effective clinical trials.[4] There is still no clear explanation of the mechanisms by which manipulation relieves LBP, although many suggestions have been made, including vertebral malposition or subluxation, reduction of disc bulge/herniation, the freeing of adhesions around a disc or facet joints, repositioning of "meniscoid structures" or torn articular cartilage within facet joints, enhanced reflex responses, and the mechanical stimulation of nociceptive joint fibers.[17, 24]

Mobilization

The rationale for the use of mobilization is more soundly based in theory than is the rationale for manipulation. The repetitive, low-stress, and small-amplitude movements of mobilization allow effective synovial fluid distribution over and through articular cartilage, disc, and partial stretching of the ligamentous joint structures, events that are necessary on a regular basis for the efficient functioning and repair of the structures involved.[5, 14, 16] In this regard, its effects on the joints and associated tissues are similar to those of exercise that have been previously described. Mobilization is usually performed in a non–weightbearing position, allowing good joint lubrication and the efficient functioning of synovial and cartilaginous joints as previously described.

Although most of the clinical trial studies have primarily considered manipulation, a small number have examined the influence of mobilization on back pain syndromes.[4] Of the four studies of acute LBP that have directly compared mobilization with manipulation, three showed an advantage for manipulation, with one finding in favor of mobilization.[12] However, mobilization is a relatively gentle procedure, its physiologic effects on joints are similar to those of active exercise, and its results would be expected to correspond more closely to those observed in studies of passive movement. For these reasons, mobilization would be expected to have a greater effect on subacute and chronic LBP rather than acute pain. Frank et al[5] clearly showed the value of passive joint motion in joint pain and dysfunction problems and point to the use of passive motion as a powerful and reliable orthopedic tool.

Manipulation

Di Fabio,[4] in an analysis of the literature on clinical trials of manipulation, identified 11 valid studies, all demonstrating the efficacy of manipulation in the treatment of the LBP. There were three other valid studies of spinal manipulation, two for the cervical and one for the sacral region, two of which showed positive results of manipulation, while one (for the cervical spine) was negative. There have been a number of other controlled studies of manipulation showing negative or equivocal results, but all of these have demonstrated major methodologic difficulties.[4] The valid trials primarily point to immediate and short-term symptomatic relief of LBP for the manipulated group as the significant advantage of the treatment, while the long-term effects of the manipulated and control groups did not differ significantly.

Meade et al,[9] in a major multicenter trial of manipulation in Great Britain, compared chiropractic care with conventional hospital outpatient management in a large group of patients and demonstrated a significant advantage for those treated by chiropractic manipulation. However, this research has been criticized in that those patients receiving chiropractic had 44% more treatments than the hospital outpatients, the chiropractic treatment was in a private clinic while the hospitalization was in a socialized system with long waiting lists, and the hospital treatment was not consistent in its form or structure. The more structured, controlled study of Hadler et al was able to demonstrate rapid pain reduction and increased mobility in those patients receiving manipulation. These latter results are typical of the "valid" studies, i.e., that pain reduction appears to be more rapid when mobilization is used and that manipulation generally fares better in the short term in comparison with other conservative treatments.

Techniques of manipulation vary considerably, not only between the different professions that practice them but also within an individual profession. Many of the clinical trials that have been conducted have been severely criticized because descriptions of the techniques used do not allow for the study to be easily replicated. In some instances, the types of techniques are not described at all, other than by the word *manipulation,* whereas with other trials the description is so vague as to be useless. The more recent and better designed clinical studies show a tendency toward better description of the manipulations for the lumbar spine, with most of the procedures listed being rotational.[4] Most studies of the effects of any treatment on LBP are qualified by problems of patient selection. There is still not complete agreement on the use of diagnostic labels, the inclusion and exclusion criteria used in trials varies widely, and the use of randomization of subjects or "blind" assessors are other factors that affect the results. Nevertheless, a close scrutiny of the best research into the effects of manipulation emphasises an important role for it in the early treatment of some forms of LBP.

Although there are recorded instances of mortality and morbidity associated with cervical manipulation, lumbar spinal manipulation appears to be relatively benign. There are recorded instances of increases in LBP and functional disorder after lumbar manipulation, and an instance of a herniated lumbar disc that may have been due to manipulative procedures, but such reports are rare. Most complications, when they do occur, follow poor diagnoses that miss conditions such as spinal osteoporosis, fracture, or a bony tumor.[7] Under these situations, lumbar manipulation is potentially very dangerous.

This relatively benign nature of lumbar spinal manipulation is demonstrated in a recent study by Cherkin et al,[19] which examined the relative cost-effectiveness of chiropractic manipulation, McKenzie therapy, and an educational booklet as treatment for LBP. They showed that manipulation and McKenzie therapy have similar effects and costs that provide only marginally better outcomes than the use of an educational booklet. While this is by no means the "last word" on the subject, it does provide therapists with considerable food for thought. Other similar recent studies are equivocal.[23]

OVERVIEW

The evidence of previous studies clearly shows a role for manipulation of the lumbar spine for acute LBP where there is restriction to a range or ranges of motion. It is important to emphasize that although most patients with acute back pain recover spontaneously, mobilization and manipulation are particularly useful in speeding up the process of recovery and return to activity.[17] Manipulation for chronic LBP appears to have a lesser chance of success, although a study by Meade et al[9] infers a stronger role in this regard. There is no doubt that there is widespread acceptance of this conservative treatment, that it will continue to be the choice of treatment of many people, and that while research on the issue has improved in both quality and quantity in recent years, the definitive research is yet to be done and the scientific community might wish to consider this research as a matter of priority.[19] Such research should not be left solely in the hands of those with a vested interest in the widespread and repeated use of their variation of manipulation as the only valid methodology for all kinds of back pain.

On the other hand, evidence for the use of exercise in the treatment of LBP and rehabilitation is overwhelming.[20] Exercise is essential for all components of the musculo-skeletal system, throughout the whole of the life cycle. The tissues of the vertebral column require the stresses of exercise, even under conditions of back pain. There are now numerous studies that show the damaging effects of disuse on the spinal tissues; that show that exercise does not usually increase low back pain, and that as lumbar function improves during an exercise regimen, the levels of LBP decline.[8,17,18] For these reasons, low-stress mobility exercises have an important role in the early treatment of acute LBP in ensuring the integrity of the musculoskeletal system. Exercise also has a most important role in the management of chronic LBP, and Mayer's studies[8] clearly show the necessity of rigorous, consistent, and aggressive exercise and work hardening to assist functional improvement and a return to work. Thus Saal and Saal's retrospective cohort study[13] considered the functional outcome of an aggressive physical rehabilitation program in patients with a diagnosis of herniated lumbar discs. Their study showed that 90% of the patients subjected to the vigorous exercise regimen had a good or excellent outcome based on measurement criteria and there was a 92% return to work. Four of the six unsuccessful patients who went to surgery were found to have spinal stenosis. The study represents a good model for the use of conservative exercise therapy, even when there is a clear diagnosis of a condition such as disc herniation. It may be that back surgery should be reserved for those patients in whom function has not been improved by an intensive physical exercise rehabilitation program.

REFERENCES

1. Cyriax J: Textbook of Orthopaedic Medicine (7th Ed.). Balliere Tindall, London, 1978
2. Deyo RH, Diehl AK, Rosenthal M: How many days of bed rest for acute low back pain? New Engl J Med 315(7):1064–1070, 1986
3. Deyo RA, Tsui-Wu Y-R: Descriptive epidemiology of low back pain and its related medical care in the United States. Spine 12(3):264–268, 1987
4. Di Fabio RP: Efficacy of Manual Therapy. Phys Therapy 72(12):853–864, 1992
5. Frank C, Akeson WH, Woo SL-Y, et al: Physiology and therapeutic value of passive joint motion. Clin Orthop Related Res 185:113–125, 1984
6. Hadler NM, Curtis P, Gillings DB, et al: A benefit of spinal manipulation as adjunctive therapy for acute low-back pain: A stratified controlled trial. Spine 12(7):703–706, 1987
7. Haldeman S: Spinal manipulative therapy: A status report. Clin Orthop Related Res 179:62–70, 1983
8. Mayer TG, Gathcel RJ, Kishino N, et al: Objective assessment of spine function following industrial injury. Spine 10(6):482–493, 1985
9. Meade TW, Dwyer S, Browne W, et al: Low back pain of mechanical origin: Randomised comparison of chiropractic and hospital outpatient treatment. Br Med J 300:1431–1437, 1990
10. Menard D, Stanish WD: The aging athlete. Am J Sports Med 17(2):187–196, 1991
11. McQuade KJ, Turner JA, Buchner DM: Physical fitness and chronic low back pain. Clin Orthop Related Results 233:198–204, 1988
12. Nwuga VCB: Relative therapeutic efficacy of vertebral manipulation and conventional treatment in back pain management. Am J Phys Med 61:273–278, 1983
13. Saal JA, Saal JS: Non operative treatment of herniated lumbar intervertebral disc with radiculopathy: An outcome study. Spine 14:4:431–436, 1989
14. Salter RB: The biologic concept of continuous passive motion of synovial joints. Clin Orthop Related Res 242:12–25, 1989
15. Shephard RJ: Management of exercise in the elderly. Appl Sports Sci 9(3):109–120, 1984
16. Twomey LT: A rationale for the treatment of back pain and joint pain by manual therapy. Phys Therapy 72(12):885–892, 1992
17. Twomey LT, Taylor JR: Physical Therapy of the Low Back (2nd Ed.). New York, Churchill Livingstone, 1994.
18. Waddell G: A new clinical model for the treatment of low-back pain. Spine 12(7):632–644, 1987
19. Cherkin D, Deyo R, Battie M: McKenzie therapy and manipulation have similar effects and costs and provide only marginally better outcomes than an educational booklet. N Engl J Med 339:1021, 1998
20. Mayer T, Polatin PB, Gatchel RJ: Functional restoration and other rehabilitation approaches to chronic musculoskeletal pain disability syndromes. Crit Rev Phys Rehab Med 10:209, 1998
21. Bendix AF, Bendix T, Labriola M, Boek Gaard P: Functional restoration for chronic low back pain. Spine 23:717, 1998
22. O'Sullivan P, Twomey LT, Allison G: Altered patterns of abdominal muscle activation in patients with chronic low back pain. Austral J Physiother 43:91, 1997

23. Skargren EI, Carlsson PG, Oberg BE: One year follow-up comparison of the cost effectiveness of chiropractic and physiotherapy as primary management for back pain. Spine 23:1875, 1998

24. Herzog W, Scheele D, Conway PJ: Electromyographic responses of back and limb muscles associated with spinal manipulative therapy. Spine 24:146, 1999

25. Adams G, Sim J: A survey of UK manual therapists' practice of and attitudes towards manipulation and its complications. Physiother Res Internat 3:206, 1998

26. O'Sullivan PB, Twomey LT, Allison GT: Dynamic stabilisation of the lumbar spine. Crit Rev Phys Rehab Med 9:315, 1997

10

Lumbar Spinal Stenosis

Nils Schönström

The concept of spinal stenosis was first introduced more than 4 decades ago by Verbiest, who described a radiculopathy caused by a narrowing of the lumbar spinal canal.[1,2] There had been sporadic reports earlier in the literature of a peculiar disease with radiculopathy that was cured by laminectomy and where no obvious pathology was found during surgery.[3,4,5,6] With Verbiest's reports, however, a possible explanation for these early results was given, and an interest in the narrow lumbar spinal canal slowly developed. After some time the concept of the developmental narrowing of the spinal canal was accepted. A true congenital form, with a stenosis present at birth, had been described by Sarpyener[7] in 1945. The term *developmental,* chosen by Verbiest, indicated that symptoms did not develop until the mature life of the victim. This form of stenosis was characterized by a short anteroposterior diameter between the posterior part of the vertebral body and the vertebral arch.[1] Later Epstein and collaborators[8,9] described narrowing around the spinal nerve leaving the dural sac on its way down the root canal under the pedicle and out through the intervertebral foramen. This form was called lateral stenosis, in contrast to the original form of stenosis around the dural sac and the cauda equina, which was called central stenosis.

The work of Kirkaldy-Willis and collaborators,[10] among others, has shown that a common type of stenosis occurs as a consequence of degenerative processes in the three-joint complex (Fig. 10-1), i.e., the disc and the two zygapophyseal joints holding two adjacent vertebrae together. This seemed to be a different etiology for stenosis than for the type initially described by Verbiest, and it is now common to distinguish between developmental and degenerative stenosis. In two clinical reports there has been a ratio of occurrence between degenerative and developmental stenosis of about 10 to 1.[11,12] In 1976 a group of authors broadly defined stenosis as "any type of narrowing of the spinal canal, nerve root canals, or intervertebral foramina."[13]

From an etiologic point of view, we generally agree on at least seven different forms of lumbar spinal stenosis:

1. Congenital, which is present at birth.[7]
2. Developmental, with a genetic disposition presenting itself with symptoms in adult life,[1,2,14] the most pronounced being a consequence of achondroplasia.[15,16,17]

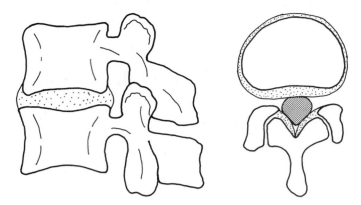

Fig. 10-1 The three-joint complex consists of the joints holding two adjacent vertebrae together, specifically the disc, which is the joint between the vertebral bodies, and the two facet joints between the posterior structures.

3. Degenerative, as a result of degenerative processes in the disc and facet joints.[8,9,10,18]

4. Metabolic, as a consequence of pathologic changes in the bone substance, e.g., Paget's disease of the bone,[19] fluorosis, and diffuse idiopathic skeletal hyperostosis.[20]

5. Iatrogenic, usually postlaminectomy.

6. Posttraumatic, with a distorted anatomy of the spinal canal as a consequence of trauma.

7. Miscellaneous, such as epidural lipomatosis[21] and cysts of the ligamentum flavum.[22]

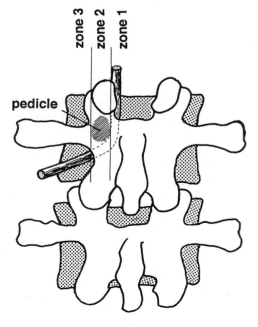

Fig. 10-2 The root canal containing the spinal nerve can be divided into three different zones in relation to the pedicle. (Adapted from Andersson GBJ, McNeill TW: Lumbar Spine Syndromes. Springer-Verlag, Vienna, 1989.)

From a morphologic point of view, lumbar spinal stenosis can be divided into central stenosis, engaging the nerve roots of the cauda equina; and lateral stenosis, disturbing the spinal nerve in the lateral recess, the nerve root canal, or intervertebral foramina. Andersson and McNeill[23] clarified the lateral anatomy in this aspect by dividing this region into three different zones related to the pedicle, which is an important landmark during surgery (Fig. 10-2). Zone 1 is the lateral recess, which is the area ventral to the superior articular process and medial to the pedicle. Zone 2 is below the pedicle, and zone 3 is lateral to the pedicle. It is questionable whether a mechanical disturbance of the spinal nerve in zone 3 should be categorized as stenosis.

PATHOANATOMY

Developmental stenosis is characterized by a short pedicle and thick lamina and usually presents at multiple levels. Its most pronounced form is seen in achondroplastic dwarfs, where it is a common finding. The stenosis in achondroplasia is different in that there is also a short interpedicular distance.[15] In the developmental form of stenosis, the emphasis is on an encroachment on the nervous structures by the skeletal structures. The central stenosis affects the roots of the cauda equina and possibly the spinal nerve in the lateral recess (zone 1). According to Verbiest, an anteroposterior diameter below 12 mm but over 10 mm is a relative stenosis in which other problems, such as a herniated disc, will lead to symptoms. If the diameter is below 10 mm, there is an absolute stenosis capable of causing symptoms by itself.[14] A few studies of skeletal collections show that these small dimensions are rare, indicating that developmental stenosis might be a rare disease.[24, 25] In Eisenstein's review of 433 skeletons, a diameter of 13 mm or smaller was present in 6.3%.

In the degenerative type of stenosis, the skeletal dimensions of each vertebra might well be within normal limits.[12] Instead, changes in the disc, ligamentum flavum, and the zygapophyseal joints lead to narrowing of the spinal canal. These changes can lead to both a central and a lateral stenosis as defined previously. These two situations will be discussed separately although it is very common that central and lateral stenosis occur together.

The central stenosis in this group has three different components, often resulting in a typical trefoil shape of the spinal canal. This trefoil shape can be present in the skeletal structure as well as the result of a deformation of the dural sac by the surrounding soft tissues. A bulging or herniated disc can give an impression in the dural sac from its anterior aspect. This can also be the result of a bony ridge in the posterior part of the vertebral body. From the posterolateral side, on both sides of the midline, enlarged zygapophyseal joints covered by a thick ligamentum flavum are causing concave impressions (Fig. 10-3). Another common contributing factor in this category is an anterior or posterior slip of one vertebra upon the next. The pars interarticularis is often intact despite the slip, and the phenomenon is referred to as pseudolisthesis or degenerative olisthesis/retrolisthesis.[18] The slip can

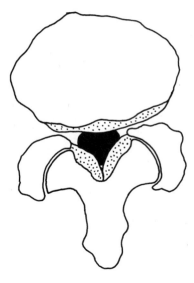

Fig. 10-3   The typical deformation of the dural sac at disc height is trefoiled.

in itself be sufficient to cause stenosis or it can significantly contribute to the deformation of the dural sac described previously as a result of soft tissue encroachment.

In the lateral type of stenosis, degenerative changes and an enlargement in one zygapophyseal joint can lead to encroachment on two consecutive spinal nerves.[26] The encroachment can occur in either the nerve leaving the dural sac in the segment above as it passes out through the intervertebral foramen, where the affected joint is the caudal limitation of the root canal (zone 2 related to the pedicle above), or the next spinal nerve as it lies in the lateral recess (zone 1 of the next pedicle) (see Fig. 10-4).

Metabolic stenosis is seen as a result of postmature growth of bone resulting in a central stenosis, a process similar to that occurring in develop-

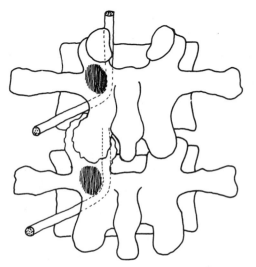

Fig. 10-4   Arthritic changes in one facet joint can lead to impingement on two different spinal nerves. The upper nerve in zone 3 and the lower nerve in zone 1.

mental stenosis. Iatrogenic stenosis is caused by previous surgery, usually resulting in three different categories of problems:

1. New bone formation from raw bone surfaces after, for example, laminectomy, or from posterior fusions.
2. Postlaminectomy membranes or cystic formations as liquor cysts.
3. Instability caused by, for example, laminectomy with a rapid progress of degeneration and accentuated slipping between adjacent vertebrae (pseudolisthesis).

PATHOPHYSIOLOGY

The Dynamic Concept in Degenerative Stenosis

The short description in the previous chapter gives a static picture of the basic changes leading to a degenerative stenosis. However, to better understand the pathophysiologic description to follow, it is helpful to adapt a more dynamic concept of degenerative stenosis.

The function of the three-joint complex, disc and facet joints, is to permit movements between the vertebrae. Normally this is achieved with the space in the spinal canal and the nerve root canals kept within a sufficient size to accommodate the nervous structures inside it. We have shown in an in vitro experiment that when a lumbar spine specimen was moved from full flexion to full extension, the size of the spinal canal seen as a transverse area was diminished by an average of 40 mm.[2, 27] The same magnitude of change in the transverse area of the spinal canal was found after a shift from 200 Newton of axial distraction to 200 Newton of axial compression. During the axial loading the spine was held in a neutral position. Because this is approximately equivalent to a shift in axial load of about 40 kg, the weight of a full-grown torso, it might represent the difference in size of the spinal canal if a subject is lying down as compared with standing up. These changes are well-tolerated with a normal canal, but as will be discussed later it can have significant implications in a spine with a narrow canal.

It has been claimed that true hypertrophy of the ligamentum flavum is extremely rare.[28] This has lead to the assumption that this ligament does not contribute to a central stenosis. However, several authors have claimed that it has been their impression during surgery that hypertrophy of the ligamentum flavum does play a role in the compression of the dural sac.[29, 30] In another experiment, we have shown that the difference in thickness of the ligamentum flavum, fully relaxed and distracted under 8 kg of load, is as an average of 2 mm.[31] This is explained by the elastic behavior of the ligamentum flavum, which can contain as much as 80% elastic fibers.[32] Thus, if the ligament becomes fully relaxed in extension, the resulting thickening of a normal ligament can contribute significantly to a further constriction of an already narrow canal, even if there is no hypertrophy.

The situation of the spinal nerve in the lateral recess (zone 1) is somewhat more static during changes of posture and load. An increase in disc bulge backward can increase the pressure on the spinal nerve because the proximal part of zone 1 is at disc height. However, a few millimeters further distally the vertebral body is the anterior limitation of this space, and here the dimensions are constant during shifts in load or posture. However, under the pedicle in zone 2, great changes occur when the spine is moved from flexion to extension. In extension the superior articular facet moves upward, toward the pedicle where the spinal nerve is situated at the very top of the foramen. In the normal situation the foramen is large enough, filled with fat and vascular structures together with the nerve, to accommodate for these changes. With a degenerative enlargement of the articular process, the difference between extension and flexion might mean the difference between encroachment and no encroachment on that spinal nerve. Also, when an axial load is applied on the spine for a longer time the creep in the disc results in a reduced disc height. The consequence of this is also a migration of the superior facet upward toward the pedicle with a risk of nerve impingement of an enlarged facet joint.

A more dynamic view on the size of the spinal canal and nerve root canals is the key to understanding why changes in posture and load are possible without problems in a normal canal and can lead to symptoms when a canal gets narrow. It also provides one explanation for the fluctuating symptoms that are so characteristic of lumbar spinal stenosis.

Experimental Data on the Size of the Canal and the Cauda Equina

Various measurements have been used to describe the available space in the lumbar spinal canal. The most common has been the anteroposterior diameter as described previously under developmental stenosis. Interpedicular distance has been proposed but not generally accepted, with the exception of stenosis in achondroplasia. The transverse area of the spinal canal, as outlined by the skeletal structures, has been used,[33] and this area will be reduced in cases of developmental stenosis. It is much less valuable in degenerative stenosis because the skeletal measurements could be normal, despite severe stenosis, as has been mentioned earlier. Based on a morphologic study on patients with central stenosis confirmed during surgery, we have found the transverse area of the dural sac to be the best measurement confirming a central stenosis on transverse sections of the lumbar spine (Fig. 10-5).[12]

What about the size of the neural elements to be accommodated in the canal? In two in vitro experiments we recorded this size expressed as the transverse area of the dural sac and its content.[34, 35] A carefully calibrated circular clamp was placed around the dural sac at the L3 level. A thin pressure-recording catheter was placed among the roots of the cauda equina inside the clamp. The clamp was tightened until the first sign of a pressure increase among the roots. The transverse area where this first pressure increase was noted was called the critical size of the dural sac. The critical size, at the L3 level, was surprisingly constant around 75 mm^2, even among different individuals with a standard deviation around 15 mm^2. The experiment was re-

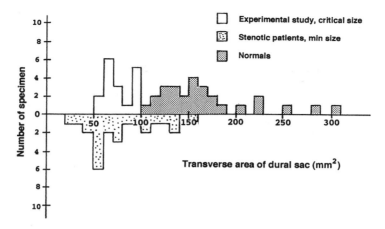

Fig. 10-5 The transverse area of the dural sac in one clinical and two experimental studies.

peated with a different clamp, a different pressure-recording system, and a different dissection technique to reach the dura, but the result was still of the same magnitude (see Fig. 10-5). To reach a further pressure increase of about 50 mm Hg among the roots, the clamp had to be tightened another 19% on average from the critical size, and to reach 100 mm Hg the area had to be reduced by an average of 26% from the critical size.

We concluded that the size of the spinal canal varies considerably among different individuals. However, when it comes to the size of its neural content the variation in size is small, and we found it possible to discuss the presence of central stenosis using the size of the dural sac on CT scans based on our experimental data. When it comes to lateral stenosis, no similar experiments have been done and one has to rely on an evaluation of the available space for the nerve on magnetic resonance imaging (MRI). Root blocks are sometimes used to confirm the diagnosis.[36]

The Effect of Pressure on Nerve Roots

The pathophysiologic response to acute mechanical pressure on the nerve roots of the cauda equina has been investigated by Olmarker and collaborators[37] in porcine experiments. A translucent pressure chamber was attached to the spine of the pig after laminectomy under general anesthesia. An acute pressure was applied to the nerve roots, using a balloon inside the chamber. Under a stepwise increase in pressure, the effect on the microcirculation of the roots was studied through the translucent chamber. The average occlusion pressure for the arterioles was slightly below the systolic pressure. It was also concluded that the flow in the capillary network was affected by venous stasis. Such venous stasis could start at a low pressure increase of only 5 to 10 mm Hg. A retrograde stasis could be responsible for disturbances of the nerve function already during venous congestion. Studying gradual decompression after initial acute compression revealed that the pressure levels had to go down to zero to get a full restitution of the blood flow. The possibility of edema formation and blocking of the axonal transport are other mechanisms that could add to the disturbance of the nerve function.

In an anatomic study on cadaver spines, Hoyland and collaborators[38] found a correlation between venous stasis in the intervertebral foramen and interstitial fibrosis in the corresponding spinal nerve. It seems possible that a chronic stasis can lead to edema, as seen in the experimental study by Olmarker et al,[37] and over time this edema could be transformed into fibrosis. Thus the fibrosis seen by Hoyland et al[38] was interpreted as the end result of chronic nerve damage.

A Model for the Encroachment on the Nerve Roots of the Cauda Equina

If we put the experimental information together, it is possible to create a hypothetic model for the pathogenesis of central stenosis of the degenerative type based on a dynamic concept. The normal spinal canal has a reserve capacity regarding the space inside the canal, a concept introduced by Weisz and Lee.[39] However, the more narrow the canal, the smaller the reserve capacity and the closer one gets to the point of the critical size. This occurs in most instances at the disc level, where the canal is made up of the two adjacent vertebrae (Fig. 10-6). The deformation of the dural sac is usually trefoiled (see Fig. 10-3). Starting the discussion from the anterior aspect of the canal, a bulging disc can easily make an impression of 2 mm as a result of axial load, based on the work of Reuber at al.[40] The posterolateral impressions are made by the enlarged facet joints, and from a dynamic point of view the encroachment is reinforced by the thickening of the ligamentum flavum, relaxed in extension, with a possible further impression of 2 mm. In a model like the one in Fig. 10-7, it has been calculated that an impression from the anterior aspect of 2 mm (disc) and 2 mm from the posterolateral sides (ligamentum flavum) will reduce the area of the dural sac around 40%, if the undeformed area is circular with 10 mm diameter.[41] Thus when the canal has reached these small dimensions (the critical size)

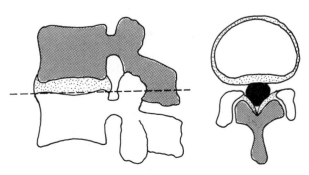

Fig. 10-6   At disc height the spinal canal is made up of two adjacent vertebrae.

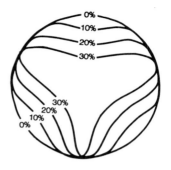

Fig. 10-7 The trefoil deformation of the initially circular dural sac can be graded in percent of the initial diameter whereby the magnitude of the deformation can be discussed.

the normal changes in disc bulge and thickness of the ligamentum flavum can reduce the available space considerably as a result of axial loading or extension of the spine. This was also confirmed in our experiment with spine specimens in various postures and axial loads, as described earlier.[27] If the cauda equina already has reached the critical size in flexion, when the canal size is at its maximum, a further reduction of the available space by 40% as a result of extension could easily result in an acute pressure increase of over 100 mm Hg among the nerve roots of the cauda equina.[35] The work of Ohlmarker et al[37] showed that this could lead to pronounced acute disturbances of nerve function. The chronic effects on the nerve roots are more unpredictable, and a certain adaptation of the nervous structures to a narrow surrounding is possible. In our experiments with acute constriction of the nerve roots, we saw a creep downward with time of the initial pressure increase if the constriction was left constant.[35] One interpretation of this phenomenon could be that it was a result of a deformation over time of the nervous structures as a consequence of the sustained compression. However, with the dynamic concept described above it is justifiable to discuss also acute changes in size on top of more long-standing chronic deformations.

THE CLINICAL PICTURE

Clinical History

Spinal stenosis can be seen in all age groups, but the main category is over 60 years of age. Many patients with lumbar spinal stenosis have a long history of low back pain with typical problems during their third and fourth decade of life, as has been described by Kirkaldy-Willis,[26] including mechanical back pain and disc disease with sciatica. After a period of less-pronounced problems in the fifth decade, the symptoms of spinal stenosis typically appear with a slow onset in the sixth decade.

Although back pain is a common symptom, the clinical picture is dominated more by various disturbances in the lower extremities. This disturbance can be pain, but is more often described as discomfort in terms of numbness, paresthesia, and weakness. Often the patient has difficulty in clearly expressing the quality of the symptoms. Together with the sometimes-bizarre nature of the symptoms, this can result in the patient being accused of malingering.

The well-known symptom of neurogenic claudication is the unique feature of the disease and needs special attention when taking the history of the patient. The symptom is usually brought on by walking and relieved by rest. However, the typical feature is the influence of posture on the physical performance. In this aspect the neurogenic claudication differs from the claudication seen in peripheral arterial disease. Extension aggravates the symptoms whereas flexion facilitates the physical performance and diminishes the symptoms. Thus walking bent forward increases the maximum walking distance.[42] Riding a bike is often possible for considerable distances,[43] and leaning forward or squatting while resting relieves the discomfort faster. There is also one specific variant of the clinical pictures of the disease in which the symptoms are brought on not so much by walking or physical exercise as by the mere extension of the back, even when standing still. This led Wilson[44] to define two types of characteristic symptoms, one postural type and one claudicant type. He also stated that often motor symptoms would precede sensory changes, leading to "drop attacks" where the patient during walking gets a sudden weakness, leading to a fall. A more infrequent symptom is a chronic cauda equina syndrome with genital pain and disturbances.

The Physical Examination

The physical examination follows the same principles as for all other problems of the lumbar spine with disturbances in the legs. A few points deserve special emphasis:

1. The patient's ability to walk and to do other forms of physical performance and the influence of posture on these abilities. Often the objective findings during a physical examination are few at rest but could be more pronounced immediately after physical exercise or a period of prolonged lumbar extension.

2. The presence or absence of arterial disease. Palpation of the abdominal aorta as well as auscultation for bruits in the iliac or femoral arteries is essential. Palpation of peripheral pulses and, when necessary, recording of ankle blood pressure with doppler technique is most helpful.

3. Hip disease as degenerative arthritis is a common differential diagnosis in this age category, and examination of these joints is mandatory.[45]

Because the typical patient with lumbar spinal stenosis usually has few pathologic signs during the physical examination, the great importance of the examination is to exclude other serious diseases such as spinal tumors, neurologic problems with demyelinating or peripheral nervous disease, hip disease, and vascular problems. One should also bear in mind that, in this age category, it is quite possible to have combinations of for example spinal stenosis and hip disease or vascular disease.

Morphologic Examination of the Spinal Canal

A morphologic examination of the spinal canal is essential if the diagnosis has to be confirmed. On a plain x-ray of the lumbar spine the morphologic prerequisites for the disease can be identified. It is also important to look for signs of destructive skeletal processes such as metastasis of malignant tumors or infections. If any form of surgical intervention is contemplated, or if other neurologic disease is suspected, a more detailed analysis of the spinal canal and nerve root canals has to be instituted.

Since Verbiest's initial description of the syndrome, myelography has been the method of choice for analysis of the dimensions of the canal and to visualize any encroachment on the nerve roots. This investigation has provided us with substantial knowledge on the dynamic behavior of the spinal canal under normal and stenotic conditions, as well as a very good overview of the whole lumbar spine.[46, 47] Introduction of modern imaging techniques such as computed tomography (CT scanning) and MRI have now given us tools to investigate the spinal canal and the nerve roots both as an overview and in great detail without the disadvantage of an invasive procedure. Therefore, in most centers today, myelography is not part of the standard morphologic evaluation of lumbar spinal stenosis and is used only under special circumstances to capture dynamic changes.

Computed tomography (CT scans) provides cuts perpendicular to the long axis of the spine, with excellent opportunities for a detailed analysis of the size and shape of the spinal canal and nerve root canals. With an appropriate window setting of the machine, it is usually possible to visualize encroachment on the nervous structures by the soft tissues, such as the disc and ligamentum flavum. It is easy to appreciate the importance of the soft tissues in this respect by looking at Fig. 10-8, which is a tracing from the CT scans from a patient with a degenerative central stenosis. Under certain circumstances the analysis concerning the soft tissues can be very difficult on CT scans, for example, with very obese patients or after previous surgery in the area. In patients with previous surgery in the area, MRI is the method of choice.

In terms of central stenosis the measurements of the critical size of the dural sac can be helpful in establishing whether there is a prerequisite for a stenosis. However, CT is still not suitable for dynamic investigations, and one has to remember that the patient is lying down, taking the axial load of the spine. Furthermore, to help the patient to lie still so that distortion from movements can be avoided, the patient is told to assume the most comfortable position. This means that he/she tries not to provoke the nerve roots so that in borderline cases the diagnosis can be missed. These deductions can be drawn from the concept of dynamic stenosis discussed above.

The development in the field of MRI has been tremendous, and the potential for further development is even greater. Although CT scanning is generally believed to be better in depicting the skeletal structures, MRI will give a detailed analysis of the soft tissues, and it has the advantage of giving both overview and detailed analysis along the axis of the spine and perpendicular to it. Surprisingly, one of the major contraindications for MRI is claustro-

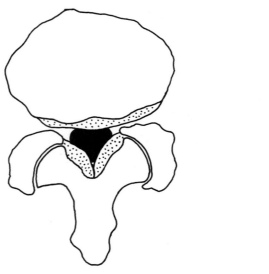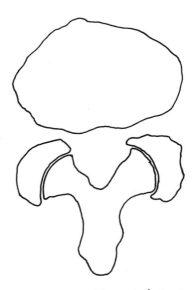

Fig. 10-8   Tracings from preoperative CT scans from a patient with central stenosis. The tracings are made with and without the soft tissues to emphasize the importance of the soft tissues in the deformation of the dural sac.

phobia. Others are metal implants in the patient, especially cardiac pacemakers. MRI has not been suitable for dynamic investigations in different postures or axial loads. However, in recent works by Willén at al[48] a method has been developed to axially load the spine with the patient still lying down. The load is applied on the shoulders using a special vest and registered as the force on a footplate. This is done to capture the dynamic events of a spinal stenosis described above, both regarding central and lateral stenosis. MRI has made a significant contribution to the analysis of lateral stenosis, with great detail of the intervertebral foramen. Together with the good overview this has made MRI the routine method for evaluation of spinal stenosis in many centers. With roots blocks, as has been described by Van Ackerveken,[36] the affected root in lateral stenosis can be confirmed. This is of importance in planning surgery so that the surgical trauma can be kept to a minimum.

The Diagnostic Synthesis

The diagnostic analysis is based on the clinical history. The clinical examination reinforces the diagnosis, mainly by excluding other reasons for the symptoms but also by helping to decide the level in lateral stenosis with rhizopathy. The morphologic evaluation of the spinal canal confirms the diagnosis and forms the basis for the planning of surgical intervention, if that is contemplated. One cannot warn too much against relying only on the morphologic analysis. A narrow lumbar canal without an appropriate clinical history does not justify the diagnosis of spinal stenosis! Even with an appropriate history and a narrow canal, it is absolutely essential to exclude other reasons for the symptoms, such as neurologic disturbances of other kinds, hip disease, and vascular problems. Certainly, if major lumbar surgery is contemplated with its attendant risks, it must be based on a sound clinical diagnosis and not just a morphologic confirmation of a narrow canal.

TREATMENT

As with most forms of low back pain, with or without sciatica, treatment is based on a correct clinical diagnosis and starts with conservative measures. A mild degree of numbness or weakness combined with a gait where the patient prefers to walk somewhat bent forward, is considered by many people to be a natural consequence of a high age. However, quality of life is an important issue, and even a mild form of lumbar spinal stenosis is often a reason for a medical consultation. Usually it is a well-motivated anxiety about possible serious disease, or a rapid deterioration in physical ability that is the reason for the visit. Therefore it is important, even in the milder forms, to make reasonable efforts to secure the diagnosis and exclude more serious disease. If this is done, sometimes the information about the spinal stenosis, and some advice on how to live with it, is all that is needed. However, if the symptoms progress, a more active strategy is required. Considering that the symptoms are brought on by encroachment on the cauda equina or the spinal nerves by the walls of the spinal canal or nerve root canals, it could seem natural to contemplate surgical intervention at an early stage when the symptoms have reached a certain level. However, as will be mentioned further on, surgery for this disease is not without risks. Furthermore, not all patients get relief from an operation, and there is a risk of recurrence. It is therefore well worth discussing the conservative, nonoperative alternatives as well as the surgical ones.

It has been shown by Johnsson and collaborators[49] that even with clinical and radiologic signs of lumbar spinal stenosis the prognosis was not bad, even when surgery was not performed and the patients were followed for at least 4 years. The reasons for this are still obscure; one assumes that the degeneration responsible for the stenosis is likely to progress with time. It emphasizes the importance of knowing the natural history of a disease, particularly when major surgery is contemplated. Surgery has a well-established position in the treatment of spinal stenosis, and when symptoms are severe and progressive, surgery is often the best solution. However, there is almost always time to consider a period of conservative treatment and to evaluate its effectiveness.

Principles of a Conservative Strategy

Bedrest and Reduced Physical Activity

This should be contemplated only in acute situations with severe back pain and sciatica. It is important to bear in mind that these are often patients at a relatively high age where inactivity implicates special risks. Bedrest for a maximum of 2 to 3 days can be an effective way of diminishing the pain of sciatica. The reason can be a reduced disc pressure, an increased size of the spinal canal with reduction of the irritation of the nerve roots, and increased blood flow after a reduction of the pressure on the roots. However, with this kind of treatment, reduced physical capacity and mental inactivity comes rapidly. It is in that respect a potentially dangerous treatment but can be effective if the pain is severe.

Corsets and Braces

The motive for this kind of treatment is to limit the motion of the different segments of the lumbar spine, thereby achieving a symptomatic relief. Whether or not a reduction in motion really is achieved by these devices can be argued, but in some cases they provide relief. In a study from 1985, Willner et al[50] showed a positive effect of a rigid plastic brace on the symptoms of spinal stenosis and spondylolisthesis. A rationale could be that it helps to avoid extension, thereby avoiding some of the insult on the nervous structures. It should be noted that they used a special jig to custom-fit the brace to the patient so that the best possible posture for symptomatic relief was obtained. This protocol also helped to exclude patients not suitable for treatment with a brace. If this could be an alternative to the short bed rest described above, the hazards of bed rest could be avoided.

Physical Exercise

Different forms of physical exercise programs have for many years been part of the standard repertoire in the treatment of low back pain. Two main reasons have been advocated. First, to strengthen the muscles controlling the movements of the lower back, thereby achieving a better control of the motion segment; second, to increase the feeling of comfort and physical security that a general exercise program can give. Sometimes this has been claimed to be the result of an increased level of endorphins reducing the pain level.

Because this is mainly a geriatric clientele, exercise programs should be individualized and monitored to avoid an increase in pain level as a result of the program. As has been mentioned, the symptoms are usually aggravated by extension, and in my opinion extension exercises should be avoided in spinal stenosis. Riding a properly adjusted bicycle is usually a good way of getting proper exercise and also gives a method of alternative transportation when walking is difficult. Restoring and strengthening the physical function while educating the patients how to use their bodies to avoid irritation of the nerve roots is certainly worthwhile.

Drug Therapy

In an acute exacerbation of back pain with sciatica, drug therapy is often a good alternative if the nerve roots or spinal nerves have been irritated by repeated mechanical and circulatory insult. According to the work of Cornefjord and collaborators edema and inflammation in the nervous structures is part of the disturbance caused by acute compression, especially in combination with a disc herniation.[51] A period of 3 to 4 weeks of anti-inflammatory treatment, usually with nonsteroidal antiinflammatory drugs (NSAIDs), can sometimes reduce the symptoms. If a reduction of an edema could be achieved, the space needed for the nerve roots would be smaller. This is important in the case of a narrow canal, where the dynamic factors described above play an important role. As always, one must make sure that there are no contraindications to that form of treatment.

It is usually a good policy to use simple analgesics such as paracetamol instead of more potent drugs that carry a risk of making the patient dependent on the drug. Spinal stenosis is a more-or-less chronic condition, and long-standing medication with analgesics is always a problem and should be instituted only together with other conservative treatment modalities and be carefully monitored with very precise instructions on dose and length of medication from the treating physician.

Back Schools and Other Education

Knowledge about the disease and the mechanisms behind the symptoms helps the patient to deal with the problems of the disease. Whether this information is delivered by the treating physician, the physiotherapist, or in organized form as a back school is not the main issue. In my experience the physiotherapist has the best ability to give this kind of information, which can be done under very practical forms together with an individualized physical exercise program. Sometimes a geriatric patient responds better to individual instruction, even if group exercises could be more stimulating. The goal is to make the patient aware of how to deal with symptoms already existing and how to avoid acute exacerbations by adjusting life-style, without reducing activity level or quality of life if possible.

The conservative treatment strategy is based on whether the patient presents during an acute exacerbation or not. If acute problems are present, a few days of bedrest combined with a suitable drug treatment could be a good start. If it is not an acute problem, a change in life-style to avoid harmful postures, combined with an individualized and carefully monitored exercise program, should be instituted. If necessary a period with a rigid brace, individually fitted according to the principles of Willner et al,[50] could be of help. A good conservative program together with some expectancy often leads to a significant improvement.

Surgical Alternatives

If conservative treatment fails in achieving a tolerable level of discomfort or progressive neourogical deficit threatens the activities of daily life for the patient, surgical treatment can be contemplated.

The aim is to relieve the discrepancy in size between the spinal canal and the size of the neural content to be accommodated within it. This is achieved by removing certain parts of the wall of the spinal canal or nerve root canals. The main procedures are laminectomy in central stenosis or laminotomy, in which the whole or parts of the lamina are removed. After that the ligamentum flavum is removed. In a few instances the disc is decompressed by a discectomy. There are variants in the procedures in which the laminae are merely opened and hinged outward on a lateral attachment and left in that position. It has also been suggested that the lateral portion of the ligamentum flavum should be saved and a decompression of the skeletal structures carried out posterior to it, to provide a soft tissue barrier between the raw bone surfaces and the nerve roots. To achieve a good decompression it is often necessary to sacrifice the inner third of the facet joint.

In lateral stenosis a decompression by foraminotomy has been the method of choice. Various forms of undercuts, taking only the most anterior part of the superior articular facet, have been developed to save as much as possible of the zygapophyseal joint and avoid secondary instability.

It is common to perform a combination of both types of procedures. In both cases there is a delicate balance between achieving a good decompression without causing significant instability. Secondary instability is a common finding, and therefore various types of fusions of the decompressed segment have to be considered. The development of transpedicular screw fixation has provided the surgeon with many alternatives for a mechanical stability during the phase of developing a solid bony fusion of the stabilized segment. In cases with radiologic signs of potential instability, such as olisthesis, fusion is usually recommended.

Despite the combination of decompression and fusion there is always a risk for a recurrence of the symptoms after surgery. Two common factors are new bone formation from the raw surfaces after resection and a progression of the degenerative changes often responsible for the disease in the first place. Postsurgical instability can significantly contribute to these problems. However, with a successful outcome of the surgery, there is a good relief of the symptoms with a dramatic improvement in the quality of life for the patient.

REFERENCES

1. Verbiest H: A radicular syndrome from developmental narrowing of the lumbar vertebral canal. J Bone Joint Surg 36-B:230–237, 1954
2. Verbiest H: Further experiences on the pathological influence of developmental narrowness of the bony lumbar vertebral canal. J Bone Joint Surg 37-B:576–583, 1955
3. Baily P, Casamajor L: Osteoarthritis of the spine as a cause of compression of the spinal cord and its roots; with report of 5 cases. J Nerv Ment Dis 38:588–609, 1911
4. Elsberg CA: Experiences in spinal surgery. Obsevations upon 60 laminectomies for spinal disease, Surg Gynecol Obstet 16:117–132, 1913
5. Kennedy F, Elsberg CA, Lambert CI: A peculiar and undescribed disease of the nerves of the cauda equina. Am J Med Sci 147:645–667, 1914
6. Sachs B, Fraenkel J: Progressive ankylotic rigidity of the spine. J Nerv Ment Dis 27:1–15, 1900

7. Sarpyener MA: Congenital stricture of the spinal canal. J Bone Joint Surg 27:70–79, 1945
8. Epstein JA, Epstein BS, Lavine LS, et al: Sciatica caused by nerve root entrapment in the lateral recess: The superior facet syndrome. J Neurosurg 36:584–589, 1972
9. Epstein JA, Epstein BS, Lavine LS, et al: Lumbar nerve root compression at the intervertebral foramina caused by arthritis of the posterior facets. J Neurosurg 39:362–369, 1973
10. Kirkaldy-Willis WH, Wedge JH, Yong-Hing K, et al: Pathology and pathogenesis of lumbar spondylosis and stenosis. Spine 3:319–328, 1978
11. Getty CJM: Lumbar spinal stenosis. The clinical spectrum and results of operation. J Bone Joint Surg 62-B:481–485, 1980
12. Schönström NSR, Bolender NFr, Spengler DM: The pathomorphology of spinal stenosis as seen on CT scans of the lumbar spine. Spine 10:806–811, 1985.
13. Arnoldi CC, Brodsky AE, Cauchoix J, et al: Lumbar spinal stenosis and nerve root entrapment syndromes: Definition and classification. Clin Othop Rel Res 115:4–5, 1976.
14. Verbiest H: Neurogenic intermittent claudication in cases with absolute and relative stenosis of the lumbar vertebral canal (ASLC and RSLC), in cases with narrow lumbar intervertebral foramina, and in cases with both entities. Clin Neurosurg 20:204–214, 1973.
15. Gelman MI: Cauda equina compression in acromegaly. Radiology 112:357–360, 1974.
16. Lutter LD, Lonstein JE, Winter RB, et al: Anatomy of the achondroplastic lumbar canal. Clin Othop Rel Res 126:139–142, 1977.
17. Lutter LD, Langer LO: Neurologic symptoms in achondroplastic dwarfs—surgical treatment. J Bone Joint Surg 59-A:87–92, 1977.
18. MacNab I: Spondylolisthesis with an intact neural arch: The so-called pseudo-spondylolisthesis. J Bone Joint Surg 32-B:325–333, 1950.
19. Weisz GM: Lumbar spinal canal stenosis in Paget's disease. Spine 8:192–198, 1983.
20. Johnsson KE, Petersson H, Wollheim FA, et al: Diffuse idiopathic skeletal hyperostosis (DISH) causing spinal stenosis and sudden paraplegia. J Rheumatol 10:784–789, 1983
21. Lipson SJ, Haheedy MH, Kaplan MM, et al: Spinal stenosis caused by lipomatosis in Cushing's syndrome. N Engl J Med 302:36, 1980.
22. Abdullah AF, Chambers RW, Daut DP: Lumbar nerve root compression by synovial cysts of the ligamentum flavum. Report of four cases. J Neurosurg 60:617–620, 1984.
23. Andersson GBJ, McNeill TW: Lumbar Spine Syndromes. Springer-Verlag, Vienna, 1989
24. Eisenstein S: The morphometry and pathological anatomy of the lumbar spine in South African Negros and Caucasoids with specific reference to spinal stenosis. J Bone Joint Surg 59-B:173–180, 1977.
25. Postachini F, Ripani M, Carpano S: Morphometry of the lumbar vertebrae. Clin Orthop Rel Res 172:296–303, 1983.
26. Kirkaldy-Willis WH: Managing Low Back Pain. Churchill-Livingstone, New York, 1983.
27. Schönström NSR, Lindahl S, Willén J, et al: Dynamic changes in the dimensions of the lumbar spinal canal. J Orthop Res 7:155–121, 1989
28. Yong-Hing K, Reilly J, Kirkaldy-Willis WH: The ligamentum flavum. Spine 1:226–234, 1976

29. Towne EB, Reichert FL: Compression of the lumbosacral roots of the spinal cord by thickened ligamenta flava. Ann Surg 94:327–336, 1931

30. Yamada H, Ohya M, Okada T, et al: Intermittent cauda equina compression due to narrow spinal canal. J Neurosurg 37:83–88, 1972

31. Schönström NSR, Hansson TH: Thickness of the human ligamentum flavum as a function of load. An in vitro experimental study. Clin Biomechan 6:19–24, 1991

32. Nachemson AL, Evans JH: Some mechanical properties of the third human lumbar interlaminar ligament. J Biomech 1:211–220, 1968

33. Ullrich CG, Binet EF, Sanecki MG, et al: Quantitative assessment of the lumbar spinal canal by computed tomography. Radiology 134:137–143, 1980

34. Schönström NSR, Bolender NFr, Spengler DM, et al: Pressure changes within the cauda equina following constriction of the dural sac. An in vitro experimental study. Spine 9:604–607, 1984.

35. Schönström NSR, Hansson TH: Pressure changes following constriction of the cauda equina. An experimental study in situ. Spine 13:385–388, 1988.

36. Van Akkerveken PF: Lateral stenosis of the lumbar spine. A new diagnostic test and its influence on management of patients with pain only. Thesis. University of Utrecht, 1989

37. Olmarker K: Spinal nerve root compression. Nutrition and function of the porcine cauda equina compressed in vivo. Acta Orthop Scand Suppl 242:1–27, 1991

38. Hoyland JA, Freemont AJ, Jayson MIV: Intervertebral foramen venous obstruction. A cause of periradicular fibrosis. Spine 14:558–568, 1989

39. Weisz GM, Lee P: Spinal canal stenosis. Concept of spinal reserve capacity: Radiologic measurements and clinical applications. Clin Orthop Rel Res 179:134–140, 1983

40. Reuber M, Schultz A, Denis F, et al: Bulging of lumbar intervertebral disks. J Biomech Engineering 104:187–192, 1982

41. Schönström NSR: The narrow lumbar canal and the size of the cauda equina in man. (Thesis). University of Göteborg, 1988.

42. Dyck P: The stoop-test in lumbar entrapment radiculopathy. Spine 4:89–92, 1979

43. Dyck P, Doyle JB: "Bicycle test" of Van Gelderen in diagnosis of intermittent cauda equina compression syndrome. Case report. J Neurosurg 46:667–670, 1977

44. Wilson CB, Ehni G, Grollmus J: Meurogenic intermittent claudication. Clin Neurosurg 18:62–85, 1971

45. Bohl WR, Steffe AD: Lumbar spinal stenosis. A cause of continued pain and disability in patients after total hip arthroplasty. Spine 4:168–173, 1979

46. Schumacher M: Die Belastungsmyelographie. Fortschr Röntgensrt 145:642–648, 1986

47. Sortland O, Magnaes B, Hauge T: Functional myelography with metrizamide in the diagnosis of lumbar spinal stenosis. Acta Radiol Suppl 355:42–54, 1977

48. Willen J, Danielsson B, Gaulitz A, et al: Dynamic effects on the lumbar spinal canal. Spine 24:2968–2976, 1997

49. Johnsson KE, Rosén I, Udén A: The Natural Course of Lumbar Spinal Stenosis. Clin Orthop Rel Res 279:82–86, 1992

50. Willner S: Effect of a rigid brace on back pain. Acta Orthop Scand 56:40–42, 1985

51. Cornefjord M, Katsuhiko S, Olmarker K, et al: A model for chronic nerve root compression studies. Spine 9:946–957, 1997

11

Control of Low Back Pain in the Workplace Using an Ergonomic Approach

Margaret I. Bullock
Joanne E. Bullock-Saxton

Epidemiologic studies show that lifetime prevalence of low back pain can be as high as 60% to 80%,[1,2] and it is not surprising that low back pain (LBP) is the most common cause of disability for people under the age of 45, accounting for almost one in every five injuries and illnesses in the work place.[3] Workers in many occupations complain of tension in the shoulders and in the upper and lower back, which interferes with their workplace performance.

Although most people with low back disorders return to function within 4 weeks, it is likely that 5% to 10% will have pain persisting for 6 months or more. Nachemson & Bigos[4] advise that it is this group with chronic low back pain that accounts for 80% of the total cost of treating the disorder. This group also has the worst functional outcome.

According to Rowe,[5] 85% of LBP sufferers have intermittent attacks of disabling pain every 3 months to 3 years and, as work absence is often related to industrial injury, this high incidence is costly to industry. Yu et al[6] have drawn attention to the economic consequences of LBP. According to some estimates, in a plant with 1000 employees, an absenteeism rate of 5% would cost about $1 million per year. The high prevalence of LBP associated with work also has important implications for the comfort and future of the person involved.

Back pain may arise from many causes, including those related to pathologic problems elsewhere in the body, or to a traumatic incident in which some component of the vertebral system is injured. Many of the work-related causes of low back pain are due to sprains and strains or to disk damage. Where back pain develops unexpectedly without disruption of the normal daily pattern of activity, it might be assumed that local degenerative changes or conditioning from previous postural or vibratory stress increased the person's susceptibility to a sudden onset of symptoms.

Individual differences are important in considering cause and effect. Personal characteristics such as age, physical conditions, and associated disease can modify the response of the body to stressful exertions. Gender differences also exist, and Biering-Sorensen[2] has shown that although the prevalence rate for men decreases after 50 years, it increases for women in this age group.

The continuing incidence of work-related low back pain and back injury and the associated costs of health care, absence from work, and worker's compensation costs have spurred an increasing interest in their prevention. This relies on an understanding of the factors that may contribute to that pain, the implication of those factors for the production of LBP, and an appreciation for the rationale of use and the relative effectiveness of different approaches that may be taken to control risk factors.

Many variables may be involved in the cause of LBP. These include physical characteristics, the experience of the worker, the demands of the task, organizational, social and cultural influences, the characteristics of the work environment, and the outcomes of the injury. Furthermore, causes of LBP are not necessarily physical. The back pain experienced by the worker may be based on a mixture of organic and psychologic causes, as well as social disturbances that may be influenced by the cultural background of the person. Such a multifactorial problem demands resolution through a variety of measures and often by a group of people with differing but complementary skills. A physiotherapist is one of such a team. The physiotherapist's role includes both therapeutic activities and rehabilitation and prevention of injury, and concern with the latter process implies an understanding of the objectives and principles of ergonomics.

Ergonomics is concerned with ensuring that the work place is designed so that work-induced injuries, disease, or discomfort are controlled and safety is ensured while efficiency and productivity are maintained or increased. Work-stress problems at home, school, or place of employment need attention and often require the cooperative activity of representatives of a number of disciplines, including engineering, psychology, medicine, and physiotherapy, to provide suitable solutions. The ability of physiotherapists to analyze body movements in detail and to evaluate postural abuse during dynamic situations makes them ideal as members of a team concerned with the design of equipment and work areas to match the physical capabilities of the user.

Bullock[7,8] has described the scope of the role of the physiotherapist, which includes responsibilities such as job analysis, work posture monitoring, task design, personnel selection and placement, education, supervision of work methods, influencing the person's motivation, and attitudes, and provision of appropriate activity breaks, exercise, and physical fitness programs. Although only those physiotherapists with further education in the practice of ergonomics are likely to act as consultants to industry, all physiotherapists have a part to play in health promotion and in the control of injury or reinjury of clients under their care.

The development of appropriate strategies for injury prevention, including the application of scientific studies to the development of guidelines, has become a special focus of attention for ergonomists. This chapter discusses the influence of some physical workplace factors on low back injuries, with special attention being paid to work postures, the influence of sustained positioning, and the demands of heavy work. The way in which risk factors may be identified and evaluated and the implementation of effective risk control measures is outlined.

WORKPLACE FACTORS INFLUENCING LOW BACK PAIN

Although it is often difficult to determine causation, workplace factors that have been found to be associated with LBP include jobs with high physical demand, including frequent heavy lifting in combination with stooped postures (in flexion and rotation), occasional heavy lifting, sudden unexpected movements, sustained postures involving bent-over working positions, prolonged sitting, prolonged standing, and vibrational conditions.[9] Manning and Shannon[10] suggest three possibilities to explain how these factors could produce pain in the low back: abnormal strain on a normal back, normal stress on an abnormal back, or normal stress on an unprepared normal back.

Manual Handling and Lifting

Work-related low back disorders have been linked to the physical demands imposed in industry. Manual materials handling (MMH), which refers to lifting, lowering, pushing, pulling, carrying, and holding, is a constant hazard in the industrial environment and is an important etiologic factor in musculoskeletal disorders and LBP. Workers with back pain lose more days from work when their jobs involve heavy loads[11] and, because pre-existing lumbar spine conditions can be aggravated by heavy loads, it follows that loads on the lumbar spine should be kept as low as possible.

The load on the spine during a lift is related to a number of factors, including the mass and bulk of the object to be lifted, the horizontal distance from the body from or to which it is lifted, the body posture of the worker, the speed of the lift, the duration or period of lifting, the frequency of lifting, and the height or vertical distance of the lift.

Injuries associated with MMH are frequently related to overexertion, where the person exceeds their own capability, or multiple exertions (described as repetitive trauma). Chaffin[12] refers to a National Institute for Occupational Safety and Health (NIOSH) study in which it was shown that overexertion was claimed as the cause of LBP by over 60% of people suffering from it, and that approximately two thirds of overexertion injury claims involved lifting loads.

Disc damage has been linked with sudden high loading of the spine, especially in flexed postures, for example, when a worker catches a heavy load. This can also occur when one of two partners loses grip on an object being lifted, so that the remaining partner unexpectedly receives an increased load. For this reason, group lifting needs careful coordination in terms of number of personnel used, size of lifters, understanding of the proposed movements, appreciation of destination, preliminary position and grip to be used, and action commands for lifting, carrying, and lowering.

Sudden unexpected and infrequent physical demands seem to cause low back pain more often than continuous heavy work. One reason for this is possibly that the person with only occasional heavy demands has not had the opportunity to learn and establish good work methods. It is important therefore that all people receive some education in correct approaches to movement. Not infrequently, goods that are less-often handled by the lifter tend to be involved in accidents leading to low back injury. Occupations involving only occasional lifting have also shown a high incidence of back pain.[13] Magora[14] claims that infrequent physical demands and sudden unexpected movements such as a rapid stretch, flexion, or rotational movement gives "more low back pain often than continuous heavy work." That this may be related to poor execution of the task is supported by the evidence that a moderate amount of daily lifting was not found to influence the rate of back ache.[14]

Other incidents that have the potential for risk of injury include loss of balance, difficulty in controlling loads or instability of the material being handled, a load falling in close proximity to the lifter, a transport cart moving unexpectedly, a thrown item not reaching the expected recipient, or space restrictions for grasping a load. In developing strategies for risk control, these factors must be taken into account. From the ergonomist's point of view, although overexertion is regarded as an important source of injury, the variety of causes of lifting-related injury demands a more global view to risk control.

Speed of lifting and handling is also important, for if the movement is not adequately under muscular control, additional stress may be suddenly imposed upon the spinal ligaments and a sprain may occur. Work demands that require rapid transfers of weights should be avoided.

Chaffin and Park[15] have asserted that the stresses induced at the lower back during weight lifting are due to a combination of the weight lifted and the person's method of lifting. The latter may be due to the person's approach or to work situations that impose restrictions on the way a lift may be performed. Physiotherapists need to give some consideration to lifting methods in their prevention program, and they need to be aware of the potential hazards of the various approaches to lifting. Advice about manual handling depends on many factors, but in particular, must be approached in terms of the individual person's capacities and movement abilities.

Gravitational forces acting upon the load held in the hand and the person's body mass create rotational moments or torques at the various articulations of the body. The skeletal muscles are positioned to exert forces in such a manner that they counteract these torques. The amount of torque at any joint is dependent on the product of the force tending to rotate the segments and the moment arm of that force (i.e., the distance from the joint to the force vector measured normal to the force vector), as shown in Fig. 11-1. The magnitude of the moment arm varies with the person's posture. If the load lifted is held close to the body, the moment arms are small and the resulting torques at the joints are small. If the load is held away from the body,

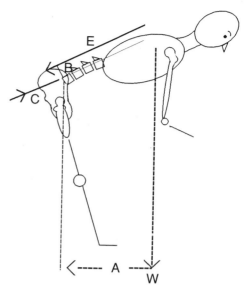

Fig. 11-1 Extensor muscle force in a stooped position:

$$\frac{E}{(=-C)} = \frac{W \times A}{B}$$

E, extensor muscle force; *W,* weight of upper body and load; *A,* moment arm of body weight; *B,* moment arm of the extensor muscle force; and *C,* compressive force acting longitudinally through the vertebral bodies and discs.

the large moment arms will cause large torques. This emphasizes the importance of positioning the body close to the load and also has implications for both access and the bulk of the object.

Studies have shown that during weight lifting, the bending moment at the lumbosacral junction can become quite large.[16] To counteract this torque, the muscles of the low back region, primarily the erector spinae group, must exert correspondingly high forces because they operate on small moment arms. The high forces generated by the low back muscles are the primary source of compression forces on the lumbosacral disc.

In lifting, the greatest stresses occur at the beginning, when the inertia of the weight has to be overcome and the load accelerated. This is why it is important for the person to be in a position to move freely into the upright posture with the load. It is not wise to start a lift in an awkward position, which will prevent a smooth lift. Storage of items and arrangement of the workplace are important factors in this respect.

The trunk extensor muscles act strongly around the vertical but they do not work when the back is fully flexed and only commence their activity after 30 degrees of extension. Electromyographic (EMG) studies[17,19] have demonstrated the electrical silence of the erector spinae in the fully flexed position, the activity of hip extensors as the trunk begins to rise, and the later vigorous activity of the erector spinae as the load nears the vertical. That is, return to the upright position from a flexed posture is begun by the hip extensor muscles rather than the lumbar spine extensors so that the posterior part of the disc, intervertebral disc, and the posterior vertebral ligament are not protected by actively contracting trunk muscles during the early stages of lifting from a flexed position. The likelihood of damage is therefore greater if load is placed on the trunk in this position. This emphasizes the value of initiating a lift through movement of the legs rather than the trunk. Further, where a stooping position is prolonged, muscles fatigue and their supporting function is decreased. Again, this poses a greater demand on the posterior aspect of the intervertebral disc and the posterior ligaments. It has been argued that continued work from a flexed posture could ultimately produce strain and could predispose a person to LBP.

Positional Influences

Many authors believe that an association exists between certain work postures, tasks, and degenerative process[20, 21] and maintain that the postural and physical demands of certain occupations produce greater "wear and tear" on the back, making these workers more susceptible to further injury. Injury due to microtrauma may accumulate and in time produce a "spontaneous" onset of pain.[23] It is also generally accepted that certain occupational and postural stresses on an already inflicted back will produce further episodes of pain.[13, 15, 24] Occupations involving light work with sustained bent-over postures are also reported to have a high incidence of backache.[25, 27] Further, Andersson[9] suggests that prolonged sitting and driving of vehicles seem to carry an increased risk of low back pain and, as Mandal[38] has noted, each day people sit for many hours hunched over tables in postures extremely harmful to the back. Many authors[29, 31] have noted the importance of frequent changes in sitting postures to avoid backache.

The interest in posture during work is in whether the posture assumed creates a load for muscles that must maintain it. Spinal stress in a given posture is influenced by gravitational forces acting on the body and from the forces that arise from the muscular activity needed to maintain the posture. Problems exist when muscles must work for sustained periods against the pull of gravity or the additional weight of an object being held or handled. Troup[24] believes that if the spine is subjected to postural stress for a lengthy period, it stiffens as well as shortens, and the neuromuscular control of spinal posture may be modified. Wickstrom[22] considers that poor posture may lead to the development of muscle imbalances and hence to back injury associated with lifting.

Based on a review of research studies, Chaffin and Andersson[33] have suggested that although most men and up to 90% of women are able to maintain a trunk flexion posture of 20 degrees throughout the day, there is an increased risk of injury if trunk flexion, side bending, or trunk rotation exceeds 20 degrees. The difficulty in tolerating the more-angled posture relates to the rapid increase of load-moment for each degree of torso inclination above 20 degrees.

The stresses of vertical compression, horizontal shear, rotary torque, or a combination of these are determined by the initial, final, and intermediate postures of the person, the velocity of movements, and the load carried by the subject during the task performed.[34] Nachemson et al[35] consider that mechanical stress has at least some role to play in the etiology of the LBP syndrome. For many years, the compressive force on the lumbar spine, and in particular at the L5-S1 junction, has been considered to be one of the primary causes of spinal stress during lifting activities. However, the significance of shearing stresses must be recognized. Vertical loading of the lumbar spine as judged by intradiscal pressure recorders is much less when lifting or carrying is performed with the spine upright. However, in this position the lumbar lordosis causes obliquity of the lower lumbar discs, and therefore vertical spinal loading produces a shearing stress at these levels.[36] This is the so called "lumbar thrust." If the lordosis is exaggerated, then the shearing force is increased and abnormal stresses are taken through the posterior ligaments, including those of the zygapophyseal joint, particularly at the lumbosacral level, and this can lead to lumbosacral strain. Such people are often overweight, which tends to enhance the lordosis.[36]

Nachemson's[37] calculations of the compressive load on the lumbar discs in different positions of the body revealed an increase in load from lying, to standing to sitting, with forward leaning increasing the load. Nachemson[37] considered that these high stresses within the lumbar disc may possibly play a role in the occurrence of posterior annulus ruptures and that dynamic forces would increase the magnitude of the stresses on the annulus.

Physiotherapists need to be aware of the implications of postural load for LBP and the importance of providing relevant advice to reduce postural stress. In considering the work features influencing postural load, special attention needs to be given to the demands for sustained positions, bent-over work postures, and the influence on posture and activity of the seated position.

Sustained Positions

A high incidence of backache has been associated with occupations involving light work with sustained postures.[27] Magora's[38] study found that the incidence of back ailments was extremely high in occupations involving prolonged sitting of longer than 4 hours or sustained standing in one place.

The sustained holding of a posture entails the isometric contraction of groups of muscles to maintain the position of a body part against the pull of gravity. This is sometimes related to the assumption of a certain posture (e.g., forward bending of the upper trunk and head) or to the maintenance of a particular limb position to ensure effective use of terminal joints (e.g., shoulder, elbow, and wrist position to facilitate finger movement). Whether the sustained isometric contraction of a muscle group creates the conditions for development of a musculoskeletal disorder such as low back pain depends on a variety of factors, such as (1) the load of the body part, (2) the duration of the sustained position, (3) the frequency of rest pauses and (4) the magnitude of the load of any object being held or moved while the postural position is maintained. In a strong static contraction, blood supply is impaired and waste products accumulate in the muscles, often resulting in acute pain in the static preloaded muscle.[39] With frequent repetition over long periods, chronic pains may result from pathologic changes in muscles, and the connective tissue of tendons, joint capsules, and joint ligaments. This process may play a part in the postural backache suffered by workers who are not able to carry out normal movement during their working day. Corlett and Manencia[40] have argued that because many muscle groups are involved in maintaining a posture, their relative contribution to the total supporting force required may change during the period for which the posture is held. This emphasizes the importance of avoiding or reducing the duration of static muscle stress.

Bent-over Work Postures

Pain following unaccustomed and long-continued stooping is a familiar event, and postural fatigue is generally recognized as an important element in the production of LBP.[25, 41] Even the maintenance of a relatively constant posture throughout the day can lead to muscular fatigue. Such postural fatigue is more disabling in people with established lumbar spinal disorders. Nachemson and Elfstrom[42] found that intradiscal pressure is increased considerably when the trunk is bent forward compared with standing in an upright position.

When the lumbar spine is flattened, as in the stooped position, the zygapophyseal joints are less able to resist compressive forces, and the majority of the intervertebral compressive force must be resisted by the disc. Kisner and Colby[43] attribute postural pain to the mechanical stresses on various structures when a faulty posture is maintained for a lengthy period. Twomey et al[44] have explained how the process of creep in flexion occurs when the spine is loaded in full flexion for a sustained period. These authors have pointed out that if such loads are prolonged beyond 1 hour, with minimal activity into another position, as may occur in some occupations, there may be a considerable degree of extrusion of fluid from the intervertebral discs, the articular cartilage of the zygapophyseal joints, and the spinal ligaments. Twomey and Taylor[45] suggest that it may take many hours of rest for fluid to be reabsorbed into the soft tissues and their shape re-established. These considerations reinforce the need to maintain the natural forward curve in the lumbar region during working activities and explains why it is inadvisable for those with LBP to sit leaning over a desk. Furthermore, opportunities for a change of position should be provided.

Seated Postures and Sedentary Work

Physiologic and epidemiologic studies have demonstrated that prolonged sitting can cause low back pain.[46] Further, investigations have shown that those who sit for half of the time or more on their jobs have about a 60% to 70% increased risk of developing back pain compared with those who sit for less than half the time. Janda[47] has attributed this sedentary life-style and associated decrease in movement to the development of muscle imbalances which, he considers, often predispose workers to low back pain. Backache when sitting still is a prevalent symptom, particularly in those who have been disabled by back and sciatic pain before. It is important, therefore, that careful thought be given to sitting posture.

In studying the alterations of the lumbar curve related to posture and seating in various positions, Keegan[48] noted that the reduction of the lumbar curve in some positions tends to force the central portion of the lower lumbar discs posteriorly by hydraulic pressure from anterior wedging. Such flattening of the lumbar curve could be caused by the tightening of the posterior thigh and gluteal muscles during hip flexion, due to their attachment to the ischium, the sacrum, and the ilium. Keegan's results[48] emphasize the fact that sitting with a 90 degree angle at the hip joints causes considerable strain at the lumbosacral junction, which would be increased by further hip flexion. Bogduk and Twomey[49] have explained how in sitting, due to the decrease in lumbar lordosis, the intervertebral discs are compressed. Flattening of the lumbar spine also occurs in the sitting position when the legs are stretched out in front of the body. This can occur when a seat is too deep. If the person sits well back to make use of the leg rest, the knees do not reach the edge and the legs must be extended further than normal. This causes tension in the posterior thigh muscles, tilting the pelvis backward and flattening the lumbar spine. Sitting with the legs stretched out because the seat is too low has a similar effect. Selecting a chair that is the correct height and depth and has a low back support to encourage forward movement of the pelvis and maintain the lumbar curve is therefore critical in ensuring comfort and safety.

Driving a vehicle, which involves prolonged sitting, also presents a risk for LBP. Kelsey[50] observed that driving for long periods often requires prolonged sitting in a seat with insufficient support for the low back and with legs extended, in a position subject to the vibration from the road and mechanical stress from starting and stopping. The absence of power steering in such circumstances can create a substantial risk to the operator, where the application of pushing and pulling forces on the steering wheel could induce major spinal stresses.

Andersson et al[51] found that lifting the lower limb to place the foot on the pedal placed stress on the lumbar spine due to the contraction of the psoas major muscle, and intradiscal pressure of the third lumbar disc was found to increase markedly during the depression of the clutch. Nachemson[52] had previously found that myoelectric activity in the psoas muscle corresponded with an increase in the intradiscal pressure in the lumbar spine. This suggests that a clutch pedal that requires greater activity of the psoas muscle (due to a high location above the floor) may produce more stress in the lumbar spine than a lower-placed pedal.

Such findings support those of Bullock,[53,54] who determined the optimal relationship of a pedal to the operator in terms of minimal spinal movements. Among her recommendations was the use of a pedal that required minimal hip flexion and abduction to reach it. Advice to drivers with LBP should include recommendations either for selection of trucks or tractors with suitably designed pedal locations or for incorporation of appropriate modifications to the seat/pedal relationship to avoid excessive lumbar movement during pedal use.

Vibration

Workers such as bus and truck drivers and heavy equipment operators are subjected to continuous vibration. The effect of vibration on height, implying spinal load, has been demonstrated by a number of researchers,[55,56] and exposure to whole body vibration is listed as one of the factors causing LBP at work.[57] Kakosky[39] has asserted that "vibration transferred from a machine to the human body may cause discomfort, a reduction in performance or even injury," and Troup[24] suggests that the risk of back trouble is increased with time spent driving.

The high frequency of low back complaints among truck drivers and drivers of work machines has focused interest on a possible relationship between LBP and vibration. Indeed, pathologic spinal changes have been identified in drivers of vehicles such as trucks, buses, tractors, taxis, and locomotives, as well as in helicopter pilots and drivers of heavy construction vehicles. Wilder et al[59] have advised that in practice, few vehicles impart a pure sinusoidal input to the driver; most vehicles transmit a complex vibration containing many impact shocks. These authors found that the amount of vibration transmitted to the driver was influenced by his working posture and that this was significantly reduced when subjects sat with a back rest inclined at an angle greater than 105 degrees from the horizontal. Minimization of vibrational conditions is an important aspect of risk control in industry.

The greatest dynamic load on the trunk and probably on the spine occurs when it is vibrated at its natural frequency. Stress is therefore likely to be greatest when the seated body is vibrated vertically in the range of 4 to 8 Hz. In a truck, vertical vibration is the dominant vibratory mode and occurs in the range of 2 to 15 Hz.[24] To prevent vibration in the range of 4 to 8 Hz, firm cushions should be supplied and the seat should be suspended to give it a natural frequency of less than 1.5 Hz.[24]

The Influence of Other Musculoskeletal Injuries and Muscle Imbalance on Low Back Pain

The LBP syndrome may sometimes present a wide variety of neuro-orthopedic signs.[14] Some of these manifestations are the result of the underlying process causing low back pain, while other clinically objective signs may be related either directly or indirectly to the actual cause of the LBP. For example, lumbosacral postural disorders, affections of the hip and knee joints, foot deformity, unequal length of the lower limbs, or muscle contractures have all been found to be accompanied by LBP.[60,62] The interrelationships between the lumbar vertebrae, sacrum, pelvis, and femur are prime factors in standing posture as well as during activity, and it is not surprising that strains in one area can lead to stresses in another.[63]

The influence of injuries in the lower limbs on the development of LBP must be considered by those concerned with prevention. Slipping and tripping are common industrial accidents, and the incidence of associated ankle and knee sprains should alert the attending physiotherapist to the possibility of future LBP, so that appropriate preventive measures may be taken. Bullock-Saxton[64] has demonstrated that the function of muscles around the hip and low back changes significantly after ankle sprain and has recommended attention to normalizing muscle imbalances and then the application of sensory-motor programs, such as those advocated by Janda and Vavrova.[65] Such an approach would ensure maintenance of kinetic control and stability. This recognizes that the maintenance of the correct upright posture depends upon the coordinated activity and endurance of many muscles and that muscle control is largely automatic. However, as Roberts[66] pointed out, altered neural activity reaching the central nervous system is likely to influence the automatic mechanisms for muscle control after injury or during disease. In time, the person may develop new patterns of muscle activity and this in turn may lead to muscle imbalance, unusual postures or to interference with the capacity to carry out certain movements. Much can often be learned about the nature and location of an injury from the changes in posture and movement patterns that follow it. Unfortunately, such new patterns may persist long after the original injuries have healed, leaving abnormalities of gait and posture attributable to habit.[66]

Active programs for prevention of LBP should include proper consideration of the long-term implications for areas remote from the site of injury and should include comprehensive assessment and management of the musculoskeletal system following lower limb injuries.

Muscle weakness and muscle imbalance may also develop as a result of injury, through poor postural habits or through overactivity or underactivity of certain groups of muscles involved in work or play. Janda and Schmidt[67] consider that once an imbalance has developed, the changes in muscle function play an important role in precipitating painful conditions of the motor system, such as LBP syndromes. These authors argue that the activity of individual muscles is not as important as their coordinated activity within different movement patterns. They have observed clinically that certain muscles appear to respond to pain by tightness and shortening, while others react by inhibition, atrophy, and weakness.

Imbalance between muscles often starts to develop in the pelvic-hip complex,[67,68] between shortened and tight hip flexors and trunk erectors in the lumbar region on the one hand and weakened gluteal and abdominal muscles on the other. Muscles that become tight or hypertonic are readily activated in most movement patterns, which is reflected by their earlier recruitment during movement. The changes in muscle length and recruitment patterns are considered to lead to anteversion of the pelvis, together with lumbar hyperlordosis and slight flexion in the hip. This may cause unfavorable changes of pressure distribution on the discs, joints, and ligaments in the lumbar region and hip joints. The possibility of muscle imbalances needs to be recognized by the physiotherapist involved in designing activity exercise programs for individual clients or for groups in industry.

According to Farfan et al,[69] muscular coordination is necessary to protect the intervertebral disc. During many dynamic activities, the abdominal muscles work exceedingly hard to balance harmful shearing, bending, or torsional stresses due to moments set up by the lumbar spine extensor muscle.[70] When rotary movements in particular take place, the abdominal musculature provides protection against harmful torsion on the lower lumbar joints via coordinated activity of the contralateral external and internal abdominal oblique muscles. Repeated minor trauma to the intervertebral disc poorly protected by the abdominal musculature could hasten degeneration of the annular fibers of the disc. The balance of activity in the flexor and extensor muscles of the lumbar spine could be affected by a life-style that places little stress on one muscle group at the expense of another. Carlsoo[71] considers that there may be an indirect link between weakness in the extensors and proneness to injury, because patients with low back disorders are prone to recurrences of pain, and those with low back soreness may demonstrate weakness in their trunk muscles. However, Carlsoo[71] argues that it is not possible to tell whether a real or apparent weakness is being measured. He suggests that patients with LBP may be unable to or unwilling to make a maximal effort during strength tests, and that this inhibition may occur consciously or unconsciously.

ERGONOMIC APPROACHES TO CONTROL OF RISKS FOR LOW BACK PAIN

Because LBP is a multifactorial problem, a team approach is necessary to provide adequate management, and approaches need to be varied according to individual circumstances.

The physiotherapist's efforts to minimize the effect of sensory or physical impairment upon movements may resolve immediate problems, but if restoration of the individual's working capacity is an aim, that approach must be supplemented by methods to improve the working environment.[75] Such programs incorporate mechanisms commonly used in ergonomics to control risks for injury.

Risk control in ergonomics relies on the identification of risk factors associated with injury, evaluation of those risks, and implementation of controls that take those risks into account. Following a job analysis, corrective and preventive measures can include advice and education in ergonomic principles; a program of instruction for newcomers to the workplace; redesign of equipment and the work environment; changes in organization and work methods; relaxation and exercises; stress relief; and appropriate assessment and treatment should symptoms occur.

Job Analysis

Ergonomic analysis is used to identify particular problems in the workplace. Through a process of systematic recording of specified aspects of the work done or of the effects on the person of that work, those aspects of the work situation that represent a risk to the worker can be identified and assessed, so that areas of risk can be placed in order of priority.

Discussion with the personnel involved often helps to reveal problem areas. Because of their intimate knowledge of the work site and the particular task to be performed, the person at risk for musculoskeletal injury has information on potential hazards that may not be apparent to management until after an accident occurs. The concept that the worker should be involved in identifying work problems and in suggesting solutions to them is not new. The practice of using a participative approach to ergonomics is growing in many countries throughout the world. Today, many ergonomists are involved in projects in which the basic idea of implementing ergonomic principles in a company is to share the responsibility with employees through increased knowledge, by which they might develop their own proposals for ergonomic improvements.[76]

Where control of LBP is the focus, the analysis includes an assessment of the work place and the work environment and the likelihood of injury within it, together with a survey of the load imposed on the worker, a comprehensive evaluation of the worker's method of performing the task, and the person's capacity to cope with the particular demands of the task.

Job analysis should refer to a classification of job activities. This allows specification of job requirements that will then be linked with demands on the person and, subsequently, their abilities. The system of job analysis may be broadly based or job specific.

Review of statistics such as incidence of accidents and injuries can reveal where and in which jobs specific injuries have occurred. The frequency and severity of injuries relative to the number of employees, the hours worked, or the areas of work can be examined. Injury incidence relative to location, occupation, or task can be determined to reveal areas of priority for risk assessment and risk control.

The approach to work analysis has been well described by Luopajarvi.[77] Surveys and observations at the work place may be carried out using simple checklist approaches or by implementing more complex procedures. Checklists provide a focus for examining specific problem areas and may deal with general issues, or more specifically with the type of handling task or the methods of carrying out a task by the operators. Checklists may provide a basis for appraising design of equipment, work space, or the environment and may also be used to review the approach to supervision and work organization.

Physiotherapists can contribute to risk assessment by focusing on three aspects: the workers, the work, and most importantly, the interaction of the worker with the work (in which postures demanded by the work, the method of performance of the task by the worker, and the consideration of individual differences in workers and their ability to cope with the work are of prime concern).

From the point of view of physical risk factors that may lead to LBP, analyses of work load that relate to observation of work postures and movements are most relevant. Data can be gathered by direct visual observations, in which postures adopted by the worker are recorded, or by more advanced methods of incorporating computerized data recording. Photography and videotaping may also be used. Using work sampling methods, the postures may be observed at predetermined intervals, so that a profile of the work demands may be gained. Analyses can reveal the frequency of stressful postures or movements that could lead to LBP. Special attention should be paid to the availability of adequate space for the worker's operation, the availability of access for the worker to equipment and storage areas, and the height relationships between the worker and the work surface, which could influence the degree of static work posture.

Physiotherapists should apply their understanding of body mechanics to analyze the dynamic posture, movement sequences, and body stability of the person during performance of their activity and any potential for injury. Details of the duration, range, direction of, and resistance to specific movements could be determined. These appraisals would help to clarify the operational demands on the musculoskeletal system, leading to the development of suitable modifications to ensure posturally safe working conditions.

Ergonomists frequently evaluate quantitatively the effects of a physical activity on a person by estimating the forces and moments acting on the musculoskeletal system during the activity. Biomechanical risks associated with lifting tasks may be investigated by collecting displacement-time data as the task is performed. The data collection is often costly because of the expense of motion analysis systems, and the processing of data can be time consuming. Biomechanical simulation can be used to reduce these constraints. However, computerized dynamic biomechanical simulation models for lifting need to be evaluated themselves for validity and reliability. To be useful to ergonomists, the simulation of human lifting must be shown to accurately predict variables commonly used in ergonomic evaluations. Variables that could be analyzed include peak vertical velocity and acceleration of the load and the total distance travelled by the load, these three variables relating to the goal or the task.

To provide realistic guidance, such biomechanical assessment needs to relate to the three cardinal planes of the body during a dynamic lifting task. Marras et al[78,79] have devised a model that collectively considers the five workplace factors of torso-twisting velocity, torso sagittal bending, torso lateral velocity, frequency of lifting, and load moment in predicting a probability that a particular job is at high risk for occupationally related low back disorders. For this model, Marras et al[79] defined risk as a combination of the incidence of low back disorder, restricted time, and lost time associated with the job. Validation studies have shown that the risk model provides a means to identify and subsequently have the potential to control risk for work-related low back disorder.

Granata and Marras[80] studied the influence of velocity and movement in the three cardinal planes of the body on the loads on the lumbar spine. They showed that when velocity is introduced, compression and shear forces on the spine increase significantly. They explain that motion on its own does not increase spinal loading but that the trunk motion accentuates antagonistic muscle co-activation, which leads to increased spinal loading. Granata and Marras[80] note that failure to predict muscle co-activation results in spine-loading estimates that could be in error by as much as 70% during dynamic exertions. They assert that to facilitate assessment of spinal load, EMG-assisted models of the trunk musculature must be used. Spinal loading (compression, lateral shear, and anterior shear forces) were calculated by Granata and Marras[80] from the vector sum of validated muscle forces. Force plate measures were used to calculate the moments imposed about the spine during a lift.

Risk Management

When risks have been identified through job analysis, the results of the various measures must be compared with recommended values and standards if they are available. This allows more satisfactory decisions to be made about the selection of control measures. It also establishes a basis for physiotherapists to provide input to the design of work layouts and tasks which, by incorporating ergonomic principles, can help to control the incidence of injury.

The health care approach for employees who have sustained injuries is primarily to promote healing, but it should also improve their level of functioning at work and at home and assist them to manage their own health and to learn methods of preventing further injury. Workers need to be encouraged to take some responsibility for minimizing the factors presenting risks for injury. Recommendations for the control of risk factors must be feasible in terms of costs and their effect on production. Proposed solutions should be evaluated for their acceptance by the workers and employers and for their effectiveness in controlling risks before firm recommendations are made.

Education and Training

Perhaps more subtle than the effects of physical factors on the worker is the potential risk associated with lack of knowledge in relation to work demands. Here, the adequacy of communication, education, and teaching is important. Within the overall program of risk control, employee education has been shown to reduce lost work time.[81] Assisting workers to recognize and avoid hazards during manual work, to improve coordination and handling skill, and to develop an awareness of their capacity for handling or tolerance for postural stress without LBP can be of value.[82]

However, poor techniques established after years of habit are very difficult to break. Strategies must be developed to encourage learning. In the workplace, people have a need for different types of learning: about facts, skills, and new attitudes. Education programs in industry should be related to workers' specific needs and must highlight design problems within the work station. Participants are then able to identify potential hazards and relate ergonomic principles to their own working environment. The programs should be presented in a way that matches the participants' educational level because personal problem solving is considered to be an essential part of the educational program. An interactive approach between educator and participant is most likely to have positive results.

Bullock[83] has outlined the objectives and possible content of educational programs that may be used for the various categories of worker in industry and has highlighted the need to use different approaches in educating work supervisors and managers, so that all personnel understand their role in prevention. Objectives for education vary according to participants and type of work, but in most cases the educational programs need to address the concept of ergonomics, the mechanism of injury relevant to that workplace, and approaches to injury prevention applicable to it. Participants would also be encouraged to question the suitability of their own environment[83] and to examine the work situation itself before considering how to cope with a particular lift or handling approach.

Educating manual workers in lifting methods is common practice, and many large firms find such programs commercially expedient. However, too little emphasis is placed on educating children, young people, and women in the correct methods of lifting.

Advice about manual lifting depends on many factors and must be approached in terms of the individual person's capacities and movement abilities. It is recommended that workers be shown those positions and movements that could be potentially hazardous in their own working environment. They should also be given the opportunity to develop sensible and safe methods of handling and lifting under guidance. They should be taught how to use their own body power in an appropriate way and advised to strengthen key muscles if weak. Special attention needs to be given to the education of new employees in an industry or of workers transferred to new manual tasks. Early training in appropriate approaches to movement and to safe working techniques with specific strength programs could help to control back injury.

The choice of approach to lifting varies with circumstances, individual preferences, an appreciation of risks and hazards, and other environmental factors. However, any lifting techniques selected need to be effective and efficient, with the lifter gaining good control of the load and maintaining balance. Preliminary planning should include consideration of the content of the load, its mass, the location of its center of gravity, the robustness of the object and possibly its wrapping, the destination of the lifted object, and the goal of the lift. The lifter needs to determine the most appropriate technique for the situation and to be flexible enough to allow adjustments in handling or body position that might be necessary during movement of the load. If stacking or storing is involved, then the lifter must consider both the method of lift and the manner in which the object will be positioned. Overall, the lifters must realize the need to protect their own physical well being while satisfying the needs of the job.

For biomechanical reasons, the load should be positioned close to the body, and the person should be in a position to move freely into the upright posture with the load. Thus there must be sufficient space in which to move and room in which to place the feet and to coordinate the total movement of feet, body, arms, and load during a transfer. It is not wise to start a lift in an awkward position that will prevent a smooth lift. Storage of items and arrangement of the workplace are important factors in this respect. Wherever possible, the grip should be diagonal, to allow a better estimate of mass and location of center of gravity and to enable the lifters to make adjustments more rapidly.

Because of the factors influencing safe and effective lifting from either the squat position or the stoop lift position, individual persons should be encouraged to find the posture that is energy efficient for them and in which the lumbar lordosis can be maintained but kept to a minimum. For the normal uninjured person without pain, there are few indicators to emphasize the value of one position or the other. However, for the person who experiences LBP, the nature of the injury and the way the stresses of injury affect the symptoms will influence the choice of method. Strength and endurance of the back extensors is important for those with LBP, and the role of the multifidus must also be noted. Mattila et al[84] showed that the multifidus was deconditioned in individuals with sedentary employment. The importance of this muscle as a stabilizer has been emphasized by the work of Hides et al.[74]

For those persons with a low back injury, lifting should be avoided initially. To avoid exacerbating pain, any posture that stresses the injured tissue should not be used. Different techniques can be attempted slowly and with caution, and postures for light lifting activities used only when they do not exacerbate symptoms. Low-level lifting of loads should be avoided.

One question associated with the squat lift is whether the person has sufficient strength in the extensors of knees and hips to raise the load. These muscles work most efficiently and effectively when the joints are at 90 degrees flexion. If the person squats before lifting, the extensor muscles are placed in a position of mechanical disadvantage, and it may be difficult for the person to raise to standing. This highlights the need to provide hip and knee extensor exercises in a prevention program.

Noting the challenges to the validity of the recommended lifting method with bent knees[15] and to the practical utility of such a method,[85] Parnianpour et al[86] applied a lifting stress calculator to individualize and optimize the lifting technique and to take clinical complaints into account. Parnianpour et al[86] reported that this model showed variability of knee joint and back joint angles for different loading conditions, but they emphasized that although the idea of distributing loads between the knee and the back according to a patient's symptoms may be appealing, there is a limited number of postures that can be assumed to carry out a lift in view of the physical characteristics of that load. These experimenters could find no single "safe" method of lifting, supporting previous assertions of the inadequacy of training in proper lifting techniques in reducing LBP and the possibility for greater success in risk control through redesign of the task or workplace.

When physical demands are high, and automation or mechanization is not feasible, appropriate mechanical aids should be provided to reduce the stresses imposed on the worker by lifting and handling loads. Mechanical aids should provide a mechanical advantage. Such implements can include cranes, hoists, hand-trucks, overhead handling equipment, articulated arms, and vacuum lifting devices. However, Resnick and Chaffin[87] have highlighted the fact that while mechanical aids do eliminate repetitive lifting components of industrial jobs, they have introduced a new set of concerns for the ergonomist. These devices require the operator to transfer the load horizontally by pushing or pulling. In this way, forces exerted by the operator are altered, as are the biomechanical stresses on the spine, because the inertia of the load-assist devices and any frictional resistance effects must be overcome as the worker manipulates the load. It is also important to remember that when using these devices, movements are dynamic, so postures and forces must change rapidly during the exertion.

There is little experimental evidence to date that so-called assistive devices such as lifting belts or braces provide real protection from injury for healthy workers carrying out lifting and handling activities.

Exercise and Fitness

Emphasis is usually given to loads that are beyond the capacity of the worker. However, it should be noted that too little activity may also be an eventual cause of LBP. Advice about exercise has been shown to be important in risk control. For example, Kellett et al's evaluation of the effect of a weekly exercise program on number of sick leave days[88] established that within the exercise group, the number of episodes of back pain was reduced, as was the number of sick leave days (by over 50%). In this study, 81% of participants in the exercise program reported a subjective improvement of back pain. Baun et al[89] and Lynch et al[90] also showed that where workers were participating in a general fitness program, they were absent less frequently than those who did not exercise, and that their health care costs were significantly lower than those of the nonexercising workers.

It is important when considering the use of exercise and fitness programs that the activities included within that program are relevant to the requirements of the job. Any research reports referring to evaluation of effectiveness of fitness programs should be assessed for the validity of the program evaluated. Where manual handling forms part of the daily activity, the type of exercise included in the program must match the demands for strength, endurance, and coordination required for lifting and handling.

In general, exercise programs should include education in movement, advice on methods of general and specific relaxation, exercises to provide active work for muscles maintained in a state of static contraction during the work period, specific exercises to strengthen muscles concerned with lifting and handling, and exercises for general physical fitness. Particular attention should be paid to the correction of muscle imbalances and to the strengthening of postural muscles. Stretching exercises for the femoral and pelvic muscles may be needed to ensure proper pelvic and spinal posture. For sedentary workers, exercises for the upper back extensors are usually helpful.

Activity programs should also emphasize the importance of changing both position and work activity during the working hours. Opportunities for job rotation that allow a change in muscle activity should be encouraged.

Back School

The introduction of "back schools" within industrial settings, as established at Danderyd Hospital, Stockholm in 1970,[91] aimed to increase the worker's ability to take care of their back by providing education about the source and management of low back pain. Zachrisson-Forssell[91] used ergonomics and education as the main elements of this Swedish program. The back school aimed to enable patients to play an active part in improving their working environment to reduce their back problem and to provide increased knowledge and enhanced understanding to minimize the risk of inappropriate therapy and reduce the demand for social, medical, and economic resources that can result from avoidable back pain. Through their controlled study, Berqguist-Ullman and Larsson[13] demonstrated a reduction in days lost from work through use of the Swedish Back School, which emphasized the application of ergonomic principles.

Nevertheless, overall these programs have not been found to be effective in the long term. After a short period of improvement, the incidence rate of LBP tends to return to normal. The variability in success of back school programs may reflect the great diversity in physical, psychologic, and social factors influencing people with LBP as well as the nature, intensity, and duration of pain and the educational level of the participants. Responsiveness of clients to particular approaches may depend on whether the components of the program match individual needs, can elicit a reaction, or can motivate the client. Education can only be seen as an adjunct to other forms of back injury control. One important feature is the need for reinforcement of advice and safe practices.

Design

Recognizing the limitations of educational programs, ergonomists have emphasized the importance of design changes in the work place and of modifications to work organization. It is considered that the most important way in which ergonomic principles may be applied for control of injury is through design, in which all factors affecting the performance of a task are considered and solutions recommended that are aimed at avoiding risks to the health and safety of the worker.

The physiotherapist must involve the worker in discussions about design needs and improvements that would contribute to work safety and effectiveness. Frequently in a work situation, more than one aspect of the work layout could have a potential for injury. It is important, when involving the worker in decision making about work postures and body positions during activity, that all risks are appreciated and that the choice of one position for the sake of comfort does not place another body part at risk. It is possible that sensations of discomfort at one site may influence the person's acceptability of the task, when injury could occur at a more vulnerable site even though no discomfort is experienced.

Good job design reduces the worker's exposure to the hazards of manual handling, and so reduces the medical and legal problems of selecting the worker for the job. It also places less reliance on the worker's willingness to follow established training procedures, such as lifting properly. However, good job design depends on a knowledge of worker capabilities and limitations and of the factors that may contribute to production of low back pain.

Knowledge of the characteristics of the workers and the task are of prime consideration in planning the workplace. Body size is an important factor to consider. Either the workplace is designed to fit a certain percentile range of the population, and operators outside this range are given another job; or it should be made adjustable. The wide range of body sizes that exist in a workplace must be recognized, and the area must be roomy enough to accommodate the large person and allow him or her to move comfortably, yet confined enough to allow the small person to be able to work and reach all controls easily. For this purpose, basic requirements of size and shape should be established, noting the relative height of the equipment and the workplace to the operator, so that the design ensures that posture is adequate, and excessive static muscle work of the head, trunk, or shoulder girdle is avoided.

An important aspect of the ergonomic approach is the careful specification of the worker-task relationship within the design, so that the load on the locomotor system is reduced and peak strains and static loads are avoided. Adverse handling stresses should be minimized, vibratory stresses reduced, and the cause of postural backache identified and removed. Tasks and equipment should be modified to reduce the effects of biomechanical stress on the worker. This may involve modifying both the work layout and the work techniques so as to avoid extensive reaching, bending, twisting, heavy lifting, repetitive motions, or forceful exertions.

Although appropriate job design minimizes many of the factors associated with LBP, much of the responsibility for protection of the back must rest with the person. Back pain and back injuries occur not only in the working environment but also away from work. It is important that everyone receive some education in ergonomic design, and also in correct approaches to movement, so that they may apply them to their leisure activities, whether it be sport, gardening, or sitting as a spectator.

To minimize load on the back through bent-over work postures, the head and neck should be able to be held erect and no prolonged trunk flexion should be required. Controls should be within comfortable reach and should not be in positions demanding twisted, cramped, or contorted positions for their operation. The working surface should be at the correct height and, where the work position is likely to be maintained for long periods, the work surface should be inclined toward the worker to reduce the need for stooping. Opportunities for a change of position should be provided. In particular, those already suffering backache should not continue working in a position that demands a sustained, stooped, sitting posture.

To avoid some of the musculoskeletal problems associated with poor positioning in sitting, attention has been given to seat and table specifications. The dual requirement for good postural support and a capacity for adequate reach and vision introduces complexity into chair and workplace design.[12] In sitting, the line of gravity passes anterior to the thoracic spine. The weight in front of the thoracic spine therefore exerts a bending moment on the spine, tending to increase the thoracic kyphosis, with the site of maximum stress being in the lower thoracic spine. Design features ensure maintenance of the normal relationship between the thorax and the pelvis. This may be achieved through use of a back rest positioned between T9 and L1.

In selecting a chair of correct height and depth for that person, a low back support, a slightly inclined seat surface to maintain the lumbar curve, and support for the feet are critical factors in ensuring comfort and safety. Use of a seat wedge could be considered because this shifts the weight onto the ischial tuberosities and encourages spinal alignment.

The relationship of the seat to work bench or desk is also important in prevention of back pain. A bench that is too high requires that the arms be raised to do the work, and this is likely to increase the lumbar lordosis. A too-low bench encourages stooped working positions. It should be noted that when using a computer, the work level to be considered is the top of the keyboard, not that of the table.

Functionally, bench height should be within about 5 cm of elbow height when sitting and standing. Platforms of varying heights for standing on can ensure appropriate relationships. Where a person is involved in continuous work at a bench or desk (e.g., in a laboratory) comfortable changes of position from standing to sitting should be possible. In such cases, use of a high stool with back rest, and a foot stool is more appropriate than using a chair. It is usually recommended that sitting not be continued for more than an hour, and standing for not more than 30 minutes at a time.

The design of activities carried out in the sitting position also needs careful consideration. For example, prolonged and repetitive pedal use in sitting, whether in industry, agriculture, or general transport, can be a risk factor for LBP. Where the line of action of the pedal is vertical, the hip extensor muscle activity needed for pedal depression may demand excessive stabilization forces in the trunk. As a result of extensive experimentation, Bullock[92] recommended that for the seated operator, a pedal path should be at 45 degrees to the horizontal and continuous with the "hip to foot on the pedal" line. Troup[24] also recommended that the line of action for pedal depression should pass from the foot through the hip joint and that the back rest should firmly resist the tendency of the pelvis to rotate.

Ergonomic guidelines have been provided for designing various aspects of work. For example, McCormick and Sanders[93] and Chaffin and Andersson[94] have outlined guidelines for the maximum holding time of a static forceful exertion, and Eastman Kodak Company,[95] McCormick and Sanders,[93] and Grandjean[96] have offered ergonomic guidelines for lifting. Dul and Hildebrandt[97] have reviewed the ergonomic guidelines relevant to protection of the back. They argue for validation and emphasize the need to extend knowledge of the relationships between back load variables such as EMG signals of trunk muscle activity, biomechanical torques or forces, intra-abdominal pressure, intradiscal pressure, and the long-term incidence of LBP. These authors have emphasized the need to develop guidelines that focus specifically on the control of LBP.

In 1981, NIOSH developed a guide[98] based on the assumption of multiplicative effects of various lifting risk factors. More recent revision of this guideline, as reported by Waters et al[99] has added two new factors for limit setting: asymmetry and coupling. Under this new equation, the recommended weight limit (which is a task-specific value defining the load weight considered safe for nearly all healthy men and for at least 90% of women) has been set at 23 kg under ideal conditions. However, it is recognized that many task-related variables exist and that, in reality, the recommended lifting limit should be below 23 kg. According to Waters and Putz-Andersson,[100] the revised NIOSH equation provides a unique set of evaluation parameters that include intermediate task-related multipliers defining the extent of physical stress associated with individual task factors, the NIOSH–recommended weight limit, and the NIOSH lifting index (LI), which gives a relative estimate of overall physical stress associated with a specific manual lifting task. However, Jager et al[101] assert that when maximum values are being recommended to limit overexertion risk to the lumbar spine during lifting and handling tasks, current knowledge must be considered and a comprehensive review of reports of recent studies undertaken. These authors advocate the application of age and gender of the workers to the development of a load limit, noting that with increasing age, lower disc or vertebral compression limits should be applied and that the limits relating to women should be lower than those relating to men.

Organizational Change

Ergonomic advice that relates solely to workplace design or education is unlikely to have a full effect on risk control. The revision of work organization and changes to the mental and social environment are also priority measures. Poor work scheduling, the demands created by peaks of activity, the time allowed for carrying out an activity, and the availability of assistance for or relief from heavy work demands can be controlled by suitable organizational procedures.

To be effective, a risk control strategy should be focused on the organizational change necessary to ensure that design solutions can be implemented once problems are identified. A work environment must be created that will ensure participation of the workers and the proper coordination of all preventive measures, encourage both the development of skills and the observance of principles relating to safe manual handling, and integrate injury prevention with work procedures and work organization. It is probable that in the past, some programs have been unsuccessful because they have placed too much emphasis on specific lifting technique instructions, given too little consideration to the coordination needed between functions affecting occupational health and safety, and had too little involvement from administrators and management in the prevention process.

Economics is an important factor in developing a strategy to convince management of the need to apply ergonomic principles within the company. Documentation of the real costs associated with accidents and poor safety may provide an effective argument to persuade managers of the value of introducing ergonomics. Managers must be made aware of potential costs of litigation and of reduced production and insurability resulting from human injury. By expressing ergonomics in terms of costs, risks avoided, and benefits gained, the value of ergonomics becomes more obvious. Strong evidence of management commitment to ergonomics, commencing with a policy statement, positively influences the attitude of supervisors and workers at the work site. If management can encourage the idea of working as a total team toward a safer working environment and can introduce appropriate education together with a participatory approach to discussion of change, then a positive approach to the introduction of change should pervade the work site.

Rehabilitation Ergonomics

The effectiveness of a man-machine system depends on the way in which the mechanical design of the equipment and work place match the capacities of the operator. This applies for all workers but is particularly important for workers who have already sustained injury. Those concerned with cost-effective rehabilitation of the injured worker should gain an appreciation of the various demands placed on the body so that they can provide advice about modifications to the work environment or the work method that would acknowledge any limitations of the operator.

For the worker who has suffered a back injury, the long-term treatment and re-education plan must be tailored to suit the job for which the person is being rehabilitated. Because different jobs require different skills, each requires specific types of preparation. Retraining in appropriate work methods, and supervision of workers returning to work after an injury are important to minimize the likelihood of further injuries. In industry, this is ideally carried out by a physiotherapist working on the site. Decisions must be made as to whether a worker shown to be susceptible to injury should be transferred from heavy to lighter tasks, although the definition of "light" is open to debate. Studies suggest that workers with LBP who stay within heavy occupations are prone to recurrence of injury. While it may not be necessarily true that the particular occupation caused an inherent back disorder, it is generally accepted that certain occupational stresses on an already afflicted back will produce further episodes of pain. Physiotherapists concerned with the care of an LBP patient should gain an appreciation of the various demands placed on the body by work, home, or leisure activities and, through assessment of relevant attributes such as joint flexibility, muscle strength and endurance, and functional capacity, provide advice about modifications of the work environment or the work method that acknowledges any limitations of the operator.

Where the physiotherapist can visit the work site to supervise work methods, the correction of operating difficulties or potentially damaging postures reinforces good work methods and encourages consultation by the worker who may be uncertain of the correct approaches to prevention.

Assessment of Functional Capacity

To protect the person against exacerbation of injury, knowledge of their functional capacity—possibly changed by the incidence of low back pain—needs to be gained. Isernhagen[102] has emphasized that for the physiotherapist to provide correct and comprehensive information about a person's functional capacity, the appropriate design of functional capacity assessments is essential.

She points out that the best functional capacity evaluators test the total person so that all aspects of movement and movement patterns can be observed. As proposed by Janda[103] in his rule of horizontal and vertical generalization, Isernhagen[104] outlines how a dysfunction in one area (e.g., the knee) may affect normal body mechanics and lead to injuries in another area (e.g., LBP).

The importance of evaluating body movements in the context of work and life situations is also highlighted by Isernhagen.[104] This positive approach, in which the person's level of capacity is assessed, leads to specifications of activities that may still be achieved by the worker. For most physical activities, the person must develop some force, sustain it for a period, and produce a movement of the body. Characteristics important to these goals are muscle strength and endurance and joint range of motion. The back is at risk when muscles responsible for its stability become weak. Low levels of power and strength influence safety and efficiency of a lift. Loss of mobility subsequent to aging may decrease the ability to reach an object or to comfortably lift it to a required height, thus demanding abnormal movements and postures to achieve the required lift. For patients who have been injured or suffer some disability, it is important to ascertain their capacity in activities that use these three characteristics. Tests involving pinching, gripping, lifting, pulling, and pushing are among the most commonly used for assessing physical activity relevant to work activity. However, lifting ability is not only a function of body weight and muscular strength; it also relies on the skillful use of the right muscles. Lifting is, or should be, a dynamic activity. Whenever the lifting effort becomes static and is sustained, the probability of injury increases for as long as it can be held.

Functional capacity assessment provides helpful information in relation to advising the LBP patient when it is safe to return to work activity and how much can be done. Isernhagen[104] asserts that such an assessment can act as a guide to the patient to reach his or her maximum potential. She explains that later assessments provide the background to graduated return to work that is at a higher but safe functional level.

Watson et al[105] suggest that the ergonomist's approach to assessing human ability in relation to work demands is appealing in that it seeks to measure interactions between the employee and the work place through the structured, systematic examination of functional items relating to both. These authors developed the Activity Matching Ability System (AMAS), whereby criteria are identified against which measures could be set. They highlight the need for instruments or assessment techniques that measure differences in functional ability. Watson et al[105] believe that the ability assessment offers clinicians a potential instrument for identifying functional deficits and for monitoring functional outcome and change, because it implies that treatments may be focused on restoring or compensating for functions vital to work performance.

Licter[106] emphasizes that the major goal of work rehabilitation is to instill safe working habits in the worker at work. The work-site assessment often clarifies the patient's occupational needs while also revealing the need for ergonomic improvements in some job functions. The rate of progression of activities depends on the tolerance of the client in duration, frequency, speed, and power as well as in overall productivity.[106] Strength levels, flexibility, and endurance, which are also usually lost after an injury and are demanded by the job, must be regained to help in the prevention of further injury or reinjury. Chaffin et al[107] demonstrated that the incidence rates of back injuries sustained at the job increased when the job strength requirements exceeded the isometric strength of the workers.

Evaluation of the previously injured client's progress should be carried out progressively according to short-term and long-term goals. Reports on the person's task performance should be provided to the employer as vocational goals are approached. This will help with placement in the work situation. Such reports should be expressed in practical and understandable terms such as weights, frequency, and amount of materials handled and/or activities performed.

Licter[106] considers that rehabilitative care is complete when the client can perform at the full physical demand of the occupation for an 8-hour day and is ready to repeat this the next day or, alternatively, when improvement has plateaued short of the goals. Duration of care varies with the type and level of disability, the client's physical disability and intellect, and their psychologic and physiologic responses to the demands of the occupation. Approaches to resolving problems must vary according to the nature of the problem, and resolution demands a therapeutic team approach.

CONCLUSIONS

The application of the principles of ergonomics to the prevention of low back pain has considerable value to the person at risk for injury. Because of the cost benefits of controlling back pain and days lost from work, the positive outcome for productivity is beneficial for industry.

Encouragement of the worker to be aware of hazards in the work place or in leisure activities and involvement in identification of risks can help to motivate the client to participate in the control of their own environment. Education in identifying risks for injury, in methods of moving the body effectively and safely, and in minimizing or eliminating postural stress through careful design are essential components of an ergonomics program. It is also important to modify attitudes to occupational health and safety, to create an environment in which protection of the person's well-being is seen as vital by all. It is hoped that this positive attitude to risk control through ergonomics will be taken increasingly by those who are consulted by sufferers of low back pain.

REFERENCES

1. Svensson HO, Andersson GB: Low back pain in forty to forty-seven year old men. I. Frequency of occurrence and impact on medical services. Scand J Rehabil Med 14(2):47, 1982
2. Biering-Sorensen F: A prospective study of low back pain in a general population. Occurrence, recurrence and aetiology. Scand J Rehabil Med 15:71, 1983

3. Borenstein DG, Wiesel SW, Boden SD: Low back pain—Medical diagnosis and comprehensive management (2nd Ed.). WB Saunders Co, Philadelphia, 1995

4. Nachemson AL, Bigos SJ: The low back. In Cruess J, Rennie WJ (Eds.): Adult orthopaedics, Vol. 2. Churchhill Livingstone, New York, 1984

5. Rowe ML: Low back pain in industry. A position paper. J Occup Med 11:161, 1969

6. Yu T, Roht LH, Wise RA, et al: Low back pain in industry an old problem revisited. J Occup Med 26:517, 1984

7. Bullock MI: Ergonomics—a broad challenge for the physiotherapist. In Bullock MI (Ed.): Ergonomics: The Physiotherapist in the Workplace. Churchill Livingstone, Edinburgh, 1990

8. Bullock MI: The physiotherapist's role in the control of industrial injuries. Control 1:2:69, 1974

9. Andersson GBJ: Epidemiologic aspects on low back pain in industry. Spine 6:1:53, 1981

10. Manning DP, Shannon HS: Slipping accidents causing low back pain in a gearbox factory. Spine 6:1:70, 1981

11. Schultz AB, Andersson GBJ: Analysis of loads on the lumbar spine. Spine 6:1:76, 1981

12. Chaffin D: Occupational biomechanics—a basis for workplace design to prevent musculoskeletal injuries. Ergonomics 30:321, 1987

13. Berqguist-Ullman M, Larsson V: Acute low back pain in industry. Acta Orthop Scand Supp 170:1, 1977

14. Magora A: Investigation of the relation between low back pain and occupation. Scand J Rehab Med 7:146, 1975

15. Chaffin DB, Park KS: A longitudinal study of low back pain associated with occupational weight lifting factors. Am Indust Hyg Assoc J 34:513, 1973

16. Tichauer ER: The biomechanics of the arm-back aggregate under industrial working conditions. ASME Preprint 65, WA/HUF-l, 1966

17. Schultz AB, Haderspeck-Grip K, Sinkora G et al: Quantitative studies of the flexion-relaxation phenomenon in the back muscles. J Orthop Res 3:2:189, 1985

18. Kumar S: The study of spinal motion during weight lifting. Irish J Med Sci 143:2:86, 1974

19. Kumar S, Davis PR: Spinal loading in static and dynamic postures: EMG an intra-abdominal pressure study. Ergonomics 26:9:913, 1983

20. Kellgren JH, Lawrence JS: Rheumatism in miners. Part II: X-ray study. Br J Ind Med 9:197, 1952

21. Troup JDG: Relation of lumbar spine disorders to heavy manual work and lifting. Lancet 1:857, 1965

22. Wickstrom G: Effect of work on degenerative back disease. Scand J Work Environ Health 4(1):1, 1978

23. Hershenson A: Cumulative injury: a national problem. J Occup Med 21(10):674, 1979

24. Troup JDG: Driver's back pain and its prevention: a review of the postural, vibratory and muscular factors, together with the problem of transmitted roadshock. Appl Ergon 9(4):207,1978

25. Lawrence, JS: Rheumatism in coal miners : Part III. occupational factors. Br J Ind Med 12(3):249, 1955

26. Brown JR: Factors involved in the causation of weight lifting accidents. Ergonomics 8(2):117, 1958

27. Partridge RE, Anderson JAD, McCarthy JA et al: Rheumatic complaints among workers in Iran foundries. Ann Rheum Dis 27:441, 1968

28. Mandal AC: The seated man (Homo Sedens): The seated work position. Theory and practice. Appl Ergon 12(1):19, 1981

29. Kottke FJ: Evaluation and treatment of low back pain due to biomechanical cause. Arch Phys Med 42:426, 1961

30. Kroemer KHB, Robinette JC: Ergonomics in the design of office furniture. Ind Med Surg 38:115, 1969

31. Magora A: Investigation of the relationship between low back pain and occupation III. Physical requirements: sitting, standing, and weight lifting. Ind Med Surg 41:5, 1972

32. Andersson G: Low back pain in industry—Epidemiological aspects. Scand J Rehabil Med 11:163, 1979

33. Chaffin DB, Andersson G: Occupational Biomechanics. (2nd Ed.): Wiley-Interscience, New York, 1991

34. Kumar S: Lifting and Ergonomics. In Bullock MI (Ed): Ergonomics: The Physiotherapist in the Workplace. Churchill Livingstone, Edinburgh, 1990

35. Nachemson AL, Schultz AB, Berkson MH: Mechanical properties of human lumbar spine motion segments. Influences of age, sex, disc level and degeneration. Spine 4(1):2, 1979

36. Edgar M: Pathologies associated with lifting. Physiotherapy 65(8):245, 1979

37. Nachemson A: The effect of forward learning on lumbar intra-discal pressure. Acta Orthop Scand XXXV:314, 1965

38. Magora A: Investigation of the relation between low back pain and occupation. Scand J Rehabil Med 7:146, 1975

39. Grandjean E, Hunting W: Ergonomics of posture—review of various problems of standing and sitting posture. Appl Ergon 8(3):135, 1977

40. Corlett EN, Manencia I: The effect and measurement of working postures. Appl Ergon 11:1:7, 1980

41. Brown JR: Lifting as an industrial hazard. Am J Indust Hyg Assoc J, 1973

42. Nachemson A, Elfstrom G: Intravital dynamic pressure movements in lumbar discs. Scand J Rehab Med l:1, 1970

43. Kisner C, Colby LA: Therapeutic Exercises: Foundations and Techniques. (2nd Ed.). FA Davis, Philadelphia, 1990

44. Twomey LT, Taylor JR, Oliver MJ: Sustained flexion loading, rapid extension loading of the lumbar spine, and the physical therapy of related injuries. Physiother Pract 4:129, 1988

45. Twomey LT, Taylor JR: Flexion creep deformation and hysteresis in the lumbar vertebral column. Spine 7:116, 1982

46. Pope MH, Frymoyer JW, Andersson GBJ: Occupational low back pain, Praeger, New York, 1984

47. Janda V: Movement patterns in the pelvic and the hip region with special reference to pathogenesis of vertebrogenic disturbances. Habilitation Thesis, Charles University, Praha, Czechoslovakia, 1964

48. Keegan JJ: Alterations to the lumbar curve related to posture and seating. J Bone Jt Surg 35A:589, 1953

49. Bogduk N, Twomey LT: Clinical Anatomy of the Lumbar Spine (2nd Ed.). Churchill Livingstone, Melbourne, 1991

50. Kelsey JL: An epidemiological study of the relationship between occupations and acute herniated lumbar intervertebral discs. Intern J Epidemiol 4(3):197, 1975

51. Andersson BJG, Ortengrem R, Nachemson A et al: The sitting posture—an electromyographic and discometric study. Orthop Clin of North Am 6:1:105, 1975

52. Nachemson A: Electromyographic studies on the vertebral portion of the psoas muscle. Acta Orthop Scand 37:177, 1966

53. Bullock MI: The determination of an optimal pedal-operator relationship by the use of stereo photo-grammetry. Biostereometrics 290. Proceedings of the Symposium of Commission V. International Society for Photogrammetry. Washington, DC, 1974

54. Bullock MI: Musculoskeletal disorders in the workplace. In Kumashiro M, Megaw ED (Eds.): Towards Human Work. Taylor & Francis, London, 1991

55. Sullivan A, McGill SM: Changes in spine length during and after seated whole body vibration. Spine 15:1257, 1990

56. Magnussen M, Almqvist M, Broman H et al: Measurement of height loss during whole body vibrations. J Spinal Dis 5:198, 1992

57. Troup JDG: Causes, prediction and prevention of back pain at work. Scand J Work Environ Health 10:419, 1984

58. Kakosky T: Vibration disease. Clin Rheumatol 3:25, 1989

59. Wilder DG, Magnusson ML, Fenwick J, Pope MH: The effect of posture and seat suspension design on disc comfort and back muscle fatigue during simulated truck driving. Appl Erg 25(2):66, 1994

60. Stevens J: Low back pain. Med Clin North Am 52:55, 1968

61. Sypher F: Pain in the back. A general theory. J Internat Coll Surg 33:718, 1960

62. Janda V: Muscles, central nervous regulation and back problems. In Kerr IM (Ed): The Neurobiologic Mechanisms in Manipulative Therapy (1st Ed.). Plenum Press, New York, 1978

63. Clayson SJ, Newman IM, Debevec DF et al: Evaluation of mobility of hip and lumbar vertebrae in normal young women. Arch Phys Med Rehab 43:1, 1962

64. Bullock-Saxton JE: Changes in muscle function at hip and low back following chronic ankle sprain. Proceedings, 11th International Congress World Confederation for Physical Therapy 1:57,1991

65. Janda V, Vavrova M: Sensory motor stimulation: A video, presented by Bullock-Saxton JE, Produced by Body Control Systems, Brisbane, 1990

66. Roberts TDM: The mechanics of the upright posture. Physiotherapy 398:404, 1969

67. Janda V, Schmid HJA: Muscles as a pathogenic factor in back pain. Proceedings of the IFOMT Conference, New Zealand 1980

68. Jull GA, Janda V: Muscles and motor control in low back pain: assessment and management. In Twomey LJ, Taylor JR (Eds.): Physical Therapy of the Low Back, Churchill Livingstone, Edinburgh, 1987

69. Farfan HF: Mechanical instability of the lumbar spine in torsion. J Bone Joint Surg 52B:748, 1970

70. Fahrni WH: Conservative treatment of lumbar disc degeneration: Our primary responsibility. Orthop Clin North Am 6:93, 1975

71. Carlsoo S: A back and lift test. Appl Erg 11(2):66, 1980

72. Hodges P, Richardson C: Inefficient muscular stabilisation of the lumbar spine associated with chronic low back pain. A motor control evaluation of transversus abdominis. Spine 21(22):2640, 1996

73. Hodges P, Richardson C: Contraction of transversus abdominis invariably precedes upper limb movement. Exper Brain Res 114:362, 1996

74. Hides J, Richardson C, Jull G. Multifidous muscle recovery is not automatic following resolution of acute first episode low level pain. Spine:21(23):2763, 1995

75. Galvin DE: Employer-based disability management and rehabilitation programs. Ann Rev Rehab 5:173–215, 1986

76. Melin E: Occupational physiotherapy in a large industry. In Bullock MI (Ed.): Ergonomics: The Physiotherapist in the Workplace. Churchill Livingstone, Edinburgh, 1990

77. Luopajarvi T: Ergonomic analysis of workplace and postural load. In Bullock MI (Ed.): Ergonomics: The Physiotherapist in the Workplace. Churchill Livingstone, Edinburgh, 1990

78. Marras WS, Lavender SA, Leyrgans SE, et al: The role of dynamic three-dimensional trunk motion in occupationally related low back pain disorders. Spine 18(5):617, 1993

79. Marras WS, Parnianpour M, Ferguson SA, et al: The classification of anatomic-and-symptom-based low back disorders using motion measure models. Spine 20:2531, 1995

80. Granata KP, Marras WS: The influence of trunk muscle coactivity on dynamic spinal loads. Spine:20(8):913, 1995

81. Tabor M: Reconstructing the scene: back injury. Occup Health Safety Feb 16, 1982

82. Troup JDG: Bone mechanics of the vertebral column, its application to prevention of back pain in the population and to assessment of working capacity in patients with lumbar spinal disability. Physiotherapy 65(8):238, 1979

83. Bullock MI: Health education in the workplace. In Isernhagen S (Ed.): Work Injury, Management and Prevention. Aspen Publishers, Rockville, Maryland, 1988

84. Mattila M, Hurme M, Alaranta H, et al: The multifidus muscle in patients with lumbar disc herniation. A histochemical and morphometric analysis of intra-operative biopsies. Spine:11(7):732, 1986

85. Graveling RA, Simpson GC, Sims MT: Lift with your legs, not with your back: A realistic directive? In Brown ID, Goldsmith R, Coombes K, et al (Ed.): Ergonomics International 85, Proceedings of the 9th Congress of the International Ergonomics Association, Bournemouth, England, Taylor & Francis, London, 1985

86. Parnianpour M, Bejjani FJ, Pavlidis L: Worker training: the fallacy of a single, correct lifting technique. Ergonomics 30(2):331, 1987

87. Resnick M L, Chaffin DB: Kinematics, Kinetics and psychophysical perceptions in symmetric and twisting, pushing and pulling tasks. Human Factors 31(1):114, 1996

88. Kellett KM, Kellett DA, Nordholm LA: Effects of an exercise program on sick leave due to back pain. Phys Therapy 71(4):283, 1991

89. Baun WB, Bernacki EJ, Tsai SP: A preliminary investigation: effect of a corporate fitness program on absenteeism and health care cost. J Occup Med 28:18, 1986

90. Lynch WD, Golaszewski TJ, Clearle AF, et al: Impact of a facility-based corporate fitness program on the number of absences from work due to illness. J Occup Med 32:9, 1990

91. Zachrisson-Forssell M: The Swedish back school. Physiotherapy 66:4:112, 1980

92. Bullock MI: Musculoskeletal disorders in the workplace. In Kumashiro M, Megaw ED (Eds.): Towards Human Work. Taylor & Francis, London, 1991

93. McCormick EJ, Sanders MS: Human Factors in Engineering and Design. McGraw-Hill International, Auckland, 1984

94. Chaffin DB, Andersson GBJ: Occupational Biomechanics. Wiley, New York,1984

95. Eastman Kodak Company: Ergonomics design for people at work. Lifetime Learning Publications 1, Belmont, California, 1983

96. Grandjean E: Fitting the task to the man. Taylor & Francis, London, 1980

97. Dul J, Hildebrandt: VH: Ergonomic guidelines for the prevention of low back pain at the work place. Ergonomics 30(2):419, 1987

98. National Institute of Occupational Safety and Health: Work Practices Guide for Manual Lifting. Publication 81-122, Government Printing Office, Washington DC, 1981

99. Waters TR, Putz-Andersson V, Garg A, Fine LJ: Revised NIOSH equation for the design and evaluation of manual lifting tasks. Ergonomics 36(7):749, 1993

100. Waters TR, Putz-Anderson V: Ergonomic considerations for manual material handling and low back pain. In Erdil M, Dickerson OB (Ed.): Van Nostrand Reinhold, New York, 1997

101. Jager M, Luttmann A, Laurig W: Lumbar load during one-handed brick laying. Internat J Ind Erg 8:261, 1991

102. Isernhagen J: Work injury, management and prevention. Aspen Publishers Rockville, Maryland, 1988

103. Janda V: Introduction to functional pathology of the motor system. In Bullock MI (Ed.): Proceedings VII Commonwealth International Conference 3:39, 1982

104. Isernhagen J: The role of functional capacities assessment after rehabilitation. In Bullock MI (Ed.): Ergonomics: The physiotherapist in the workplace. Churchill Livingstone, Edinburgh, 1990

105. Watson H, Whalley S, McClelland I: Matching work demands to functional ability. In Bullock MI (Ed.): Ergonomics: The Physiotherapist in the Workplace. Churchill Livingstone, Edinburgh, 1990

106. Licter R: Work simulation: Putting training to work. Occup Med: State of the Art Reviews 7(1):125, 1992

107. Chaffin D, Herrin G, Keyserling W: Pre-employment strength testing: J Occup Med 20(6):403, 1978

12

Therapeutic Exercise for Back Pain

Joseph P. Farrell
Michael Koury
Caroline Drye Taylor

Because there are numerous risk factors and pathologic entities that contribute to low back pain (LBP) and associated symptoms, it is essential that the treatment of LBP should address the many causes of this disease process.[1] For decades, considerable attention has been given to exercise as a treatment of LBP. Recent studies support the premise that physical activity and exercise are beneficial for patients with back pain.[2,3,4,5] Active rehabilitation programs that emphasize exercise and patient participation not only appear to restore function but in many cases may be associated with reduction in pain[2,6,7] and improved strength, endurance, and levels of fitness.[8] Lower extremity flexibility,[9] strength, and endurance of muscle groups such as the abdominals,[10,11,12] spinal extensors,[13] latissimus dorsi, transversus abdominis, internal obliques,[14,15,16,17] and lower extremities[18] all appear important in rehabilitation of the spine. Research has shown that patients suffering from LBP who underwent an aggressive exercise program were able to avoid surgical intervention, even in the presence of herniated nucleus pulposis (HNP) with radicular and neurologic signs.[7] One study has reported improvement in pain control and function in patients suffering chronic LBP in the presence of spondylolysis and spondylolisthesis using a very specific exercise training program of the deep abdominals and mutifidus muscles.[17]

This chapter discusses the role of therapeutic exercise in the management of individuals with back pain. The following topics are emphasized:

1. The evaluation process that leads to successful exercise programs
2. Principles of therapeutic exercise training pertaining to spinal stability, strength, coordination, balance, endurance, kinesthetic awareness, and aerobic fitness
3. Progression of exercise
4. Functional training
5. Integration of exercise and overall patient management

THE EVALUATION PROCESS

Successful treatment outcomes depend on methodical patient evaluation. Physical and functional limitations should be identified by carefully interviewing the patient and by performing appropriate physical and functional examinations. These provide the basis for realistic goal setting and the development of an individualized therapeutic exercise program.

The Patient Interview

During the interview process, it is imperative that the clinician acquires an understanding of the patient's life-style and the specifics of his or her working environment and recreational activities. It is also important to determine the extent to which the patient's normal activities are restricted by LBP, if the patient's goals include resumption of all of these activities, and how much time the patient can realistically devote to a home exercise program.

Determining the behavior of the symptoms during various activities will help to identify movements or postures that increase and/or decrease the patient's symptoms. This information assists the therapist in understanding the types of exercises that may be indicated during subsequent treatments.

Patients may report problems with the position of their spine during activities (e.g., flexion vs. extension), their tolerance to axial loading (e.g., activities that increase vertical compression on the spine such as sitting or standing for long periods of time or carrying heavy objects), sensitivity to pressure against the spine, and difficulty maintaining any position for extended periods.[19] If the patient's LBP is irritated by varying degrees of spinal flexion or extension, then careful attention will need to be paid to the amount of lordosis that is maintained during exercise and functional activities. Patients who are sensitive to tasks that increase axial loading of the spine may need to avoid exercises that add to the compression of the spine. Strategies for "unloading" the spine are discussed in the Treatment section of this chapter.

Occasionally patients may not tolerate direct pressure against their spine because of acute tenderness. These patients will need to exercise in positions that decrease or avoid pressure on the spine (e.g., in quadruped or prone position over a gym ball). Finally, if symptoms increase when a certain position is maintained for extended periods, the exercise program will have to allow for frequent changes in posture.

Gathering sufficient information to understand how the problem affects the patient over the course of 24 hours is important for determining whether the patient needs instruction in sleeping positions and pacing of activity, exercise, and rest. Load-sensitive patients may need to plan to lie down at some point in the day to decrease the axial loading forces on the vertebral column.

Asking questions regarding the patient's medical history, use of medications, or the results of special tests (e.g., x-rays, magnetic resonance imaging

[MRI]) assists in identifying specific contraindications to treatment and should ensure safety in the application of the treatment program.

For the current episode of spinal pain and previous history of spinal complaints, it is important to determine if the symptoms are stable or deteriorating. Any indication of deterioration would alert the clinician that the intensity of the exercise program should be gentle until it is clear that exercise will not lead to further deterioration of the pathologic process or an increase in symptoms.

The patient who has experienced previous episodes of spinal pain should be able to describe the type(s) of treatments that he or she has received (physical therapy, chiropractic, injections, medications, etc.), the nature of the previous exercise programs (e.g., flexion or extension, aerobic, various home programs), and whether or not these interventions helped in achieving his or her goals. The patient should demonstrate their previous exercise programs because verbal descriptions may not always be accurate.

Because the interview process is subjective, the astute clinician takes into consideration the factors that may affect the information that the patient provides regarding his or her spinal problem. These factors include the patient's perception of pain, level of motivation, possible involvement with litigation or compensation,[20] and potential avoidance behaviors associated with negative aspects of his or her life-style or work environment.[20, 21, 22] All of these factors may affect the patient's compliance with the exercise program and influence the treatment outcome.

The Physical Examination

Data collected from the patient interview enables the clinician to plan and prioritize physical and functional examination procedures during the initial evaluation and subsequent treatments. Typically, all patients undergo active spinal range-of-motion (ROM) testing. Motion testing helps to identify pain-provoking and pain-easing movements and any restriction of movement. This assists the clinician in choosing the spinal position(s) that are safest and most comfortable for the initial exercise program.

The neurologic status and the presence of adverse neural tissue tension (ANTT)[23] should be assessed. Passive neck flexion, straight leg raising, passive knee bend testing, and the slump test are performed, depending on the nature of the patient's complaint.[23, 24] In our experience many clinicians are unsuccessful treating spinal patients with exercise because signs of ANTT are not identified and treated.

Standardized muscle length tests[25] of muscles that directly or indirectly affect the lumbopelvic region during functional activities should be performed. Often muscles and joints in other regions of the body may contribute to pain in the lumbar spine. For example, a golfer may lack mobility of the shoulders or thoracic spine. This contributes to an alteration of the golf swing that may lead to excess torsion forces on the lumbar spine, thus causing lower back pain. Athletes with ligamentous laxity and lower extremity overuse syndromes have been shown to be more prone to LBP.[26] Clearly, the clinician should not limit the mobility and muscle length testing to muscles that most directly affect the lumbar spine. It is important to evaluate all possible contributing factors.

It is helpful to test various functional activities that relate to the patient's functional limitations as an adjunct to specific manual muscle testing of the lower extremities and the trunk. We routinely assess activities such as single-leg or double-leg squats to test strength and endurance of the quadriceps and gluteals. The patient's ability to control the spinal column should also be observed during these tests. A simple count of the number of repetitions prior to losing control of the spine (e.g., side flexion or lateral hip shift) and/or lower extremity fatigue provides baseline data from which progress may be judged. Careful observation of these maneuvers may also confirm lower extremity joint or muscle tightness, that would be addressed by the ensuing exercise program.

If the patient must perform tasks at home or work that require repetitive pushing or pulling, then a loaded cart or pulley system can be used to document the amount of weight the patient can safely move. Other functional activities should be assessed as indicated to observe any physical restriction that may be impeding function and to determine the need for specific training in body mechanics (e.g., rising from a chair, dressing, doing laundry tasks, etc.).

Lifting is a key functional activity for nearly any individual experiencing back pain. It is important to test the specific type of lift (e.g., floor to waist or waist to shoulder level) that the patient performs at home or work. Measurement of the amount of weight, number of repetitions prior to experiencing symptoms, and distance the load is carried and observation of spinal position (e.g., flexed or extended) provide objective and inexpensive measurements of this particular functional test. Often videotaping of this test provides visual feedback for the patient to assist in learning correct lifting technique.

Specific muscle strength and endurance testing of the truncal global muscle system (e.g., rectus abdominis, external obliques, and lumbar iliocostalis) and the local muscle system (e.g., multifidus, transversus abdominis, and posterior fibers of the internal obliques) are necessary because these muscles systems each have different roles in providing dynamic stability of the lumbar spine.[27] Bergmark[27] hypothesized that the global system provides general truncal stability but does not have a direct segmental influence on the spine. The local system provides segmental stability and directly controls the lumbar motion segment.[28, 29] The clinician can record the number of repetitions prior to fatigue or time an isometric hold in the test position of the truncal muscles to document the baseline measure.

Back extensors may be tested globally through range or isometrically in prone by extending over a pillow. Fig. 12-1 shows a patient in a bridging position while the therapist applies alternating torsional forces to the pelvis. The assessment of torsional truncal resistance to activate truncal cocontrac-

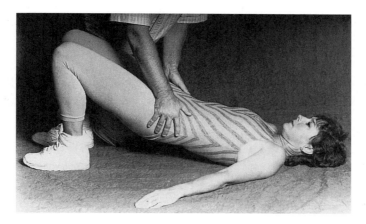

Fig. 12-1   Bridge position as therapist applies torsional force to pelvis.

tion is important because these muscles promote stability of the spinal column.[30]

The clinician should screen patients for cardiovascular risk factors before performing even a submaximal stress test (heart rate kept under 75% of the predicted maximum heart rate). The American College of Sports Medicine[31] recommends that men over 40 years and women over the age of 50 years should be evaluated by a physician prior to beginning any vigorous exercise program. Cardiovascular fitness may be measured by using a timed test on a stationary bicycle or treadmill.[31,32] The patient's heart rate and blood pressure should be monitored during the test to ensure that his or her response to exercise is appropriate for the particular age group. Timing the onset of back or leg symptoms during the cardiovascular testing provides additional baseline data from which progress may be assessed.

The final component of the physical examination is the determination of the patient's spinal functional position (SFP). Morgan[33] describes the spinal functional position as "the most stable and asymptomatic position of the spine for the task at hand." The patient is first assessed in a hook-lying position. Exploration of posterior and anterior pelvic tilting will indicate whether the patient's symptoms are increased, decreased, or eliminated at any point between spinal flexion and extension. The most comfortable position is by definition the SFP. This position is also referred to as "spinal neutral" by other practitioners.[7]

The SFP is not specifically related to the medical diagnosis; however, it is not unusual to see patients with stenosis or facet syndromes exhibit an SFP that is biased toward flexion of the lumbar spine. The critical factor is to find the most comfortable lumbopelvic position for the patient. This position may vary, depending on the posture or activity performed by the patient (e.g., supine, sitting, standing). The SFP may not be the same from day to day.[33] Identifying the SFP assists the clinician in determining the positions and the ROM in which the patient may safely begin to exercise while controlling pain. The roles of the transversus abdominis, internal obliques, and multifidus relating to the SFP are discussed in the Stabilization section of this chapter.

PRINCIPLES OF EXERCISE RELATING TO BACK PAIN

Self-Management

The major goal of any exercise program for the LBP patient is to teach the patient to control and minimize risk factors while normalizing spinal movement patterns during work, home, or recreational activities. Each patient should obtain skills needed to apply the principles of back care to problem situations that confront them on a daily basis. Encouraging patient responsibility for long-term low-back management is very important in light of health care reform, which has significantly affected the insurance industry in the United States. Many patients experience financial limitations (e.g., $1500 per year or 1 to 6 physical therapy visits per year) due to their particular insurance coverage. Therefore the patient and clinician need to plan the course of treatment based on not only the presenting physical dysfunction but also the patient's insurance resources.

Stabilization

During the past decade the term *spinal stabilization* has emerged in the literature. At times this term has been described as rigid fixation to prevent movements of vertebral motion segments. However, we agree with Morgan[33] that it is impractical and rarely necessary to train patients to maintain the spine in one lumbar position during exercise and activities of daily living. As patients improve they are encouraged to exercise within the lumbopelvic ROM that is painless; therefore, the patient is not maintaining a strict SFP throughout the treatment program.

Dynamic spinal stabilization in practice is a complex neuromuscular skill that necessitates continuous muscular adjustments to maintain a safe stable spinal position.[29,33] For example, as an individual lifts a box overhead the tendency is to extend the spine. The deep abdominals and multifidus must work in concert to counteract this tendency to extend the spine.

Porterfield[34] defines *dynamic stabilization* as the ability of the patient to be active throughout the day without increasing symptoms. A cornerstone of our approach to exercise is to make every attempt to work the patient as vigorously as possible without increasing symptoms. As patients progress in their ability to control the SFP during various exercises, there should be a corresponding increase in the ability to perform activities of daily living without increasing symptoms.

The concept of spinal stabilization has been evolving recently. Many authors contend that the neuromuscular system becomes disrupted with patients suffering from LBP.[28,29,35,36] These disruptions have been shown to relate to patterns of recruitment and segmental changes within the muscles.[29,36,37,38]

Hodges and Richardson[29] used electromyographic (EMG) analysis of abdominal, deltoid, and multifidus muscles during movements of the upper limb in normal subjects and patients with chronic LBP. They found in the control group that the transversus abdominis was the first muscle activated, and that activity was present prior to limb movement. The transversus abdominis, in patients with LBP, was delayed and failed to be active before the deltoid in all directions. They hypothesized that the transversus abdominis is an important stabilizer of the spine, and that people with chronic LBP have a deficit with control of contraction of transversus abdominis.

Hides et al[39] compared two groups of subjects with first episodes of LBP using real time ultrasound imaging of the multifidus. One group was instructed in bed rest for 1 to 3 days, absence from work, and prescribed medications. The other group was trained in specific stabilization exercises using a cocontraction of the transverse abdominis and multifidus muscles. The exercises were based on the approach of Richardson and Jull.[28] They found at the end of a 4-week period there was no difference in either group in terms of pain, disability, or ROM, but the exercise group had a more rapid and complete recovery of the multifidus muscle. They concluded that multifidus recovery does not occur automatically with resolution of pain and disability and suggested they may be predisposed to further injury and recurrence of LBP. O'Sullivan et al[17] found favorable results with spondylosis and spondylolisthesis patients using similar cocontractions of deep abdominal muscles and multifidus. The exercise group showed a statistically significant reduction in pain intensity and functional disability levels at a 30-month follow-up.

Due to the apparent latent response of the transversus abdominis and muscle changes in the multifidus in patients with LBP, we initially instruct our patients to cocontract the transversus abdominis and multifidus (see Chapter 8 for specifics) in hook-lying, quadruped, prone, and standing postures. We refer to this as *abdominal setting*. After patients master this cocontraction, we assist them in finding their spinal functional position (SFP). However, with some patients we find it is helpful to locate the SFP prior to initiating abdominal setting when pain is the dominant variable. This is especially true for those patients who tend to be biased toward a more flexed SFP (e.g., stenosis).

Proprioception in the Lower Back

Degenerative changes in the lumbar region, such as osteophytes and traction spurs, are visible pathologic effects of vertebral motion segment instability. Bony and ligamentous structures provide static stability, while muscular function supplies dynamic stability. Brooks[40] suggests that dynamic stability requires more than force generated by muscle tension. The force must be coordinated during a precise movement or alteration of a specific task that requires a balance between antagonist and agonistic forces. The ability to learn and refine this sort of skill is defined as proprioception.[40]

Parkhurst and Burnett[41] explored the relationship between injury and proprioception in the lumbar region. They reported that impaired proprioception was associated with an increase in the number of lower back injuries. Therefore, restoring proprioception skill in patients experiencing back pain should be a goal of all exercise programs.

Clinically, the patient must be re-educated to coordinate the spine during functional activities. When the patient is able to recognize small changes in movement patterns and control the SFP, then they have begun to learn how to control their spine and body in space. Repetition of these movements enhances the neurophysiologic learning process.[42] The goal is to develop engrams for these activities and diminish repetitive trauma to the spine due to poor proprioception.[43]

Recently several studies[29,44,45,46] have reported specific dysfunction of the multifidus and deep abdominals in the chronic LBP population. This specific dysfunction results in altered patterns of coordination between truncal muscles, which leads to the global muscle system having a tendency to substitute and dominate over the impaired local muscle system.[28] Thus the importance of specific training of the local muscle system as it relates to functional tasks is important in back rehabilitation and in reducing the risk of recurrence.

Endurance and Strength

Numerous researchers have observed a decrease in muscular endurance of truncal muscles that was proportional to the degree of chronicity of LBP.[45,46] Clinically, it is critical that the patient is rehabilitated to the point at which he or she has the strength and endurance to return to the rigors of specific lifestyle or work environments.[7,13] Thus, as the patient progresses during an exercise training program, it is critical to exercise at an intensity that will improve truncal endurance to the point that he or she is able to maintain dynamic stability throughout the day.

Exercise During the Pain Phase

To begin the exercise portion of the rehabilitation program, patients must first learn the limits of their SFP so that they may gain an appreciation of the lumbopelvic positions to be avoided due to pain. Initially the patient may not have the strength or proprioceptive ability to prevent painful movements. Prepositioning the spine to prevent movement out of the SFP is often necessary. Morgan[33] describes two methods of prepositioning the spine. Passive prepositioning uses body and/or limb placement to avoid movement of the lumbopelvic region into painful positions. Minimal muscular effort is required, and assistive devices (Fig. 12-2) help the patient to maintain a safe, painless SFP. Even during the pain control phase of rehabilitation the patient is then able to exercise the abdominals and upper extremities fairly vigorously (Fig. 12-3) with minimal risk of aggravating LBP.

Active prepositioning is used[33] as the patient learns to control the SFP. If the SFP is biased toward flexion, the patient will be instructed to actively maintain a posterior pelvic tilt while concurrently contracting the tranversus abdominis.

When proprioception and pain control improves, other techniques are used to challenge the patient while maintaining a safe SFP. Alternating iso-

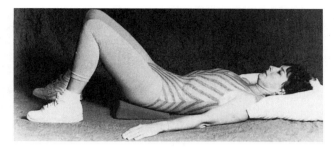

Fig. 12-2   Passive prepositioning of the lumbar spine in flexion to maintain a safe SFP.

metric exercises and rhythmic stabilization techniques[47] are employed to facilitate truncal muscles in an isometric manner because movement through range often provokes pain during the pain control phase (Fig. 12-4). As range of movement improves and the excursion of painless lumbopelvic motion increases, the vigor of the program is progressed.

Treatment Progression

After the patient learns the limits of the SFP in hook-lying, prone, side-lying, quadruped, and standing positions, exercises can be performed in any or all of the developmental postures. The need to develop proximal stability (e.g., truncal) as a base for distal mobility (e.g., superimposing movement of the extremities) is a key concept in the sequencing of exercises.[33, 47] Ultimately the patient must develop the skill to control movement of the spine during complex total body movements. Many options are employed to strengthen the trunk and extremity musculature through this developmental sequence.

Exercises usually begin in hook-lying position. Once the patient is able to actively preposition and control the spine in the hook-lying position, arm movements and lower extremity movements are added to challenge the patient's ability to maintain the SFP and transversus abdominis contraction. To

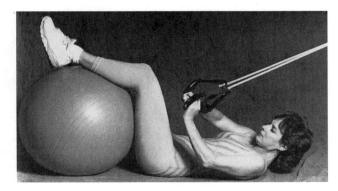

Fig. 12-3   Diagonal pulls to exercise the abdominals and upper extremities while patient is passively prepositioned.

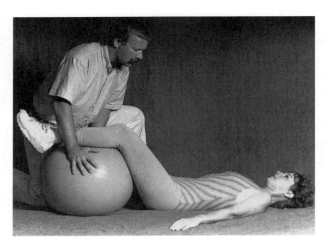

Fig. 12-4   Rhythmic stabilization technique, prepositioning using gym ball. Resistance to trunk is provided indirectly through gym ball.

facilitate coordination while maintaining the SFP, contralateral arm/leg movements are used (Fig. 12-5). The further the patient extends the upper or lower extremities (Fig. 12-6), the more difficult it is to maintain the SFP. The addition of cuff weights on ankles and wrists further challenges the patient in terms of truncal strength. An increase in the number of repetitions of the "dead bug" exercise facilitates endurance and enhances coordination through repetition. An advanced patient may be able to perform difficult trunk stabilization exercises such as the one depicted in Fig. 12-7. These exercises require a significant amount of deep abdominal strength to maintain the SFP.

Other exercises for abdominals traditionally include abdominal curls (rectus abdominis) and abdominal oblique curls while maintaining the SFP. As the patient advances, the performance of abdominal curls on a gym ball further challenges balance and proprioception and increases the range through which the abdominals must contract (Fig. 12-8).

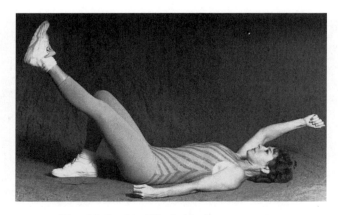

Fig. 12-5   Modified deadbug exercise.

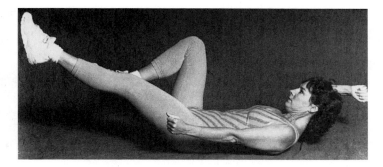

Fig. 12-6 Advanced deadbug exercise: bicycling action of the lower extremities with alternating shoulder flexion.

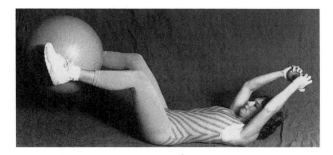

Fig. 12-7 Gym ball between legs with weights in hands moving in opposite directions.

Fig. 12-8 Abdominal curl on the ball starting in spinal extension. **B,** End position for abdominal curl on the gym ball.

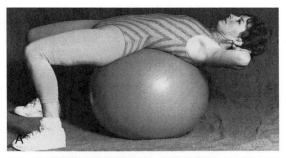

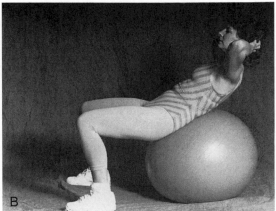

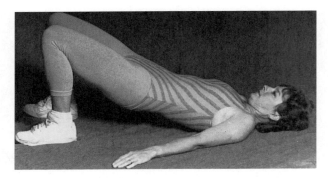

Fig. 12-9   Bridge position to strengthen spinal extensors, gluteals, and hamstrings.

To begin exercising spinal extensors, gluteals, and hamstrings, the bridging position (Fig. 12-9) is used initially. The same principles of maintaining a painless SFP is encouraged. The patient may begin with a simple gluteal set and progress to the point where the bridge position is maintained while superimposing leg movements (Fig. 12-10) or arm movements (Fig. 12-11), or in a bridge position on a gym ball. To exercise upper trunk extensors the patient can lie prone over a ball (Fig. 12-12) and extend the trunk within the pain-free range. Endurance can be facilitated by maintaining the spine in extension and superimposing numerous repetitions of upper extremity movements using weights (Fig. 12-13) or in a bridge position on a ball (Fig. 12-14).

When the patient has mastered bridging activities on the floor, a gym ball can be used to challenge balance and proprioception and to facilitate recruitment of the spinal stabilizers. By bridging with the feet on the ball (Fig. 12-15) while maintaining an SFP, the patient trains the back extensors and gluteals quite vigorously. Bridging with the heels or toes dug into the ball also increases the vigor and balance required of the exercise. To facili-

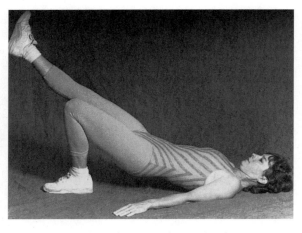

Fig. 12-10   Extending one leg in bridge position.

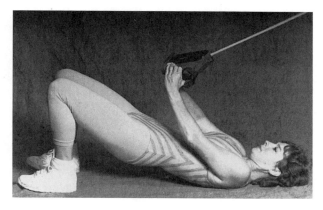

Fig. 12-11 Bridging while using a Sportcord.

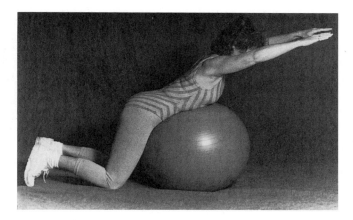

Fig. 12-12 Upper spinal extension over a gym ball.

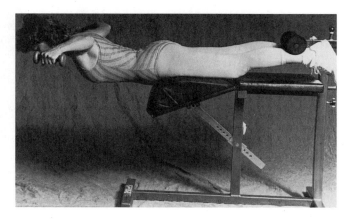

Fig. 12-13 Superimposed arm movements when isometrically holding back extension position on "Roman chair."

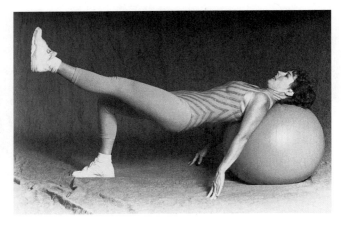

Fig. 12-14   Maintaining a bridge position on gym ball, alternately extending legs.

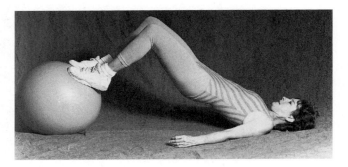

Fig. 12-15   Bridging with feet on ball.

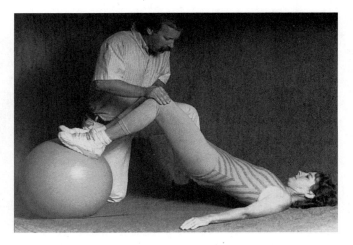

Fig. 12-16   Rhythmic stabilization technique in bridging position with feet on the ball.

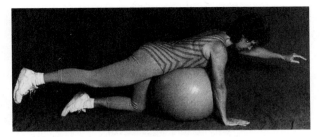

Fig. 12-17 Quadruped position with support of the gym ball.

tate coactivation of the truncal muscles the physical therapist can perform rhythmic stabilization techniques (Fig. 12-16). This requires advanced skill and challenges fine neuromuscular adjustments to maintain the SFP. This exercise also develops a faster reaction time for the muscle to react to external forces. According to Taimela et al,[48] improving slow psychomotor speed of reaction is important to decrease the risk of recurrence of LBP. These authors also reported that patients presenting with chronic LBP had slow truncal reaction speeds.

Stabilization training in the quadruped position requires increased balance and proprioception. Recently, Gill and Callaghan[49] demonstrated that patients with LBP lacked normal proprioception in the quadruped position. Coactivation of the transversus abdominis and multifidus in quadruped has been show to improve spinal stability.[17] If the patient has difficulty maintaining the quadruped position initially, a gym ball can be used to support the trunk (Fig. 12-17). As the patient progresses, arm or leg motions can be superimposed while maintaining the SFP (Fig. 12-18). To further challenge the patient, weights can be used on the ankles and wrists. Finally, foam rollers in quadruped may be used to fully challenge proprioception and balance (Fig. 12-19).

The duration of the treatment program depends on the chronicity of the spinal dysfunction and whether the treatment regimen is changing treatment goals. For chronic LBP it is suggested that to affect chronic deconditioning and poor movement patterning, 2 to 3 months of intensive treatment may be required before functional improvement is noted.[50]

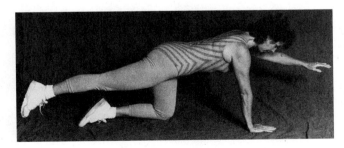

Fig. 12-18 Contralateral arm and leg movements in unsupported quadruped position.

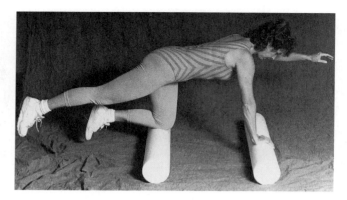

Fig. 12-19   Quadruped position using foam rollers to challenge proprioception and balance.

Unloading the Spine

Many patients are sensitive to axial loading through the spine during activities of daily living and exercise. When this is the case, an attempt should be made to control the axial load that the spine must bear during exercise or to allow intermittent "unweighting" throughout the day. Various traction devices can be used to provide distraction of the spine or in an inclined position before, during, or after exercise. Prone-lying over a gym ball also provides gentle distraction. Providing for upper extremity support during upright exercises such as squats, walking on a treadmill, sitting, or cycling decreases spinal loading (Fig. 12-20).

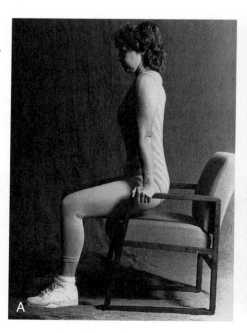
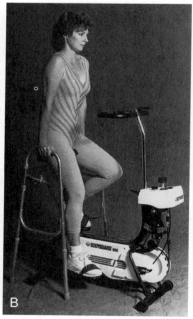

Fig. 12-20   A, Unloading the spine while sitting. **B,** Unloading when riding the bicycle.

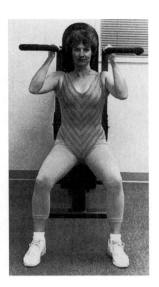

Fig. 12-21   Novak pulldown to unload.

When pulley systems or overhead weights are used to provide resistance to the upper extremities during stabilization training, there is an axial force upward on the spine that helps to counteract the compressive forces generated when the abdominals and extensors are cocontracting to stabilize the spine (Fig. 12-21). This type of exercise allows the load-sensitive patient to exercise more vigorously without increasing symptoms.

Functional Training

One reason for poor results of many exercise programs is failure to adequately train the patient in functional activities.[51] Various methods of improving the strength and coordination of truncal muscles have been presented as a precursor to functional training of the patient. Through carefully planned movement training patients are taught how to perform tasks that are pertinent to their daily function. Patients are instructed in how to perform functional activities in a manner that is safe for the spine and that no longer aggravates the symptoms. Repetition of the task (e.g., lifting) helps the patient learn new movement patterns and breaks substitution patterns that put the spine at risk. For example, most back patients must lean over a sink to wash their faces or remove groceries from a grocery basket, which usually facilitates truncal flexion. To teach the patient to eliminate flexion-dominated movement patterns, we can teach the patient to maintain the SFP in standing, and then advance to transitional movements such as half-bending. With the use of a wooden stick and a mirror for visual feedback, the patient is instructed to bend from the hips (hip hinge) while maintaining the SFP (Fig. 12-22). The spine is actively positioned in a pain-free position, and the patient is taught to move the spine much like the arm of a crane. More complex spinal control is required to combine the hip hinge with lower extremity movements in standing (Fig. 12-23). The squat with the hip

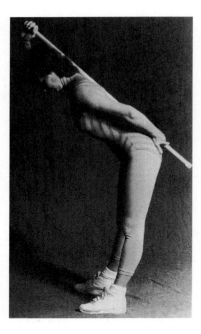

Fig. 12-22 Standing hip hinge.

hinge allows the patient to pick up a box or get an object out of a grocery cart (Fig. 12-24).

In preparation for training in lifting the patient can strengthen and improve the endurance of the truncal and lower extremity muscles by maintaining the squat position and performing various arm movements with weights (Fig. 12-25). If the goal is to repetitively lift 40 lb boxes, then the patient needs to gradually start lifting loads (e.g., 5 to 10 lbs), progressing the weight and number of lifts toward the demands of the work environment. When the patient is able to meet the lifting requirements of their job in the physical therapy gym, then he or she is ready to return to work.

Fig. 12-23 Combined hip hinge with squatting.

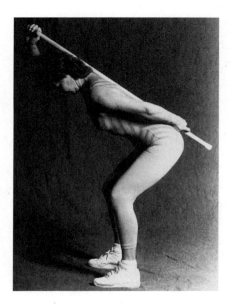

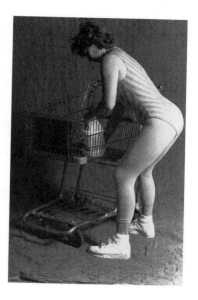

Fig. 12-24   Using hip hinge to get an object out of a cart.

Cardiovascular Conditioning

Aerobic activity in a painless manner is encouraged early in the treatment program. Ideally, we want to find an aerobic activity that the patient will continue indefinitely when physical therapy is discontinued. If walking decreases pain, then a walking program is initiated on the treadmill and at home. If the patient is load sensitive, he or she is instructed to walk on a treadmill while taking weight off the spine by using safety rails of the treadmill or with the use a traction harness.

Flexibility Training

Flexibility training usually begins at the outset of an exercise program. Stretching exercises may be needed to address mobility of the spine and

Fig. 12-25   Arm activities superimposed on a squat position.

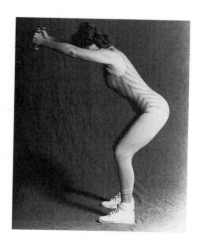

other joint restrictions. The most common muscle restrictions are found in the length of the hip rotators, adductors, iliopsoas, rectus femoris, hamstrings, gluteals, gastrosoleus, and back extensors. The patient is instructed in pre- and postexercise stretching routines as needed.

Static stretching is easy and safe because the patient is in control of the stretch. The patient positions the body part to be stretched and gradually increases the stretch for a 30-second count.[52] Proprioceptive neuromuscular facilitation techniques (e.g., hold-relax) have also been shown to be effective methods of muscle stretching.[53]

Exercises such as press-ups and knees to chest help to increase sagittal spinal ROM. It is important to note that many patients will not tolerate direct stretching of the spine during an acute episode of back pain. It is best to allow these patients to exercise and function in a restricted ROM until they have an increased range of their SFP. Continuous assessment will help the clinician know when it is safe to resume direct spinal stretching exercise. The reader is encouraged to review McKenzie's principles[54] for the application of flexion and extension exercises to different lumbar syndromes.

When muscles of the spine and extremities are stretched, nerves and fascia are also being stretched. Stretching the hamstrings of back patients in the presence of "adverse neural tissue tension"[23] warrants caution. Breig and Troup[55] have shown that internal rotation and adduction in straight leg raising increases the tension on the lumbosacral nerves. It is usually safest to begin stretching the limb in a position that decreases tension on the neural system (e.g., in some hip abduction, external rotation position). As the neural tension sign decreases, the muscle stretching may be progressed toward hip adduction and internal rotation to affect the lateral hamstrings. Because of the effect of stretching on neural structures, the patient's neurologic status should be monitored at regular intervals throughout treatment.

Home Exercises and Patient Management

Patients usually begin a home exercise program within the first treatment visit to reinforce the importance of taking an active part in rehabilitation. We carefully instruct patients in the number of repetitions and sets of each exercise as well as the amount of weight to use. When patients are discharged, they should understand the role of exercise in the ongoing management of spinal pain. They should also be able to apply principles of ergonomics to new tasks they will encounter in the work, home or recreational environments.

We encourage our patients to continue to exercise indefinitely. If the patient will not be seen again for quite some time we also provide instruction in ways to progress the level of difficulty of the program. Instruction is given not only in self-treatment techniques but also in when it is appropriate to seek professional advice for an exacerbation of back and/or leg pain. It is suggested that patients with chronic spinal dysfunction have their exercise programs re-evaluated periodically (e.g., every 3 to 6 months) to modify the program to meet new goals and to ensure compliance.[56]

SUMMARY

Therapeutic exercise is one of the most important components in the rehabilitation of the patient with LBP. A thorough examination is necessary to identify the patient's unique needs and to set realistic treatment goals. A carefully planned treatment program must be continually assessed to ensure that the treatment goals are being achieved. The exercise and functional training program should be task and/or job specific. It should involve detailed training in spinal proprioception, truncal (local and global muscle systems) and lower extremity strengthening, flexibility, endurance, aerobic conditioning, coordination, and specific functional skills. The exercise program should be individualized and challenging to the patient. The home exercise program should be similar to the program that was performed in the physical therapy gym. Adjunctive exercise equipment such as gym balls, rubber tubing, foam rollers, and cuff weights are inexpensive investments that allow patients to perform exercise programs on an ongoing basis at home.

ACKNOWLEDGMENTS

The authors wish to acknowledge Michael Moore, PT; Tim McGonigle, PT; Dennis Morgan, PT, DC; and Eileen Vollowitz, PT, for many conceptual ideas presented in this chapter. In addition, we wish to thank Edie Farrell, PT, for serving as our model and Chris Chenard for producing the photographs.

REFERENCES

1. National Institute for Occupational Safety and Health (NIOSH). Work practices guide for manual lifting. National Institute for Occupational Safety and Health, DHHS Publication NO. NIOSH 81, 1981
2. Mayer TG, Gatchell RJ, Kishino N, et al: A prospective short-term study of chronic low back pain patients utilizing novel objective functional measurement. Pain 25:53, 1986
3. Edwards BC, Zusman M, Hardcastle P, et al: A physical approach to the rehabilitation of patients disabled by chronic LBP. Med J Aust 156:167, 1992
4. Mitchell RI, Carmen GM: Results of a multicenter trial using an intensive active exercise program for the treatment of acute soft tissue and back injuries. Spine 15:514, 1990
5. van Tulder MW, Koes BW, Bouter LM: Conservative treatment of acute and chronic nonspecific low back pain. A systematic review of randomized controlled trials of most common interventions. Spine 22(18):2128, 1997
6. Smith S, Mayer TG, Gatchell RJ, Beck TJ: Quantification of lumbar function. Part I: isometric and multispeed isokinetic trunk strength measures in sagittal and axial planes in normal subjects. Spine 10:757, 1985
7. Saal JA, Saal, JS: Nonoperative treatment of herniated lumbar intervertebral disc with radiculopathy. An outcome study. Spine 14:431, 1989
8. Lindstrom I, Ohlund C, Ckaes E, et al: Mobility, strength and fitness after a graded activity program of patients with subacute low back pain. Spine 17:641, 1992

9. Saal JS: Flexibility training. Phys Med Rehabil: State Art Rev 1:537, 1987

10. Mc Neil T, Warwick D, Andersson G, Schultz A: Trunk strengths in attempted flexion, extension and lateral bending in healthy subjects and patients with low back disorders. Spine 5:529, 1980

11. Rissanen A, Kalimo H, Alaranta H: Effect of intensive training on the isokinetic strength and structure of lumbar muscles in patients with chronic low back pain. Spine 20:333–340, 1995

12. Hides J, Richardson C, Jull G. Multifidus muscle rehabilitation decreases recurrence of symptoms following first episodes of low back pain. In Proceedings of the 1996 National Physiotherapy Congress of Australia, Queensland, Australia, 43, 1996

13. Smidt GL, Herring T, Amundsen L, et al: Assessment of abdominal and back extensor functions. Spine 11:29, 1983

14. Bogduck N, MacIntosh J: The applied anatomy of the thoracolumbar fascia. Spine 9:164, 1984

15. Gracovetsky S, Farfan H, Hellew C: The abdominal mechanism. Spine 10:317, 1985

16. Hodges P, Richardson C: Inefficient muscular stabilisation of the lumbar spine associated with low back pain: A motor control evaluation of the transversus abdominis. Spine 21:40, 1996

17. O'Sullivan PB, Twomey LT, Allison GT: Evaluation of specific stabilizing exercise in the treatment of chronic low back pain with radiologic diagnosis of spondylolysis or spondylolisthesis. Spine 22(24):2959, 1997

18. Saal JA: General principles and guidelines for rehabilitation of the injured athlete. Phys Med Rehabil: State of the Art Rev 1:523, 1987

19. Vollowitz E: Furniture Prescription. Top Acute Care Rehabil 2:18, 1988

20. Hildebrandt J, Pfingsten M, Saur P, Jansen J: Prediction of success from a multidisciplinary tretment program for chronic low back pain. Spine 22:990, 1997

21. Greenough GC, Fraser RD: The effects of compensation on recovery from low back injury. Spine 14:947, 1989

22. Polatin PB, Gatchell RJ, Barnes D, et al: A psychosociomedical prediction model of response to treatment by chronically disabled workers with low back pain. Spine 14:956, 1989

23. Butler D: Mobilization of the Nervous System. Churchill Livingstone, New York, 1991

24. Maitland GD: Vertebral Manipulation (5th Ed.). Butterworths, London, 1986

25. Janda V: Muscle Function Testing. Butterworths, London, 1983

26. Nadler SF, Wu KD, Galski T, Feinberg JH : Low back pain in college athletes: A prospective study correlating lower extremity overuse or aquired ligamentous laxity with low back pain. Spine 23:828, 1998

27. Bergmark A: Stability of the lumbar spine. A study in mechanical engineering. Acta Orthop Scand 230(suppl 60):20, 1989

28. Richardson C, Jull G. Muscle control-pain control. What exercises would you prescribe? Man Therapy 1:2–10, 1995

29. Hodges P, Richardson C, Jull G: Evaluation of the relationship between laboratory and clinical tests of transversus abdominus function. Physiother Res Internat 1:30–40, 1996

30. Richardson C, Jull G, Toppenberg R, Comerford M: Techniques for active lumbar stabilisation for spinal protection. A pilot study. Aust J Physiol 38:105, 1992

31. American College of Sports Medicine: Guidelines for exercise testing and prescription (4th Ed.). Lea & Febiger, Philadelphia, 1991

32. Astrand PE, Rodahl K: Textbook of Work Physiology: Physiological Bases of Exercise (3rd Ed.). McGraw-Hill, New York, 1986

33. Morgan D: Concepts in functional training and postural stabilization for the low back injured. Top Acute Care Trauma Rehabil 2:8, 1988

34. Porterfield JA, DeRosa C: Mechanical Low Back Pain: Perspective in Functional Anatomy. WB Saunders, Philadelphia, 1990

35. O'Sullivan PB, Twomey L, Allison GT: Dysfunction of the neuro-muscular system in the presence of low back pain—Implications for physical therapy management. J Man Manip Therapy 5(1):20, 1997

36. Byl N, Sinnott P: Variations in balance and body sway in middle aged adult subjects with healthy backs compared with subjects with low back dysfunction. Spine 16(3):325, 1991

37. Mattila M, Hurme M, Alaranta H, et al: The multifidus muscle in patients with lumbar intervertebral disc herniation. A histochemical and morphometric analysis of intraoperative biopsies. Spine 11(7):733, 1986

38. Zhu X-Z, Parnianpour M, Nordin M, Kahanovitz N: Histochemistry and morphology of the erector spinae muscle in lumbar disc herniation. Spine 14(4):391, 1989

39. Hides J, Richardson C, Jull G: Multifidus recovery is not automatic following resolution of acute first episode of low back pain. Spine 21:2763, 1996

40. Brooks VB: Motor control: How posture and movement are governed. Phys Therapy 63:664, 1983

41. Parkhurst TM, Burnett CN: Injury and proprioception in the lower back. JOSPT 19(5):282, 1994

42. Harris FA: Facilitation techniques and technological adjuncts in therapeutic exercise. In Basmajian JV (Ed.): Therapeutic Exercise (4th Ed.). Williams & Wilkins, Baltimore, 1984

43. Saal JA: The new back school prescription: Stabilization training II. Occup Med State Art Rev 7:33, 1992

44. Hides J, Stokes M, Saide M, et al: Evidence of lumbar multifidus muscle wasting ipsilateral to symptoms in patients with acute and subacute low back pain. Spine 19:165, 1994

45. Suzaki N, Endo S: A qualitative study of trunk muscle strength and fatiguability in the low back pain syndrome. Spine 8:69, 1984

46. Cooper R, Stokes M, Sweet C, et al: Increased central drive during fatiguing contractions of the paraspinal muscles in patients with chronic LBP. Spine 18(5):610, 1993

47. Knott J, Voss DE: Proprioceptive neuromuscular facilitation (2nd Ed.). Harper & Row, New York, 1968

48. Taimela S, Osterman L, Alaranta H, Kijala AS: Long psychomotor reaction times in patients with chronic LBP. Arch Phys Med Rehab 74:1161, 1993

49. Gill KP, Callaghan MJ: Measurement of lumbar proprioception in individuals with and without low back pain. Spine 23:371, 1998

50. Manniche C, Lundberg E, Christenson I, et al: Intensive dynamic back exercises for chronic low back pain: a clinical trial. Pain 47:53, 1991

51. Estlander A, Mellin G, VanHaranta H, Hupli M: Effects and follow-up of a multimodel treatment program including intensive physical training for low back patients. Scand J Rehabil Med 23:97, 1991

52. Bandy WD, Irion JM, Biggler M: The effect of time and frequency of static stretching on flexibility of the hamstring muscles. Phys Therapy 77:1090, 1997

53. Sody S, Wortman M, Blanke D: Flexibility training: Ballistic static or proprioceptive neuromuscular facilitation. Arch Phys Med Rehabil 63:261, 1982

54. McKenzie R: The Lumbar Spine. Spinal Publications, Waikenei, New Zealand, 1980

55. Breig A, Troup J: Biomechanical considerations in the straight leg raising test. Spine 4:242, 1979

56. Reilly K, Lovejoy B, Williams R, Roth H: Differences between a supervised and independent strength and conditioning program with chronic low back syndromes. J Occup Med 31:547, 1989

13

Psychologic Aspects of Back Pain: Implications for Physical Therapists

Dennis C. Turk
Akiko Okifuji
Jeffrey J. Sherman

Back pain is ubiquitous in western countries. The yearly prevalence of back pain in working adults in the United States is 50% and accounts for over 156 million lost work days for employed individuals. Of those in the United States with back pain, 15% to 20% will seek medical care.[1] In the United States it is estimated that there are 5.2 million people disabled by persistent back pain, with 2.6 million permanently disabled. The costs of back pain to the economy are staggering, with estimated health care expenditures at $20 billion and indemnity costs, lost tax revenue, and lost productivity at least three times as expensive. Although these are U.S. figures, there is no reason to believe that these statistics would be very different in most industrialized countries. Regardless, these figures do not do justice to the incalculable human suffering associated with chronic back pain.

By any criteria, back pain most be viewed as a significant problem that has reached epidemic proportions with few signs that the epidemic is abating. This state of affairs seems paradoxic given the major advances in knowledge of sensory physiology, anatomy, and biochemistry along with the development of potent analgesic medications and other innovative medical and surgical interventions. Despite these advances, pain relief for many back pain patients remains elusive. It seems reasonable to ask, how can a problem as prevalent, costly, and devastating as pain be so poorly understood and managed?

Support for the preparation of this manuscript was provided in part by grants from the National Institute of Arthritis and Musculoskeletal and Skin Diseases (R01 AR44724) and the National Institute of Child Health and Human Development (HD33989) awarded to the first author and National Institutes of Health/Shannon Director's Award (R55 AR44230) awarded to the second author.

351

This chapter discusses a number of issues that may help to clarify the factors that contribute to the apparent paradox of increasing numbers and modest outcomes at the time of advanced knowledge. However, first a self-test is presented to orient you to some of the topics that are addressed and sensitize the reader to some important issues that may contribute to the problem of treating people with chronic pain successfully.

SELF-TEST

True   False

1. Pain is directly proportional to tissue damage.
2. Pain without any pathology indicates that the patient is malingering.
3. Psychologic factors are unimportant for those patients who have known pathology for their pain.
4. Patients who do not follow a therapeutic regimen must be ignorant or have personality problems.
5. Motivating patients is not a physical therapist's responsibility.

Although you may not have selected the response *true* for each of these questions, these are commonly held stereotypes of chronic low back pain (LBP), LBP patients, and clinical responsibility. The primary objective of this chapter is to describe the various psychologic factors relevant to understanding and treating chronic pain patients and, in particular, to indicate the importance of these factors for physical therapists in treating chronic LBP patients. First, we describe traditional, unidimensional models of chronic pain because the models clinicians hold have an important influence on how patients are viewed, evaluated, and treated. We then discuss specific psychologic factors (behavioral, emotional, and cognitive) that are most relevant to the assessment and treatment of chronic LBP patients, emphasizing the implications of these factors for physical therapists in their treatment of these patients. We then describe some efforts to develop comprehensive, multidimensional models that integrate physical and psychologic factors. Finally, we describe a general approach to treatment (cognitive-behavioral) of chronic pain patients that follows from these integration models. We describe some techniques (especially, motivational interviewing) that have been developed and that may augment usual physical therapies and thereby facilitate successful outcome.

Our central objective is to encourage you to think about and behave differently toward patients. In short, we hope to convince you that how you think about your patients (e.g., not as "pain patients" but rather as "people with pain"), engage them in treatment (attending to their beliefs, expectations, and concerns; focusing on and building motivation), and interact with them (collaboratively; positively reinforcing their efforts as well as achievements) should be given as much attention as the time given to deciding whether to use McKenzie or Williams exercises, transcutaneous electrical nerve stimulation (TENS), and ice packs or hot packs.

UNIDIMENSIONAL CONCEPTUALIZATIONS OF CHRONIC PAIN

We can contrast two types of models or conceptualizations: unidimensional ones that focus on single causes of the symptoms reported, and multidimensional ones that suggest the importance of a range of factors that influence patients' experiences and reports of pain. We begin with a brief overview of the unidimensional conceptualizations (i.e., biomedical, psychogenic, motivational) and then describe a set of relevant psychologic factors and follow this discussion with a description of integrated, multidimensional conceptual models.

Biomedical Model of Chronic Pain

The traditional biomedical or somatic view is reductionistic. This perspective assumes that every report of pain must be associated with a specific physical cause. As a consequence, the extent of pain reported should be directly proportional to the amount of detectable tissue damage. Health care providers may spend inordinate amounts of time and effort (often at great expense) attempting to establish the specific link between tissue damage and the pain complaint. The expectation is that once *the* physical cause has been identified, appropriate treatment will follow. Treatment will focus on eliminating the putative cause(s) of the pain or chemically or surgically disrupting the pain pathways.

There are, however, several perplexing features of persistent reports of back pain that do not fit neatly within the traditional biomedical model, with its suggestion of an isomorphic relationship between tissue pathology and symptoms. A particular conundrum is the fact that pain may be reported even in the absence of identified pathologic process. For example, in 80% to 85% of the cases, the cause of back pain is unknown.[2] Conversely, diagnostic imaging studies using computed tomography (CT) scans and magnetic resonance imaging (MRI) have consistently noted the presence of significant pathology in up to 35% of asymptomatic individuals.[3,4] Thus there may be reports of severe pain in the absence of identifiable pathology, and pathology in the absence of any reported pain. Furthermore, the same medical, surgical, or physical intervention performed to correct identical pathologic "causes" of pain and performed in the same manner may lead to disparate results.

Psychogenic Model of Chronic Pain

As is frequently the case in medicine, when physical explanations prove inadequate to explain symptoms or when the results of treatment are inconsistent, psychologic etiologic alternatives are proposed as explanations. If the pain reported is deemed to be "disproportionate" (the criteria for proportionate is based on the subjective opinion of the health care provider) to objectively determined pathologic process, or if the complaint is recalcitrant to "appropriate" treatment that should eliminate or alleviate the pain, then it is assumed that psychologic factors must be implicated in the reported pain. The psychogenic view is posed as an alternative to a biomedical model. From this perspective, if the patient's report of pain occurs in the absence of, or is disproportionate to, objective physical pathology, then the pain reports must have a psychologic etiology and thus are "psychogenic."

Assessment based on the psychogenic perspective is directed toward identifying the personality factors or psychopathologic tendencies that initiate and maintain the reported pain. Once identified, treatment is geared toward helping the patient gain insight into the maladaptive, predisposing psychologic factors. The assumption is that once the patient becomes aware of these psychologic causes of symptoms he or she will be able to develop better methods for dealing with them and thus the symptoms will be relieved. The goal of treatment is to foster insight, after which pain will resolve. Unfortunately, to date, insight has not been shown to be effective in reducing symptoms of the majority of patients with chronic back pain.

Motivational Model

The motivational conceptualization is an alternative to the psychogenic model. From this perspective, reports of pain in the absence of or in excess of physical pathology are attributed to the desire of the patient to obtain some benefit such as attention, time off from undesirable activities, or financial compensation. In contrast to the psychogenic model, in the motivational model the assumption is that the patient is consciously attempting to acquire a desirable outcome. Simply put, the complaint of pain in the absence of pathologic process is regarded as fraudulent.

Assessment of patients from the motivational model focuses on identifying discrepancies between what patients say they are capable of doing and what they actually can do. From this perspective a high degree of discrepancy between what the patient says about his or her pain and disability and performance on more objective assessment of physical functioning are taken as evidence that the patient is exaggerating or fabricating his or her symptoms to obtain a desired outcome. Thus, repeated performance of functional capacity testing that identifies discrepancies (sometimes referred to as the "index of congruence") in performance has been used to label patients as malingerers at worst or symptom magnifiers at best. Surveillance is also used as an assessment method, again looking for discrepancies between the patient's complaints and objective performance. Thus a patient who indicates that he cannot lift weights over 5 lbs might be videotaped lifting groceries out of his car. The ability to lift bags of groceries is taken as an indication that the patient is capable of lifting. Thus the report of the inability to lift, in the light of the observation of lifting groceries, is viewed as an instance of fabrication.

The treatment from the motivational perspective is simple—denial of disability claims in the absence of pathologic process when there is a high degree of discrepancy between what the patient claims and what he or she is observed to do. The assumption is that denial of disability will lead to prompt resolution of the reported symptoms. Although this view is prevalent, especially among third-party payers, there is little evidence of dramatic cure of pain following denial of disability claims.

The biomedical, psychogenic, and motivational views are unidimensional where the report of pain is ascribed to *either* physical *or* psychologic factors. Rather than being categorical, either somatogenic or psychogenic, both physical and psychologic components may interact to create and influence the experience of pain. There has been a tremendous number of studies examining the role of behavioral, emotional, and cognitive factors in chronic pain patients. The next section reviews the most prominent psychologic factors shown to play an important role in influencing not only the report of symptoms but also patients' responses to rehabilitation efforts. Thus an understanding of the psychology of pain is important for physical therapists if they hope to optimize their efforts in facilitating patients' rehabilitation.

PSYCHOLOGY OF PAIN

For the individual experiencing chronic back pain, there is a continuing quest for relief that remains elusive and leads to feelings of frustration, demoralization, and depression, compromising the quality of all aspects of their lives. Patients with chronic back pain confront not only the stress of pain but also a cascade of ongoing problems (e.g., financial, familial). Moreover, the experience of "medical limbo" (i.e., the presence of a painful condition that eludes diagnosis and that carries the implication of either psychiatric causation or malingering on the one hand, or an undiagnosed potentially disabling condition on the other) is itself the source of significant stress and can initiate psychologic distress.

Biomedical factors, in the majority of cases, appear to instigate the initial report of pain. Over time, however, psychosocial and behavioral factors may serve to maintain and exacerbate the level of pain, influence adjustment, and contribute to excessive disability. Following from this view, back pain that persists over time should not be viewed as solely physical or solely psychologic; the experience of pain is maintained by an interdependent set of biomedical, psychosocial, and behavioral factors.

Consider the following scenario. A patient with back pain becomes inactive, leading to preoccupation with his or her body and pain, and these cognitive-attentional changes increase the likelihood of amplifying and distorting pain symptoms. Patients may then perceive themselves as being disabled. At the same time, due to fear, the pain sufferer limits his or her opportunities to identify activities that build flexibility, endurance, and strength without the risk of pain or injury. To the pain sufferer, hurt is often viewed as synonymous with harm. Thus, if an activity produces an increase in pain, the chronic pain sufferer terminates the activity and avoids similar activities in the future. Indeed, chronic pain sufferers often develop negative expectations about their own ability to exert any control over their pain. The negative expectations lead to feelings of frustration and demoralization when "uncontrollable" pain interferes with participation in physical and social activities.

Pain sufferers frequently terminate efforts to develop new strategies to manage pain and, instead, turn to passive coping strategies such as inactivity, medication, or alcohol to reduce emotional distress and pain. They also absolve themselves of personal responsibility for managing their pain and, instead, rely on family and health care providers. The thinking, or "cognitive activity," of back pain patients has been shown to contribute to the exacerbation, attenuation, or maintenance of pain, pain behaviors, affective distress, and dysfunctional adjustment to chronic pain.[5,6]

Significant others also may unwittingly contribute to the pain and disability observed in chronic back pain patients. For example, if a patient's complaint about his back pain results in his wife giving him more attention, then the positive attention may reward and thereby increase the likelihood of more complaint to obtain the desired attention. The physical therapist who responds to the patient's complaints of increased pain by terminating exercise may also be promoting complaints as a means for the patient to avoid pain produced by use of deconditioned muscles during exercises. We discuss the role of rewards and attention in more detail in the next section.

If psychologic factors can influence pain in a maladaptive manner, then they can also have a positive effect. Individuals who feel that they have a number of successful methods for coping with pain may suffer less than those who feel helpless and hopeless.

In the case of chronic back pain, health care providers need to consider not only the physical basis of pain (the nociceptive, sensory component) but also patients' mood, fears, expectancies, coping resources, coping efforts, and response of significant others, including themselves. Regardless of whether there is an identifiable physical basis for the reported pain, psychosocial and behavioral factors will interact to influence the nature, severity, and persistence of pain and disability. In particular, behavioral, emotional, and cognitive variables should be addressed. We now consider the specific psychologic principles and variables and show how they may influence pain perception, reports of pain, and response to treatment.

Behavioral Factors

Pain is an unavoidable part of human lives. No learning is needed to activate nociceptive receptors. However, pain is a potent and salient experience for humans. We all attempt to avoid, modify, or cope with pain. There are three major principles of behavioral learning that help us understand acquisition of adaptive as well as dysfunctional behaviors associated with pain.

Classical (Respondent) Conditioning

Classical conditioning is widely known as Pavlovian learning from the seminal research of Russian physiologist, Ivan Pavlov. In his classic experiment,

Pavlov found that a dog could be taught, or "conditioned," to salivate at the sound of a bell by pairing the sound with food presented to a hungry dog. Salivation of dogs to food is a natural response; however, by preceding the feeding with the sound of a bell, Pavlov's dogs learned to associate the bell with an imminent feeding. Once this association was learned, or "conditioned," the dogs were found to salivate at the mere sound of bell *even in the absence of the food.* That is, the dogs were conditioned to anticipate food at the sound of a bell.

The influence of classical conditioning can be often be observed in humans. For example, cancer patients receiving chemotherapy often suffer from extreme gastrointestinal symptoms (nausea and vomiting) resulting from the pharmacologic effects of chemotherapy. The nausea has been shown to be classically conditioned to neutral cues paired with the chemotherapy, such as doctors, nurses, the hospital, and even patients' clothes.[7] Once acquired, learned responses tend to persist over long periods. It is not uncommon to observe cancer patients long in remission who report nausea as soon as they see their doctor's face, even years after the completion of the treatment.

Although we hope that the effects of classical conditioning are not so pronounced with physical therapists, they are certainly not immune to such learning, and they may become a potent cue for back pain patients to respond in certain ways. Table 13-1 illustrates the way in which physical therapists may evoke a conditioned fear response in the patients they are treating.

A patient, for example, who received a painful treatment from a physical therapist may become conditioned to experience a negative emotional response to the presence of the physical therapist, to the treatment room, and to any contextual cues associated with the nociceptive stimulus. The negative emotional reaction may lead to tensing of muscles, and this in turn may exacerbate pain and thereby strengthen the association between the presence of the physical therapist and pain.

Once an acute pain problem persists, fear of motor activities becomes increasingly conditioned, resulting in avoidance of activity. The avoidance of pain is a powerful rationale for reduction of activity, whereas muscle soreness associated with exercise functions as a justification for further avoidance. Thus, although it may be useful to reduce movement in the acute

Table 13-1 Classical Conditioning: Example with Pain–PT Association

Step 1: Natural Consequence of Pain—Fear

    Pain ➡ Fear

Step 2: Pairing

    PT Session

     | ➡   Fear

    Pain

Step 3: Conditioned Fear

    PT ➡ Fear

pain stage, limitation of activities can be chronically maintained not only by pain but also by anticipatory fear that has been acquired through classical conditioning.

In chronic pain, many activities that are neutral or pleasurable may elicit or exacerbate pain and are thus experienced as aversive and are avoided. Over time, more and more activities (e.g., people, physical locations, physical exercise) may be expected to elicit or exacerbate pain and will be avoided. Fear of pain may become associated with an expanding number of situations and behaviors. Avoided activities may involve simple motor behaviors but may also involve work, leisure, and sexual activity. Anticipatory fear and anxiety also elicit physiologic reactivity that may aggravate pain. Thus, psychologic factors may directly affect nociceptive stimulation and need not be viewed as only reactions to pain. We will return to this point later.

Insofar as activity-avoidance succeeds in preventing pain aggravation, the conviction that patients should remain inactive will be difficult to modify. By contrast, repeatedly engaging in behavior that produces significantly less pain than was predicted (corrective feedback) will be followed by reductions in anticipatory fear and anxiety associated with the activity. These adjustments will be increasingly followed by appropriate avoidance behavior, even to elimination of all inappropriate avoidance. Such transformations add support to the importance of a quota-based physical therapy program, with patients progressively increasing their activity levels despite fear of injury and discomfort associated with renewed use of deconditioned muscles.

Operant Conditioning—Environmental Contingencies of Reinforcement

As long ago as the early part of the twentieth century, the effects of environmental factors in shaping the experience of people suffering with pain were acknowledged. A new era in thinking about pain began in 1976 with Fordyce's[8] extension of *operant conditioning* to chronic pain. The main focus of operant learning is modification in frequency of a given behavior. If the consequence of the given behavior is rewarding, the likelihood of its occurrence increases; if the consequence is aversive, the likelihood of its occurrence decreases (see Table 13-2). Thus, only preexisting behaviors are operantly conditioned.

Behaviors associated with pain, such as limping and moaning, are called "pain behaviors." When an individual is exposed to a stimulus that causes tissue damage, the immediate behavior is withdrawal in an attempt to escape from noxious sensations. Such pain behaviors are adaptive and appropriate. According to Fordyce,[8] these behaviors can be subjected to the principles of operant conditioning. For example, pain behaviors such as avoidance of activity and help seeking effectively prevent or withdraw aversive results (i.e., pain). This negative reinforcement makes such behaviors more likely to occur in the future. The operant view proposes that acute pain behaviors such as avoidance of activity to protect a wounded limb from

Table 13-2 Operant Schedules of Reinforcement

Schedule	Consequences	Probability of the Behavior Recurring
Positive reinforcement	Reward the behavior	More likely
Negative reinforcement	Prevent or withdraw aversive results	More likely
Punishment	Punish the behavior	Less likely
Neglect	Prevent or withdraw positive results	Less likely

producing additional noxious input may come under the control of external contingencies of reinforcement (responses increase or decrease as a function of their reinforcing consequences: see Table 13-2) and thus develop into a chronic pain problem.

Pain behaviors are conceptualized as overt expressions of pain, distress, and suffering. As we noted earlier, these behaviors may be positively reinforced directly, for example, by attention from a spouse or health care providers. The principles of learning suggest that behaviors that are positively reinforced will be reported more frequently. Pain behaviors may also be maintained by the escape from noxious stimulation by the use of drugs or rest, or the avoidance of undesirable activities such as work. In addition "well behaviors" (e.g., activity, working) may not be positively reinforced, and the more rewarding pain behaviors may therefore be maintained.

We can consider an example to illustrate the role of operant conditioning. When a back pain sufferer's pain flares up, she may lie down and hold her back. Her husband may observe her behavior and infer that she is experiencing pain. He may respond by offering to rub her back. This response may positively reward the woman, and her pain behaviors (i.e., lying down) may be repeated even in the absence of pain. In other words, the woman's pain behaviors are being maintained by the learned consequences.

Another powerful way he reinforces her pain behaviors is by permitting her to avoid undesirable activities. When observing his wife lying on the floor, the husband may suggest that they cancel the evening plans with his brother, an activity that she may have preferred to avoid anyway. In this situation, her pain reports and behaviors are rewarded by her husband providing her with extra attention and comfort and the opportunity to avoid an undesirable social obligation.

It should be noted that the pain sufferer does not consciously communicate pain to obtain attention or avoid undesirable activities. It is more likely to be the result of a gradual process of the shaping of behavior that neither she nor her husband recognizes. Thus an individual's response to life stressors as well as how others respond to the pain sufferer can influence the experience of pain in many ways, but are not the cause of the pain condition.

Health care professionals may also reinforce pain and pain behavior by their responses. The physician who prescribes medication on the patient's complaint may be reinforcing the patient's reports of pain. That is, the patient learns that his or her behavior elicits a response from the physician, and if the response provides some relief of pain, then the patient may learn to report pain in order to obtain the desired outcome. This is the case when pain medication is prescribed on a "take as needed" (PRN) basis. In this case the patient must indicate that the pain has increased in order to take the medication. If the medication provides some reduction of pain then, the attention to and self-rating of pain may be maintained by the anticipated outcome of pain relief.

Physical therapists who suggest that patients engage in some exercises until the "pain becomes too severe" are functioning in the same way as the physician. The reinforcement of reduction in activity to reduce pain will come to maintain complaints and subsequently inactivity. The alternative for the physical therapist is to prescribe exercises on a work-to-goal rather than work-to-pain basis. Termination of the exercise is then paired with completion of a designated set of exercises, not pain. Here we can see how classical and operant conditioning become related. The pairing of the neutral and pain-evoking stimuli are classically conditioned, and the reinforcement schedule established by the health care professional leads to operant learning.

The combination of reinforced pain behaviors and neglected well behaviors is common in chronic LBP (Table 13-3). The operant learning paradigm does not uncover the etiology of pain but focuses primarily on the maintenance of pain behaviors and deficiency in well behaviors. Adjustment of reinforcement schedules will likely modify the probability of recurrence of pain behaviors and well behaviors.

It is important not to make the mistake of viewing pain behaviors as being synonymous with **malingering.** Malingering involves the patient consciously and purposely faking a symptom such as pain for some gain, usually financial. In the case of pain behaviors, there is no suggestion of conscious deception but rather the unintended performance of pain behaviors resulting from environmental reinforcement contingencies. The patient

Table 13-3 Example of Operant Maintenance of Pain Behavior in Chronic Low Back Pain

Operant Conditioning Stage	Chronic Stage: Even Without Pain
Pain➡Limping➡Sympathy (positive reinforcement)	➡Limping likely to recur
Pain➡Limping➡Avoiding work (negative reinforcement)	➡Limping likely to recur
Pain➡Exercise➡Flare-up (punishment)	➡Exercise unlikely to recur
Pain➡Exercise➡Apathy from others (neglect)	➡Exercise unlikely to recur

is typically not aware that these behaviors are being displayed, nor is he or she consciously motivated to obtain a positive reinforcement from the behaviors. Contrary to the beliefs of many third-party payers, there is little support for the contention that outright faking of pain for financial gain is prevalent.

The operant view has generated what has proven to be an effective treatment for select samples of chronic pain patients. Operant technique focuses on the elimination of pain behaviors by withdrawal of attention and increasing of well behaviors by positive reinforcement. Treatment based on operant conditioning is discussed later in this chapter.

Social Learning Mechanisms

Social learning has received some attention in acute pain and in the development and maintenance of chronic pain states. From this perspective the acquisition of pain behaviors may occur by means of "observational" learning and "modeling" processes. That is, individuals can acquire responses that were not previously in their behavioral repertoire by the observation of others performing these activities. Children acquire attitudes about health and health care and the perception and interpretation of symptoms and physiologic processes from their parents and social environment. They learn appropriate and inappropriate responses to injury and disease and thus may be more or less likely to ignore or overrespond to symptoms they experience based on behaviors modeled in childhood. The culturally acquired perception and interpretation of symptoms determines how people deal with illness. The observation of others in pain is an event that captivates attention. This attention may have survival value, may help to avoid experiencing more pain, and may help to learn what to do about acute pain.

There is ample experimental evidence of the role of social learning from controlled laboratory pain studies and from some evidence based on observations of patients behaviors in naturalistic and clinical settings. Physiologic responses to pain stimuli may be conditioned during observation of others in pain. For example, children of chronic pain patients may choose more pain-related responses during stressful times than do children with healthy or diabetic parents. These children tend to exhibit greater illness behaviors (for example, complaining, days absent, visit to school nurse) than children of healthy parents.

Expectancies and actual behavioral responses to nociceptive stimulation are based, at least partially, on prior social leaning history. This may contribute to the marked variability in response to objectively similar degrees of physical pathology noted by health care providers.

Emotional (Affective) Factors

Pain is ultimately a subjective, private experience, but it is invariably described in terms of sensory and affective properties. As defined by the

International Association for the Study of Pain: "[Pain] is unquestionably a sensation in a part or parts of the body but it is also always unpleasant and therefore also an emotional experience."[9] The central and interactive roles of sensory information and affective state are supported by an overwhelming amount of evidence.[10] The affective components of pain include many different emotions, but they are primarily negative emotions. Anxiety and depression have received the greatest amount of attention in chronic pain patients; however, anger has recently received considerable interest as an important emotion in chronic pain patients.

Depression and Anxiety

Research suggests that from 40% to 50% of chronic pain patients suffer from depression.[11] In the majority of cases, depression appears to be patients' reactions to their plight, although some have suggested that chronic pain is a form of "masked depression." That is, patients' reports of pain cover for underlying depression because it may be more acceptable to complain of pain than to acknowledge that one is depressed. This acknowledgment does not necessarily occur at a conscious level. Although this may be true in a small number of cases, the research on this topic does not suggest that depression precedes the development of chronic pain.[12]

It is not surprising that a large number of chronic pain patients are depressed. It is interesting to ponder the other side of the coin. Given the nature of the symptom and the problems created by chronic pain, why is it that all such patients are *not* depressed? Turk and colleagues[13, 14] examined this question and determined that patients' appraisals of the effects of the pain on their lives and of their ability to exert any control over the pain and their lives mediated the pain-depression relationship. That is, those patients who believed that they could continue to function despite their pain, and that they could maintain some control despite their pain, did not become depressed.

Anger

Anger has been widely observed in individuals with chronic pain.[15] Pilowsky and Spence[16] reported an incidence of "bottled-up anger" in 53% of chronic pain patients. Kerns et al[17] noted that the internalization of angry feelings was strongly related to measures of pain intensity, perceived interference, and reported frequency of pain behaviors. Summers et al[18] examined patients with spinal cord injuries and found that anger and hostility were powerful predictors of pain severity. Moreover, even though chronic pain patients in psychotherapy might present an image of themselves as even-tempered, 88% of the patients treated acknowledged their feelings of anger when these were explicitly sought.[19]

Frustrations related to persistence of symptoms, limited information on etiology, and repeated treatment failures along with anger toward employers, insurance companies, the health care system, family members, and themselves, all contribute to the general dysphoric mood of these patients. The effects of anger and frustration on exacerbation of pain and treatment acceptance has not received much attention, but it would be reasonable to expect that the presence of anger may serve as a complicating factor, increasing autonomic arousal and blocking motivation and acceptance of treatments oriented toward rehabilitation and disability management rather than cure, which are often the only treatments available for chronic pain.[20]

It is important to be aware of the important role of negative mood in chronic pain patients because it is likely to affect treatment motivation and compliance with treatment recommendations. For example, the patient who is anxious may fear engaging in what they perceive as physically demanding activities; patients who are depressed and who feel helpless may have little initiative to comply; and patients who are angry with the health care system are not likely to be motivated to respond to recommendations from yet another health care professional.

Cognitive (Thinking) Factors

A great deal of research has been directed toward identifying cognitive factors that contribute to pain and disability. These studies have consistently demonstrated that patients' attitudes, beliefs, and expectancies about their plight, themselves, their coping resources, and the health care system affect reports of pain, activity, disability, and response to treatment.

Beliefs about Pain

People respond to medical conditions in part based on their subjective ideas about illness and their symptoms. Health care providers working with chronic pain patients are aware that patients having similar pain histories and reports of pain may differ greatly in their beliefs about their pain. Behavior and emotions are influenced by interpretations of events, rather than solely by objective characteristics of the event itself. Thus pain, when interpreted as signifying ongoing tissue damage or a progressive disease, is likely to produce considerably more suffering and behavioral dysfunction than if it is viewed as being the result of a stable problem that is expected to improve.

People build fairly elaborate views of their physical state, and these views or representations provide the basis for action plans and coping. Beliefs about the meaning of pain and one's ability to function despite discomfort are important aspects of expectations about pain. For example, a cognitive representation that one has a very serious, debilitating condition, that disability is a necessary aspect of pain, that activity is dangerous, and that pain is an acceptable excuse for neglecting responsibilities will likely result in maladaptive responses. Similarly, if patients believe they have a serious condition that is quite fragile and a high risk for reinjury, they may fear engaging in physical activities. Through a process of stimulus generalization, patients may avoid more and more activities, becoming more physically de-conditioned and more disabled.

Consider the case of an individual who wakes up one morning with a backache. Very different responses would be expected if he attributed the backache to muscular strain from overdoing in on the tennis court the previous day in comparison with his interpretation that the back pain signaled a herniated disc and his friend had a similar problem requiring surgery and a poor postoperative recovery. Thus, although the amount of nociceptive input in the two cases may be equivalent, the emotional and behavioral responses would vary in nature and intensity. If the interpretation was that the back pain was related to overexercise, there might be little emotional arousal, and the man might take some over-the-counter analgesics, a hot shower, and take it easy for a few days. On the other hand, interpretation of the back pain as indicating a herniated disc would likely generate significant worry and might result in a call to an orthopedist.

Certain beliefs may lead to maladaptive coping, increased suffering, and greater disability. Patients who believe their pain is likely to persist may be quite passive in their coping efforts and fail to make use of strategies to cope with pain. Patients who consider their pain to be an unexplainable mystery may negatively evaluate their own abilities to control or decrease pain, and are less likely to rate their coping strategies as effective in controlling and decreasing pain. A person's beliefs, appraisals, and expectancies regarding the consequences of an event and his or her ability, are hypothesized to effect functioning in two ways. They may have a direct influence on mood and an indirect one through their effects on coping efforts.

Low back pain patients often demonstrate poor behavioral persistence in various exercise tasks. Their performance on these tasks may be independent of physical exertion or actual self-reports of pain, but rather be related to *previous* pain reports. These patients appear to have a negative view of their abilities and expect increased pain if they performed physical exercises. Thus the rationale for their avoidance of exercise was not the presence of pain but their *learned expectation* of heightened pain and accompanying physical arousal that might exacerbate pain and reinforce patients' beliefs regarding the pervasiveness of their disability. If patients view disability as a necessary reaction to their pain, that activity is dangerous, and that pain is an acceptable excuse for neglecting their responsibilities, they are likely to experience greater disability. Patients' negative perceptions of their capabilities for physical performance form a vicious circle, with the failure to perform activities reinforcing the perception of helplessness and incapacity.

Spiegel and Bloom[21] reported that the ratings of pain severity by cancer patients could be predicted not only by their use of analgesics and affective state but also by their *interpretations of pain*. Patients who attributed their pain to a worsening of their underlying disease experienced more pain despite having levels of disease progression comparable to patients with more benign interpretations. A strong illness conviction, the firm belief that the pain is caused by physical pathologic process and requires further surgical intervention, compounded by the belief that physical activity may cause further damage, can all make compliance with a physical exercise program unlikely.

Once beliefs and expectancies about a disease are formed they become stable and are very difficult to modify. Patients tend to avoid experiences that could invalidate their beliefs and guide their behavior in accordance with these beliefs, even in situations where the belief is no longer valid. Consequently, they do not receive corrective feedback. For example, a chronic pain patient who is deconditioned may experience some muscular soreness following activity. Although the soreness does not imply further tissue damage, it nevertheless confirms the belief that he should avoid the activity. Consequently the belief may lead to avoidance of the activity in the future, perpetuating the vicious circle.

In addition to beliefs about capabilities to function despite pain, beliefs about pain itself appear to be important in understanding response to treatment, adherence to self-management activities, and disability. When successful rehabilitation occurs there appears to be an important cognitive shift from beliefs about helplessness and passivity to resourcefulness and ability to function regardless of pain, and from an illness conviction to a rehabilitation conviction.

Clearly, it appears essential for patients with chronic back pain to develop adaptive beliefs about the relation among impairment, pain, suffering, and disability, and to de-emphasize the role of experienced pain in their regulation of functioning. In fact, results from numerous treatment outcome studies have shown that changes in pain level do not parallel changes in other variables of interest, including activity level, medication use, return to work, rated ability to cope with pain, and pursuit of further treatment. If physical therapists hope to achieve better outcomes and to reduce their frustration from patients' lack of compliance with their advice, then they need to learn about, to attend to, and to address patients' concerns within this therapeutic context.

Self-Efficacy

Self-efficacy is a personal expectation that is particularly important in patients with low back pain. A self-efficacy expectation is defined as a personal conviction that one can successfully execute a course of action (perform required behaviors) to produce a desired outcome in a given situation. Self-efficacy has been demonstrated as a major mediator of therapeutic change. Given sufficient motivation to engage in a behavior, it is an individual's self-efficacy beliefs that determine the choice of activities that he or she will initiate, the amount of effort that will be expended, and how long the individual will persist in the face of obstacles and aversive experiences. Efficacy judgments are based on four sources of information regarding one's capabilities, listed in descending order of effects:

One's own past performance at the task or similar tasks

The performance accomplishments of others who are perceived to be similar to oneself

Verbal persuasion by others that one is capable

Perception of one's own state of physiologic arousal, which is in turn partly determined by prior efficacy estimation

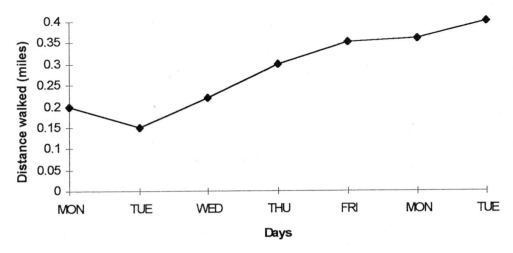

Fig. 13-1 Sample chart.

Performance mastery experience can be created by encouraging patients to undertake sub-tasks that are initially attainable but become increasingly difficult, and subsequently approaching the desired level of performance. In a quota-based physical therapy system the initial goal is set below initial performance in order to increase performance mastery. It is important to remember that coping behaviors are influenced by the individual's beliefs that the demands of a situation do not exceed their coping resources. For example, Council et al[6] asked patients to rate their self-efficacy as well as expectancy of pain related to performance during movement tasks. Patients' performance levels were highly related to their self-efficacy expectations, which in turn appeared to be determined by their expectancies regarding levels of pain that would be experienced.

Thus physical therapists need to assess patients' degree of confidence in their ability to perform specific exercises and to address the patients' concerns. Beginning exercises at an achievable level (e.g., 20% below tolerance) and then gradually increasing the exercises will lead to paced mastery as a reasonable strategy. In this way patients will achieve initial successes and build up their sense of self-efficacy. The use of exercise charts is also beneficial because these will permit patients to review their progress, and the feedback from the charts can reinforce their efforts as well as success. Charts can be quite simple, as shown in Fig. 13-1, and provide excellent avenues for delivering the types of self-efficacy–enhancing information described above.

Catastrophic Thinking

Catastrophizing—experiencing extremely negative thoughts about one's plight and interpreting even minor problems as major catastrophes—appears to be a particularly potent way of thinking that greatly influences pain and disability. Several lines of research have indicated that catastrophizing and adaptive coping strategies are important in determining one's reaction to pain. Individuals who spontaneously used more catastrophizing thoughts reported more pain than those who did not catastrophize in several acute and chronic pain studies. Turk, Meichenbaum, and Genest[22] concluded that "what appears to distinguish low from high pain tolerant individuals is their cognitive processing, catastrophizing thoughts and feelings that precede, accompany, and follow aversive stimulation . . ." (p. 197). As we shall see, these thoughts may have both direct and indirect effects on the experience of pain.

Coping

Self-regulation of pain and its effects depends on the individual's specific ways of dealing with pain, adjusting to pain, and reducing or minimizing pain and distress caused by pain; in other words, their coping strategies. Coping is assumed to be manifested by spontaneously employed purposeful and intentional acts, and it can be assessed in terms of overt and covert behaviors. Overt, behavioral coping strategies include rest, medication, and use of relaxation. Covert coping strategies include various means of distracting oneself from pain, reassuring oneself that the pain will diminish, seeking information, and problem solving. Coping strategies are thought to act to alter both the perception of intensity of pain and one's ability to manage or tolerate pain and to continue everyday activities.

Studies have found active coping strategies (efforts to function in spite of pain or to distract oneself from pain, such as activity or ignoring pain) to be associated with adaptive functioning, and passive coping strategies (depending on others for help in pain control and restricted activities) to be related to greater pain and depression. However, beyond this, there is no evidence supporting the greater effectiveness of any one active coping strategy compared with any other.[23] It seems more likely that different strategies will be more effective than others for some individuals at some times but not necessarily for all individuals all of the time.

Repeated performance of exercises can increase pain and become monotonous. If physical therapists want to increase compliance with an exercise program, they need to consider strategies that will deal with both of these. The former can be addressed by information and discussion. Moreover, relaxation exercises might be used in conjunction with the physical exercises. The issue of tedium is important because the exercises need to be performed on a regular basis over a long time without the presence of the physical therapist or other patients. Helping the patient anticipate this and working with him or her to generate strategies to cope with the monotony (e.g., doing exercises at a gym or health club, with a friend, using music) will increase the likelihood of long-term compliance.

A number of studies have demonstrated that if patients are instructed in the use of adaptive coping strategies, their rating of intensity of pain decreases and tolerance of pain increases. The most important factor in poor coping appears to be the presence of catastrophic thinking, rather than differences in the nature of specific adaptive coping strategies.

INDIRECT EFFECTS OF PSYCHOLOGIC FACTORS ON PAIN

Psychologic factors may act indirectly on pain and disability by reducing physical activity, consequently reducing muscle flexibility, strength, tone, and endurance. Fear of reinjury, fear of loss of disability compensation, and job dissatisfaction can also influence return to work.

Pain sufferers can develop ways of coping that in the short run seem adaptive, but in the long run maintain the chronic pain condition and result in greater disability. As noted earlier, one of the ways of coping is avoidance of activities because of the fear of pain or injury. For example, following an accident in which an individual hurts his back, he learned that certain movements made his pain worse. In response, he may stop engaging in activities that exacerbate his pain and restrict his movements in an attempt to avoid pain. Consequently, he may lose muscle strength, flexibility, and endurance. Here a vicious circle can be created, for as the muscles become weaker, more and more activities that cause pain may be avoided.

As the person with back pain remains inactive and becomes more physically deconditioned, this patient may not allow himself the opportunity to identify the activities that build flexibility, endurance, and strength without the risk of pain or injury. In addition, the distorted movements and postures that the individual assumes to protect himself from pain may cause further pain unrelated to his initial injury. Thus when the person limps, he protects muscles on one side of his back, but the muscles on the other side of his back become overactive and can develop into painful conditions of their own. Avoidance of activity, although it is a seemingly rational way to manage a pain problem, can actually play a large role in maintaining the chronic pain condition and increasing disability. In addition to contributing to the maintenance of the pain condition, the use of avoidant coping strategies has other negative consequences.

After having limited success in controlling pain, chronic pain sufferers can perceive pain and the factors that influence the pain to be outside of their personal control. Individuals who feel pain is uncontrollable are not likely to attempt new strategies to manage their pain. Instead, pain sufferers feel increasingly frustrated and demoralized when *uncontrollable* pain interferes with participation in rewarding recreational, occupational, and social activities. It is common for pain sufferers to resort to passive coping strategies such as inactivity, self-medication, or alcohol to reduce emotional distress and pain.

Pain sufferers who feel little personal control over their pain are also likely to *catastrophize* about the effects of situations that trigger or worsen pain as well as catastrophize about the effects of pain flare episodes. In contrast, individuals who believe they are able to control the situations that contribute to pain flare-ups are more resourceful and are more likely to develop strategies (e.g., relaxation or stress management strategies described below) that are effective in limiting the effects of the pain episodes or flare-ups and thus are able to limit the adverse effects of the pain problem.

If psychologic factors can influence pain in a maladaptive manner, they can also have a positive effect. Individuals who feel they have a number of successful methods for coping with pain may suffer less than those who feel helpless and hopeless. Later in this chapter we consider some of the psychologic interventions that have been shown to be effective in helping people with persistent pain to either eliminate their pain or, if pain cannot be eliminated, reduce their pain, distress, and suffering. These interventions are designed not only to decrease pain but also to improve physical and psychologic functioning.

DIRECT EFFECTS OF PSYCHOLOGIC FACTORS ON PAIN

Several studies have suggested that psychologic factors may actually have a direct effect on physiologic parameters associated more directly with the production or exacerbation of nociception. Cognitive interpretations and affective arousal may have a direct effect on physiology by increasing autonomic sympathetic nervous system arousal, endogenous opioid (endorphins) production, and elevated levels of muscle tension.

Effects of Thoughts on Autonomic Arousal

Circumstances that are appraised as potentially threatening to safety or comfort are likely to generate strong physiologic reactions. In patients suffering from recurrent migraine headaches, Jamner and Tursky[24] observed increased skin conductance (indicating emotional arousal) in response simply to seeing words describing migraine headaches displayed on a screen.

Chronic increases in sympathetic nervous system activation, leading to increased skeletal muscle tone, may set the stage for hyperactive muscle contraction and possibly for the persistence of a contraction following conscious muscle activation. Excessive sympathetic arousal is viewed as the immediate precursor of muscle hypertonicity, hyperactivity, and persistence. These in turn are the proximal causes of muscle spasm and pain. In is common for someone in pain to exaggerate or amplify the significance of their problem and needlessly *turn on* their sympathetic nervous system. In this way, thought processes may influence sympathetic arousal and thereby predispose the individual to further injury or otherwise complicate the process of recovery.

The direct effect of thoughts on muscle tension response was demonstrated by Flor, Turk and Birbaumer.[25] These investigators interviewed patients with back pain disorders, patients with other pain disorders, and healthy individuals. Muscle tension sensors were placed on the surface of the lower back, forearm, and forehead. At the same time as muscle activity was being monitored, patients were then asked to recall and describe in as much detail as possible the last time they experienced extreme pain and the last time they experienced severe stress. The study found that when discussing their pain or stress, the back pain patients had significantly elevated muscle tension in their back, but not in their forehead or forearm. However, when these back pain patients were resting and not discussing their pain or stress, their back muscle tension level was no higher than in the non–back pain patients or the healthy individuals. Neither the non–back pain patients nor the healthy individuals showed elevations in muscle tension when discussing severe stresses. Thus back pain patients showed pain-site–specific muscular arousal simply by talking about their pain and stress. Similar results have been observed in studies with patients with other types of pain.[23] That is, pain site-specific muscular responding to simply thinking about or talking about pain or stress.

Effects of Thinking on Biochemistry

Bandura and his colleagues[5] directly examined the role of central opioid activity in cognitive control of pain. They provided training in psychologic control of pain in which subjects received instructions and practice in using different coping strategies for alleviating pain, including attention diversion from pain sensations to other matters, engaging imagery, imaginal separation (dissociation) of the limb in pain from the rest of the body, transformation of pain as non-pain sensations, and self-encouragement of coping efforts. They demonstrated that (1) self-efficacy increased with cognitive training, (2) self-efficacy predicted pain tolerance, and (3) that naloxone (an opioid antagonist) blocked the effects of cognitive coping. The latter result implicates the direct effects of thoughts on the endogenous opioids (endorphins). Bandura et al[5] concluded that the physical mechanism by which self-efficacy influences pain perception may at least be partially mediated by the endogenous opioid system.

O'Leary et al[26] provided stress management treatment (described below) to rheumatoid arthritis (RA) patients. Degree of self-efficacy (expectations about the ability to control pain and disability) enhancement was correlated with treatment effectiveness. Those with higher self-efficacy and greater self-efficacy enhancement displayed greater numbers of suppressor T-cells (a direct effect of self-efficacy on physiology). Significant effects were also obtained for self-efficacy, pain, and joint impairment. Increased self-efficacy for functioning was associated with decreased disability and joint impairment.

INTEGRATIVE MODELS

Given our discussion of the psychologic factors that have been implicated as playing a role in pain, we can now consider how these factors can be integrated within multidimensional models of pain. Several multidimensional models have been developed, but the two most widely discussed are the gate control theory and the biopsychosocial model. These are not competing models but are actually complementary.

Pain is a complex subjective phenomenon comprising a range of factors, each of which contributes to the interpretation of nociception as pain. Thus pain is uniquely experienced by each individual. A significant factor contributing to the current situation relates to diagnostic uncertainty. The diagnosis of pain is not an exact science. A major problem in understanding pain is that it is a subjective (internal) state. There is no *pain thermometer* that can accurately measure the amount of pain an individual feels or should be experiencing. Although we all know what pain is, it can never be objectively measured; we can only infer how much pain is present from indications such as the amount of tissue damaged, verbal pain complaints, or nonverbal pain behaviors (overt expressions of pain and suffering such as limping or guarded movements). Even with tissue damage, it is impossible to specify how much pain *should be* experienced. For example, should a cut that is a half-inch long and one quarter-inch deep hurt twice as much as a cut that is a quarter-inch long and one-eighth inch deep? Nociception is a sensory process, and pain is a perceptual process that requires attention and interpretation of the nociceptive input. Thus, nociception and pain are not synonymous.

An integrative model of chronic pain and acute recurrent pain needs to incorporate the mutual interrelationships among physical, psychosocial, and behavioral factors and the changes that occur among these relationships over time. A model that focuses on only one of these sets of factors will inevitably be incomplete.

Investigators have proposed integrative models of pain, each with a somewhat different emphasis, but each of them attempting to integrate physiologic and psychologic variables in the etiology, severity, exacerbation, and maintenance of pain. The physiologic model proposed by Melzack and Wall[27] can be contrasted with the more psychologic, cognitive-behavioral (biobehavioral) model proposed by Turk and his colleagues.[22, 28, 29] Melzack and Wall focus primarily on the basic anatomy and physiology of pain whereas Turk et al emphasize the influence of psychologic processes on physical factors underlying the experience of pain. Yet both incorporate both physical and psychologic factors to account for the experience of pain.

Gate Control Theory

The first attempt to develop an integrative model designed to address the problems created by unidimensional models and to integrate physiologic and psychologic factors was the gate control theory proposed by Melzack and Wall.[27] Perhaps the most important contribution of the gate control theory is the way it changed thinking about pain perception. In this model, three systems are postulated to be related to the processing of nociceptive stimulation—sensory-discriminative, motivational-affective, and cognitive-evaluative—all thought to contribute to the subjective experience of pain. Thus the gate control theory specifically includes psychologic factors as an integral aspect of the pain experience. It emphasized the central nervous system (CNS) mechanisms and provided a physiologic basis for the role of psychologic factors in chronic pain.

The gate control theory proposes that a mechanism in the dorsal horn substantia gelatinosa of the spinal cord acts as a spinal gating mechanism that inhibits or facilitates transmission of nerve impulses from the body to the brain on the basis of the diameters of the active peripheral fibers as well as the dynamic action of brain processes. It was postulated that the spinal gating mechanism was influenced by the relative amount of excitatory activity in afferent, large-diameter (myelinated) and small-diameter (unmyelinated nociceptors) fibers converging in the dorsal horns. It was further proposed that activity in A-beta (large-diameter) fibers tends to inhibit transmission of nociceptive signals (closes the gate) while activity in A-delta and c (small-diameter) fibers tends to facilitate transmission (open the gate). The hypothetic gate is proposed to be located in the dorsal horn, and it is at this point that sensory input is modulated by the balance of activity of small-diameter (A-delta and c) and large-diameter (A-beta) fibers.

Melzack and Wall[27] postulated further that the spinal gating mechanism is influenced not only by peripheral afferent activity but also by efferent neural impulses that descend from the brain. They proposed that a specialized system of large-diameter, rapidly conducting fibers (the central control trigger) activate selective cognitive processes that then influence, by way of descending fibers, the modulating properties of the spinal gating mechanism. They suggested that the brain stem reticular formation functions as a central biasing mechanism, inhibiting the transmission of pain signals at multiple synaptic levels of the somatosensory system.

The gate control theory maintains that the large-diameter fibers play an important role in pain by inhibiting synaptic transmission in dorsal horn cells. When large-fiber input is decreased, mild stimuli that are not typically painful trigger severe pain. Loss of sensory input to this complex neural system, such as occurs in neuropathies, causalgia, and phantom limb pain, tend to weaken inhibition and lead to persistent pain. Herniated disc material, tumors, and other factors that exert pressure on or irritate these neural structures may operate through this mechanism. Emotional stress and medication that affect the reticular formation may also alter the biasing mechanisms and thus intensity of pain.

From the gate control perspective, the experience of pain is an ongoing sequence of activities, largely reflexive at the outset, but modifiable even in the earliest stages by a variety of excitatory and inhibitory influences, and by the integration of ascending and descending nervous system activity. The process results in overt expressions communicating pain and strategies by the individual to terminate the pain. In addition, considerable potential for shaping of the pain experience is implied because the gate control theory invokes continuous interaction of multiple systems (sensory-physiologic, affect, cognition, and, ultimately, behavior).

The gate control model describes the integration of peripheral stimuli with cortical variables, such as mood and anxiety, in the perception of pain. This model contradicts the notion that pain is either somatic or psychogenic and instead postulates that both factors have either potentiating or moderating effects on pain perception. In this model, for example, pain is not understood to be the result of depression or vice versa, but rather the two are seen as evolving simultaneously. Any significant change in mood or pain will necessarily alter the others. The gate control theory's emphasis on the modulation of inputs in the dorsal horns and the dynamic role of the brain in pain processes and perception resulted in the integration of psychologic variables such as past experience, attention, and other cognitive activities into current research and therapy on pain. Prior to this formulation, psychologic processes were largely dismissed as reactions to pain. This new model suggested that cutting nerves and pathways was inadequate because a host of other factors modulated the input. Perhaps the major contribution of the gate control theory was that it highlighted the central nervous system as an essential component in pain processes and perception.

The physiologic details of the gate control model have been challenged, and it has been suggested that the model is incomplete. As additional knowledge has been gathered since the original formulation in 1965, specific points of posited mechanisms have been disputed and have required revision and reformulation. Overall, however, the gate control theory has proved remarkably resilient and flexible in the face of accumulating scientific data and challenges. It still provides a powerful summary of the phenomena observed in the spinal cord and brain, and this model has the capacity to explain many of the most mysterious and puzzling problems encountered in the clinic. This theory has had enormous heuristic value in stimulating further research in the basic science of pain mechanisms as well as in spurring new clinical treatments.

The gate control theory can be credited as a source of inspiration for diverse clinical applications to control or manage pain, including neurophysiologically based procedures (for example, neural stimulation techniques, from peripheral nerves and collateral processes in the dorsal columns of the spinal cord), pharmacologic advances, behavioral treatments, and those interventions targeting modification of attentional and perceptual processes involved in the pain experience. After the gate control theory was proposed in 1965, no one could try to explain pain exclusively in terms of peripheral factors.

Biopsychosocial Model of Chronic Pain

Although the gate control model provided a conceptual basis for the role of psychologic factors in pain, it does not address the nature of the interaction in depth. Unlike the unidimensional biomedical perspective, which focuses on etiologic and pathophysiologic explanations for chronic pain, or the psychogenic view, which suggests pain as physical manifestations of psychologic difficulties, the biopsychosocial view provides an integrated model for chronic pain that incorporates purely mechanical and physiologic processes as well as psychologic and social contextual variables that may cause and perpetuate chronic pain. In contrast to the biomedical model's emphasis on the disease process, the biopsychosocial model views illness as a dynamic and reciprocal interaction between biologic, psychologic, and sociocultural variables that shape the persons response to pain.[28, 29] The biologic substrate of a disease is known to affect psychologic factors (e.g., mood) and the social context within which the person exists (e.g., interpersonal relationships).

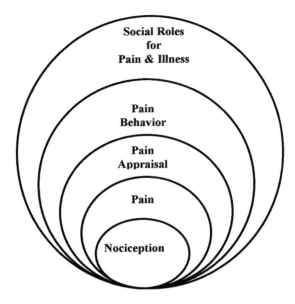

Fig. 13-2   Biopsychosocial model of pain.

The conceptual view of the biopsychosocial model is depicted in Fig. 13-2. The biopsychosocial model presumes some form of physical pathology or at least physical change in the muscles, joints, or nerves that generate nociceptive input to the brain. At the periphery nociceptive fibers transmit sensations that may or may not be interpreted as pain. Such sensation is not yet considered pain until subjected to higher-order psychologic and mental processing that involves perception, appraisal, and behavior. Perception involves the interpretation of nociceptive input and identifies the type of pain (i.e., sharp, burning, punishing, cruel). Appraisal involves the meaning that is attributed to the pain and influences subsequent behaviors. The individual may choose to ignore the pain and continue working, walking, socializing, and engaging in previous levels of activity or may choose to leave work, refrain from all activity, and assume the sick role. In turn, this interpersonal role is shaped by responses from significant others that may promote either the healthy and active response or the sick role. The biopsychosocial model has been instrumental in the development of cognitive-behavioral treatment approaches for chronic pain.

Cognitive-Behavioral Model for the Treatment of Chronic Back Pain

The cognitive-behavioral model has become the most commonly accepted and clinically useful conceptualization of chronic pain that follows from the biopsychosocial conceptualization of pain because it appears to have heuristic value for explaining the experience of and response to chronic pain. The cognitive-behavioral perspective suggests that behavior and emotions are influenced by interpretations of events, rather than solely by the objective characteristics of an event itself. Rather than focusing on the contribution of cognitive and emotional contributions to the perception of a set of symptoms in a static fashion, or exclusively on behavioral responses and environmental reinforcement contingencies, emphasis is placed on the ongoing reciprocal relationships among physical, cognitive, affective, social, and behavioral factors.

The cognitive-behavioral model incorporates many of the psychologic variables described above; namely, anticipation, avoidance, and contingencies of reinforcement, but suggests that cognitive factors—in particular, expectations rather than conditioning factors—are of central importance. The cognitive-behavioral model suggests that conditioned reactions are largely self-activated on the basis of learned expectations rather than automatically evoked. The critical factor for the cognitive-behavioral model therefore is not that events occur together in time but that people learn to predict them and to summon appropriate reactions. It is the individual patient's processing of information that results in anticipatory anxiety and avoidance behaviors.

According to the cognitive-behavioral model, it is patients' perspectives based on their idiosyncratic attitudes, beliefs, and unique representations that filter and interact reciprocally with emotional factors, social influences, behavioral responses, and sensory phenomena. Moreover, patients' behaviors elicit responses from significant others that can reinforce both adaptive and maladaptive modes of thinking, feeling, and behaving. Thus a reciprocal and synergistic model is proposed. One effective cognitive-behavioral interviewing and intervention technique is the introduction of self-monitoring records of symptoms, feelings, thoughts, and actions. Such daily diaries are useful diagnostically and clinically. They have the potential of demonstrating to the clinician and the patient the patterns of maladaptive thinking and pain behaviors that may be contributing to their pain experience. Self-monitoring records can be used for many purposes, such as allowing the therapist to know when flare-ups occur, identifying the precedents and antecedents of painful episodes, and determining target behaviors, thoughts, and feelings that should be addressed during therapy sessions.

Assumptions of Cognitive-Behavioral Treatment

There are five central assumptions that characterize the cognitive-behavioral perspective on treatment (summarized in Table 13-4). The first assumption is that all people are active processors of information rather than passive reactors to environmental contingencies. People attempt to make sense of the stimuli from the external environment by filtering information through organizing attitudes derived from their prior learning histories and by general strategies that guide the processing of information. People's responses (overt as well as covert) are based on these appraisals and subsequent expectations and are not totally dependent on the actual consequences of their behaviors (i.e., positive and negative reinforcements and punishments). From this perspective, the anticipated consequences are as important in guiding behavior as are the actual consequences.

Table 13-4 Assumptions of Cognitive-Behavioral Perspective
1. People are active processors of information rather than passive reactors to environmental contingencies.
2. Thoughts (for example, appraisals, attributions, expectancies) can elicit or modulate affect and physiologic arousal, both of which may serve as impetuses for behavior. Conversely, affect, physiology, and behavior can instigate or influence one's thinking processes.
3. Behavior is reciprocally determined by both the environment and the individual.
4. If people have learned maladaptive ways of thinking, feeling, and responding, then successful interventions designed to alter behavior should focus on each of these maladaptive thoughts, feelings, physiology, as well as behaviors and not one to the exclusion of the others.
5. In the same way that people are instrumental in the development and maintenance of maladaptive thoughts, feelings, and behaviors, they can, are, and should be considered active agents of change of their maladaptive modes of responding.

A second assumption of the cognitive-behavioral perspective is that one's thoughts (for example, appraisals, attributions, expectancies) can elicit or modulate affect and physiologic arousal, both of which may serve as impetuses for behavior. Conversely, affect, physiology, and behavior can instigate or influence one's thinking processes. Thus the causal priority depends on where in the cycle one chooses to begin. Causal priority may be less of a concern than the view of an interactive process that extends over time with the interaction of thoughts, feelings, physiologic activity, and behavior.

Unlike the more behavioral models (operant and respondent conditioning) described earlier, which emphasize the influence of the environment on behavior, the cognitive-behavioral perspective focuses on the reciprocal effects of the individual on the environment as well as the influence of environment on behavior. The third assumption of the cognitive-behavioral perspective, therefore, is that behavior is reciprocally determined by both the environment and the individual. Individuals not only passively respond to their environment but elicit environmental responses by their behavior. In a very real sense, people create their environments. The patient who becomes aware of a physical event (symptoms) and decides the symptom requires attention from a health care provider initiates a set of circumstances different from the individual with the same symptom who chooses to self-medicate.

A fourth assumption is that if people have learned maladaptive ways of thinking, feeling, and responding, then successful interventions designed to alter behavior should focus on these maladaptive thoughts, feelings, physiology, and behaviors and not on one to the exclusion of the others. There is no expectancy that changing only thoughts, or feelings, or behaviors will necessarily result in changes in the other two areas.

The final assumption of the cognitive-behavioral perspective is that in the same way as people are instrumental in the development and maintenance of maladaptive thoughts, feelings, and behaviors, they can, are, and should be considered active agents of change of their maladaptive modes of responding. Patients with chronic pain, no matter how severe and despite their common beliefs to the contrary, are not helpless pawns of fate. They can and should become instrumental in learning and carrying out more effective modes of responding to their environment and their plight.

From the cognitive-behavioral model, people with pain are viewed as having negative expectations about their own ability to control certain motor skills without pain. Moreover, pain patients tend to believe they have limited ability to exert any control over their pain. Such negative, maladaptive appraisals about the situation and personal efficacy may reinforce the experience of demoralization, inactivity, and overreaction to nociceptive stimulation. These cognitive appraisals and expectations are postulated as having an effect on behavior leading to reduced efforts and activity, which may contribute to increased psychologic distress (helplessness) and subsequent physical limitations. If one accepts that pain is a complex, subjective phenomenon that is uniquely experienced by each individual, then knowledge about idiosyncratic beliefs, appraisals, and coping repertoires becomes critical for optimal treatment planning and for accurately evaluating treatment outcome.

Biomedical factors that may have initiated the original report of pain play a diminishing role in disability over time, although secondary problems associated with deconditioning may exacerbate and maintain the problem. Inactivity leads to increased focus on and preoccupation with the body and pain, and these cognitive-attentional changes increase the likelihood of misinterpreting symptoms, overemphasizing symptoms, and perceiving oneself as being disabled. Reduction of activity, fear of reinjury, pain, loss of compensation, and an environment that, perhaps, unwittingly supports the *pain-patient role* can impede alleviation of pain, successful rehabilitation, reduction of disability, and improvement in adjustment. As has been noted, cognitive factors may not only affect the patient's behavior and indirectly their pain but may actually have a direct effect on physiologic factors believed to be associated with the experience of pain.

Patients' beliefs, appraisals, and expectations about pain, their ability to cope, social supports, their disorder, the medicolegal system, the health care system, and their employers are all important because they may facilitate or disrupt the patient's sense of control. These factors also influence patients' investment in treatment, acceptance of responsibility, perceptions of disability, adherence to treatment recommendations, support from significant others, expectancies for treatment, and acceptance of treatment rationale.

Cognitive interpretations also affect how patients present symptoms to significant others, including health care providers and employers. Overt communication of pain, suffering, and distress will enlist responses that may reinforce the pain behaviors and impressions about the seriousness, severity, and uncontrollability of the pain. That is, complaints of pain may lead physicians to prescribe more potent medications, order additional diagnostic tests, and, in some cases perform surgery. Family members may express sympathy, excuse the patient from usual responsibilities, and encourage passivity, thereby fostering further physical deconditioning. It should be obvious that the cognitive-behavioral perspective integrates the operant conditioning emphasis on external reinforcement and respondent view of learned avoidance within the framework of information processing.

People with persistent pain often have negative expectations about their own ability and responsibility to exert any control over their pain. Moreover, they often view themselves as helpless. Such negative, maladaptive appraisals about their condition, situation, and their personal efficacy in controlling their pain and problems associated with pain reinforce their experience of demoralization, inactivity, and overreaction to nociceptive stimulation. These cognitive appraisals are posited as having an effect on behavior, leading to reduced effort, reduced perseverance in the face of difficulty, and reduced activity and increased psychologic distress.

As noted in the research described earlier, the specific thoughts and feelings that patients experienced prior to exacerbation of pain, during an exacerbation or intense episode of pain, as well as following a pain episode can greatly influence the experience of pain and subsequent pain episodes. Moreover, the methods patients use to control their emotional arousal and symptoms have been shown to be important predictors of both cognitive and behavioral responses.

From the cognitive-behavioral perspective, assessment of and consequently treatment of the patient with persistent pain requires a broader strategy than those based on the previous dichotomous models described, which examine and address the entire range of psychosocial and behavioral factors, in addition to biomedical ones.

The cognitive-behavioral perspective on pain management focuses on providing the patient with techniques to gain a sense of control over the effects of pain on his or her life as well as actually modifying the affective, behavioral, cognitive, and sensory facets of the experience. Behavioral experiences help to show patients that they are capable of more than they assumed, increasing their sense of personal competence. Cognitive techniques (for example, self-monitoring to identify relationship among thoughts, mood, and behavior, distraction using imagery, and problem-solving) help to place affective, behavioral, cognitive, and sensory responses under the patients' control.

The assumption is that long-term maintenance of behavioral changes will occur only if the patient has learned to attribute success to his or her own efforts. There are suggestions that these treatments can result in changes of beliefs about pain, coping style, and reported pain severity, as well as direct behavior changes. Further, treatment that results in increases in perceived control over pain and decreased catastrophizing also are associated with decreases in pain severity ratings and functional disability.

USING PSYCHOLOGY IN PHYSICAL THERAPY: MOTIVATING THE CHRONIC PAIN PATIENT

So far, we reviewed how important and relevant the psychologic factors are to LBP. But how this can help the physical therapist treat his or her patients, since the physical therapist is not a psychologist? We believe that knowledge of the psychologic factors described previously will be helpful as therapists think about and interact with their patients. One does not need to be a psychologist to make use of the information.

We have all been confronted with the patient who, despite our best efforts, does not improve. We may face patients for whom our recommendations are met with doubting glances, furrowed brows, negative head nods, and other indications of skepticism. As in the case of cognitive-behavioral therapy, physical therapy requires a patient to be an active participant, engage in home exercises, and practice on his own. In short, motivation to change is a critical factor that may impede or promote recovery. Now we present a specific psychosocial strategy that may help therapists change patients' motivational levels.

Motivation Enhancement Techniques

Miller and colleagues[30,31] developed an approach designed to enhance a patient's motivation to change with a strong emphasis on specific clinician-patient interactions. The assumption when using motivational enhancement technique (MET) with pain patients is that how well the patient manages his pain depends on what he does. MET is based on the assumption that people vary in their degree of readiness for change. Stages depicting readiness for change are presented in Table 13-5.

Specific intervention strategies are organized to help a patient move from one stage to a more desirable stage or to keep the person in the action and maintenance stage. According to Miller and Rollnick,[31] there are several key components therapists should keep in mind:

1. Be empathetic. Judgmental attitudes by therapist are counterproductive.

2. Be specific to point out the discrepancy between what a patient wants from therapy (e.g., "I want to get well") and what he or she is doing (e.g., "I can't do my exercise because I am not well"). This should help patients organize ideas that their maladaptive behaviors are actually preventing them from obtaining their goal of getting better.

Table 13-5 Stages of Motivation

1. **Precontemplative stage:** Patient does not perceive a need to change and actively resists change
2. **Contemplation stage:** Patient begins to see a need for change and may consider making a change in the future
3. **Preparation stage:** Patient feels ready to change and makes a first concrete (behavioral) change
4. **Action stage:** Patient actively engages in behaviors consistent with regimen
5. **Maintenance stage:** Patient executes plans to sustain the changes made
6. **Relapse stage:** Some patients fail to sustain the effort

3.   Do not be argumentative. Therapist and patient should remain on the same side, not arguing against each other. Do not let the patient present a counterargument for why he or she should *not* engage in therapeutic effort.

4.   Be supportive, particularly for enhancing self-efficacy beliefs. The greater the confidence in one's ability to successfully perform therapeutic regimen, the better the outcome.

The physical therapist must determine whether the patient is ready to change. Patients who are not considering any changes in their behavior are considered to be in the precontemplative stage. Such patients do not perceive a need to change and will actively resist change. They may have a strong illness conviction and believe that something must be done to them before any improvement can occur and that any change in their behavior is superfluous to their recovery. Such patients may still be quite miserable but such misery is significantly different from a readiness to seriously contemplate specific behavioral changes necessary to feel better. During the contemplation stage the patient sees a need for change and may be considering making a change in the future. Such patients are weighing the pros and cons of change but are not yet fully committed to the idea. Although precontemplaters may make resistant, argumentative statements, contemplators usually make statements to indicate that change might be reasonable. The preparation stage involves both an intention to make changes and the initial steps toward change. During the action stage the patient is taking concrete activities (i.e., home exercise, walking, stress management) that will lead to desired change and decreased pain. Individuals in the fifth stage are maintaining those active efforts to sustain change. Finally, some individuals may *relapse* if they are unable to sustain the changes. Of course, they are free to reenter the change cycle at any point.

Some specific intervention strategies are listed in Table 13-6 to help a patient move from one stage to a more desirable stage or to keep the person in the action and maintenance stage. If the patient is in the precontemplation stage, all that may be possible is to raise the patient's doubt that not changing will only serve to continue misery. If the patient states that exercise is "out of the question!" "hurts too much," or "makes the pain worse," the goal of the therapist should be to raise doubt with the patient. The therapist should listen to the patient, acknowledge his ambivalence but encourage thoughts about the negative effects of inactivity.

During the contemplation stage, when the patient is evaluating the pros and cons of change, the therapist can tip the balance by, for example, building on comments about the negative effects of inactivity. During the preparation and action stages the patient will need assistance in developing and implementing a gradual plan for change and continued support and reinforcement of his readiness to change. Similarly, during the maintenance phase the therapist must provide considerable praise and reinforcement as well as continued assistance. Most importantly, if the patient relapses and experiences a severe pain episode, the therapist's role is to normalize the event, review the continuing process of recovery, and assist in the patients re-entry into his or her rehabilitation program.

Table 13-6 Specific Techniques Used in MET

MET Tactics	How to Do
Identify the discrepancy between patients' behaviors and goals of therapy	**Eliciting motivational statements by helping patients** • Recognize problems ("Yeah, I guess I really miss doing yard work") • Express concerns ("I worry what would happen if I don't do something to get rid of my pain") • Express interest in changing ("I could try to walk 10 minutes a day")
Strengthen patients' self-efficacy for change	• Search for evidence to be optimistic ("I guess if I limit my exercise to 20 minutes, I can do it every other day, at least") **Providing feedback**
Handle resistance to change	• Positively reinforce effort and progress **Providing reflective feedback** • Avoid confrontational argument • Provide reflection ("Sounds like you are really worried about having flare-up after exercise")
Strengthen commitment to change	• Reframe ("Sounds like management of flare-up is the key issue for you") **Planning** • Always providing free choice for patients (either 10 minutes fast walking or 10 minutes weight lifting per day) • Discussing pros and cons of planned change vs. no change
Follow-through	• Collaborating on prioritization of goals **Reviewing** • Reviewing progress, motivation, and commitment

CONCLUSION

It has become abundantly clear that no isomorphic relationship exists among tissue damage, nociception, and pain report. The more recent conceptualizations discussed view pain as a perceptual process resulting from the nociceptive input, which is modulated on a number of different levels in the CNS. In this chapter conceptual models were presented to explain the subjective experience of pain. As was noted, the current state of knowledge suggests that pain must be viewed as a complex phenomenon that incorporates physical, psychosocial, and behavioral factors. Failure to incorporate each of these factors will lead to an incomplete understanding. It is wise to recall John Bonica's comment in the preface to the first edition[32] of his volume, *The Management of Pain,* and repeated in the second edition some 36 years later[33]:

> The crucial role of psychological and environmental factors in causing pain in a significant number of patients only recently received attention. As a consequence, there has emerged a sketch plan of pain apparatus with its receptors, conducting fibers, and its standard function which is to be applicable to all cir-

cumstances. But . . . in so doing, medicine has overlooked the fact that the activity of this apparatus is subject to a constantly changing influence of the mind. (p. 12)

The range of psychologic variables that have been identified as being of central importance in pain, along with current understanding of the physiologic basis of pain, were reviewed. We now encourage you to return to the self-quiz on the first page of this chapter. You might want to have your colleagues answer the questions. You can then use the information you acquired in this chapter to educate them. After all, the best way to find out what you really learned is to try to teach someone else.

We hope that the material presented will influence your responses to the quiz, but even more will help your clinical practice with the next patient you treat. Physical therapy is a critical component of treatment for low back pain. Better understanding and incorporation of psychologic factors in physical therapy contributes to refinements in understanding of pain and advances in clinical management.

REFERENCES

1. Bigos S, Boyer O, Braen G, et al: Acute low back problems in adults. Washington, DC, US Department of Health and Human Services, 1994
2. Deyo RA: Early diagnostic evaluation of low back pain. J Gen Intern Med 1:328–338, 1986
3. Jensen M, Brant-Zawadzki M, Obuchowski N, et al: Magnetic resonance imaging of the lumbar spine in people without back pain. N Engl J Med 331:69–73, 1994
4. Wiesel SW, Tsourmas N, Feffer HL, et al: A study of computer-assisted tomography. I. The incidence of positive CAT scans in an asymptomatic group of patients. Spine 9:549–551, 1984
5. Bandura A, Cioffi D, Taylor CB, et al: Perceived self-efficacy in coping with cognitive stressors and opioid activation. J Pers Soc Psychol 55:479–488, 1988
6. Council J, Ahern D, Follick M, et al: Expectancies and functional impairment in chronic low back pain. Pain 33:323–331 1988
7. Carey M, Burish T: Etiology and treatment of the psychological side effects associated with cancer chemotherapy: a critical review and discussion. Psychol Bull 104:307–325, 1988
8. Fordyce W: Behavioral Methods in Chronic Pain and Illness. Mosby, St. Louis, 1976
9. International Association for the Study of Pain: Classification of chronic pain. Descriptions of chronic pain syndromes and definitions of pain terms. Pain 3:S1–226, 1986
10. Fernandez E, Turk DC: Sensory and affective components of pain: separation and synthesis. Psychol Bull 112:205–217, 1992
11. Romano JM, Turner JA: Chronic pain and depression: does the evidence support a relationship? Psychol Bull 97:18–34, 1985
12. Turk DC, Salovey P: "Chronic pain as a variant of depressive disease." A critical reappraisal. J Nerv Ment Dis 172:398–404, 1984
13. Rudy TE, Kerns RD, Turk DC: Chronic pain and depression: toward a cognitive-behavioral mediation model. Pain 35:129–140, 1988

14. Turk DC, Okifuji A, Scharff L: Chronic pain and depression: role of perceived impact and perceived control in different age cohorts. Pain 61:93–101, 1995

15. Schwartz L, Slater M, Birchler G, et al: Depression in spouses of chronic pain patients: the role of patient pain and anger, and marital satisfaction. Pain 44:61–67, 1991

16. Pilowsky I, Spence N: Pain, anger, and illness behaviour. J Psychosom Res 20:411–416, 1976

17. Kerns R, Rosenberg R, Jacob M: Anger expression and chronic pain. J Behav Med 17:57–67, 1994

18. Summers JD, Rapoff MA, Varghese G, et al: Psychosocial factors in chronic spinal cord injury pain. Pain 47:183–189, 1991

19. Corbishley M, Hendrickson R, Beutler L, et al: Behavior, affect, and cognition among psychogenic pain patients in group expressive psychotherapy. J Pain Symptom Manag 5:241–248, 1990

20. Fernandez E, Turk DC: The scope and significance of anger in the experience of chronic pain. Pain 61:165–175, 1995

21. Spiegel D, Bloom J: Pain in metastatic breast cancer. Cancer 52:341–345, 1983

22. Turk D, Meichenbaum D, Genest M: Pain and Behavioral Medicine: A Cognitive-behavioral Perspective. Guilford, New York, 1983

23. Flor H, Turk DC: Psychophysiology of chronic pain: do chronic pain patients exhibit symptom-specific psychophysiological responses? Psychol Bull 105:215–259, 1989

24. Jamner L, Tursky B: Discrimination between intensity and affective pain descriptors: a psychophysiological evaluation. Pain 30:271–283, 1987

25. Flor H, Turk DC, Birbaumer N: Assessment of stress-related psychophysiological reactions in chronic back pain patients. J Consult Clin Psychol 53:354–364, 1985

26. O'Leary A, Shoor S, Lorig K, et al: A cognitive-behavioral treatment for rheumatoid arthritis. Health Psychol 7:527–544, 1988

27. Melzack W, Wall P: Pain mechanisms: a new theory. Science 150:971–979, 1965

28. Turk D: Biopsychosocial perspective on chronic pain. In Gatchel R, Turk D (Eds.): Psychological Approaches to Pain Management: A Practitioner's Handbook. Guilford, New York, 1996

29. Turk D, Flor H: Chronic pain: a behavioral perspective. In Gatchel R, Turk D (Eds.): Psychosocial Factors in Pain. Guilford, New York, 1999

30. Miller W, Benefield R, Tongigan J: Enhancing motivation for change in problem drinking: a controlled comparison of two therapist styles. J Consult Clin Psychol 61:455–461, 1993

31. Miller W, Rollnick S: Motivational Interviewing: Preparing People to Change Addictive Behavior. Guilford, New York, 1991

32. Bonica J: The management of Pain. Lea & Febiger, Philadelphia, 1954

33. Bonica J: Evolution and current status of pain programs. J Pain Symp Manage 5:368–374, 1990

14

Back Pain: A Rationale for Conservative Management

James R. Taylor
Lance T. Twomey

The high prevalence of low back pain (LBP) in industrial societies is described as reaching epidemic proportions. Lifetime prevalences are generally reported to be in the range 58%–84%.[1,2,3] The peak prevalence appears to be between age 50 and 65.[4] Twelve-month prevalence, which may be a more accurate indication of the demand for treatment, is reported in the range 18% to 40%.[5,6,7] It has been claimed that most LBP is "nonspecific" and that a diagnosis of its pathologic basis or the pain source is seldom made.[8,9,10] However, studies using selective block techniques have succeeded in identifying the likely pain source in a very high proportion of unselected cases of LBP,[11] and comparison of block techniques with clinical diagnosis shows that a skilled therapist can correctly identify the same pain source as the blocks in a good proportion of cases.[12] Because some invasive interventions, such as surgical fusion, have fallen into disfavor, better conservative methods of management are being developed and tested with scientific rigor. Physical therapists are closely involved in the development of such new initiatives.

THE CHANGING SCENE

Considering the local scene, in the past 20 years there has been a virtual revolution in the postgraduate education of physical therapists in Australia. In 1981 Twomey was only the second Australian physiotherapist to graduate with a research PhD. Now, in this large country with its relatively small population, there are scores of Australian physiotherapists with research-based PhDs, hundreds with other research degrees and an even larger number who have done postgraduate study to become manipulative physiotherapists.

Physiotherapists have made and are continuing to make a significant contribution to advancement in musculoskeletal knowledge, particularly regarding the human spine. This is having an important "spin-off" in the way they practice their profession. For a long time now, Australian physical therapists have been primary contact health professions as well as providers of conservative management for back pain patients referred to them by medical practitioners. They are at the forefront in diagnosis and management of musculoskeletal conditions. The significant contribution of physical therapists to our understanding of LBP and dysfunction is reflected in many of the chapters in this book.

From its inception, the purpose of this book has been to bring together the basic sciences and clinical practice. Sometimes advances are brought about by the application of basic research findings to clinical practice. In other instances, objective testing of an established clinical model, empirically believed to be useful in practice, may provide objective evidence for its efficacy or otherwise. Unfortunately, it is often the case that traditional treatments that have never been tested are continued for want of a better method. It is important that as far as possible diagnostic and management methods should be evidence based. We are still some way from achieving that goal.

In the 12 years since this book first appeared there have been substantial changes in understanding LBP sources and mechanisms. There have also been advances in knowledge of the epidemiology and natural history of back pain that influence our approach to management.

This edition describes advances in basic knowledge and in management of LBP syndromes. In assessing a patient with chronic pain we need to take account of peripheral nociception, the heightened sensitivity of peripheral and central neurons with "central pain" and the behavioral sequelae of chronic pain. The advances in pathoanatomic knowledge should give us a more soundly based understanding of pain mechanisms and of some of the causes of pain syndromes. Awareness of the likely sources of peripheral nociceptive pain has helped us to track it to its source with more confidence by careful clinical skills and possibly to confirm it by the use of selective block techniques.[12, 13] In chronic pain syndromes the importance of central pain has been recognized,[14] and the high frequency of depression has been acknowledged (see Chapter 13). A better understanding of the interplay between chronic pain and its central and behavioral sequelae permit a better appreciation of the complexity of the patient's problem. Partly as a consequence of our realization of behavioral and central pain mechanisms, in management there has been a swing away from the indiscriminate used of spinal fusion to persistence with conservative management of LBP and also with less emphasis on ongoing passive treatments by the therapist and more emphasis on active exercise by the patient.

Until recently, the lumbar spine was a neglected field in basic science and clinical research, relative to organ systems such as the cardiovascular and gastrointestinal systems. Improved investigative methods and treatments have long been established in cardiovascular and alimentary tract diseases, but unscientific practices and empirical approaches have persisted in the diagnosis and management of LBP syndromes with the multiplication of "alternative" approaches that have no rational basis.

DIAGNOSIS

Accurate diagosis is a prerequisite for scientific management. In the spine, a segmental diagnosis can often be made on clinical grounds, and it should be possible to confirm it in many cases by other appropriate investigations. Historically, it has been an accepted principle of the medical model of pain that it has a causative pathology, as in chest pain from coronary artery spasm or abdominal pain from acute inflammation of the appendix. The pathologic cause and the pain effect is still generally accepted for these acute or recurrent painful conditions, but in the area of spinal pain, it is claimed that up to 90% of low back pain does not have a readily demonstrable pathologic basis,[10] or that an identified pathologic process is not the established cause of the pain.[15] It has therefore been suggested that the medical model should not apply, and frequently psychosocial issues or central pain are cited as the reason for the chronicity of the pain syndrome. Despite this trend away from attributing chronic back pain to local nociception in a damaged spinal structure, recent research has provided evidence that a nociceptive pain source can be regularly identified in chronic spinal pain syndromes and that successful treatment of the pain can cause abnormal psychologic profiles to revert to normal.[11, 16] Apart from skilled clinical assessment, we require an approach such as selective blocks to identify the pain source and other more sophisticated approaches, perhaps not as yet generally available, to identify the causative pathology. The trend of decrying anatomically based diagnosis of low back pain remains widespread.

Constrasting Views of Epidemiologists and Clinicians

Epidemiologic data suggest that most acute back pain resolves untreated. Medical bureaucrats, whose primary concern is to control costs, use this to claim that investigation is unwarranted and discourage efforts to achieve a scientific diagnosis of the nature of an individual patient's pain problem. Sptizer's observation[10] about the rarity of accurate diagnosis of the source of low back pain may relate to the inclusion, in prevalence studies of back pain, of large numbers of subjects with mild and transient pain episodes together with the more persistent and severe pain syndromes. The subjects with mild, short-term back pain who are not investigated are described as having "non-specific" back pain.

When this philosophy of epidemiologists and medical bureaucrats is rigidly applied, it is not surprising that many patients with chronic or recurrent low back pain remain poorly investigated and without a segmental diagnosis of the pain source. The absence of an accurate diagnosis may prove costly to both the patient and the community in the longer term. Closer cooperation between appropriately skilled physical therapists and medical practitioners could provide more accurate diagnoses in a much higher proportion of patients than in the sample cited by the Quebec Task Force.[10–13]

CHRONIC PAIN, NOCICEPTION, CENTRAL PAIN, AND DEPRESSION

The current understanding of central pain owes much to the research of Melzack and Wall.[14] However, if this is used to suggest that in chronic pain, peripheral nociception is no longer an issue and that further pursuit of accurate diagnosis of a pain source is a waste of time, it is patently wrong and may prevent the application of treatment that could resolve the patient's pain and its behavioral sequelae.[16]

It has become a common attitude, among clinicians who see patients with chronic low back pain with depressive or other behavioral features, to attribute the chronicity of the pain to psychosocial factors and to neglect persisting physical signs of nociception. A high proportion of patients with any form of chronic pain develop secondary symptoms of depression. These often become more intrusive and disruptive of the patient's life that the original nociceptive pain problem. However, the work of Bogduk, Schwatzer and their colleagues[11,13] has shown that in chronic whiplash pain or chronic low pack pain a pain source can still be identified and successfully treated and that the secondary behavioral features can return spontaneously to normal in patients whose nociceptive pain is treated successfully by physical means.[16]

We accept that central mechanisms of pain develop in chronic pain syndromes and that both peripheral and central neurons develop increased sensitivity to painful and other stimuli. This does not invalidate the concept that accurate segmental diagnosis should be a primary objective of the clinician who sees patients with chronic LBP. Physical therapists, particularly those with postgraduate training in spinal conditions, are now making a major contribution in the clinical diagnosis of the segmental origin of low back pain syndromes. In cooperation with an appropriately trained medical graduate, this diagnosis may be confirmed "objectively" by other investigative methods, including local anesthetic blocks to the nerves or joints at the painful dysfunctional level.

RELEVANT PATHOLOGY: A MORE DISCERNING APPROACH

It is a general principle of medical science that dysfunction or pain has a pathologic correlate, although an understanding of the relevant pathology in chronic pain may require an extensive knowledge of the complex relationship between structure and function, not only locally in the spine but also in the related nervous system.

The identification of symptomatic pathology in the low back remains a contentious issue. It is often emphasized that most of the pathology demonstrated by imaging, such as a bulging posterior annulus in a middle-aged person, may be asymptomatic. An example of how asymptomatic pathology may become relevant is the finding of L5 spondylolysis in a person complaining of lumbosacral pain since a recent injury. The spondylolysis may be long standing, but it may have become symptomatic following an injury to the weakened segment with the development of clinical instability. A further example would be the lumbar disc that may have been fissured for years without symptoms; however, after a lifting-twisting injury the fissure may extend by tearing into the outer, innervated third of the annulus, with acute onset of low back pain correlating either with a high-intensity zone on an MRI[17] or with reproduction of the patient's pain on lumbar discography. Such investigations may not always be justifiable on the grounds of cost or on a basis of risk as opposed to benefit. On the other hand, the patient who knows that the cause of his or her pain has been established is generally much more prepared to persist with active rehabilitation than the one who remains in the dark about the cause of chronic pain and persisting incapacity. Moreover, if the pain does not resolve with appropriate conservative measures, referral for a surgical opinion can be made with sound knowledge of the nature of the problem. It is often through the cooperation between a physical therapist with the appropriate physical diagnostic skills and a suitably trained medical practitioner that the issue of which pathology is symptomatic can be resolved.

EXERCISE, FITNESS, AND LOW BACK PAIN

It is increasingly recognized that the management of persistent low back pain requires active rather than ongoing passive treatment methods, where the patients do the work rather than the therapist.

As previously acknowledged (Chapter 9), all elements of the musculoskeletal system react adversely to rest and positively to exercise and movement. There is considerable evidence to strongly support the need for continuing high levels of exercise activity and fitness in individuals with back pain. Physical activity by patients with back pain not only restores function but also is associated with a reduction in pain.[18,19,21] In spite of this evidence, bedrest, analgesics, corsets, and avoidance of physical activity remain the most commonly prescribed forms of management.[22]

Habitual reduction in activity, especially when linked with bedrest, is inevitably associated with a decline in fitness and strength and an inability to react appropriately to changes in the environment. Patients who respond to their back pain in this way become weaker, less mobile, and more rapidly fatigued than those who maintain an adequate level of fitness through exercise. They are more likely to suffer early recurrence of their back pain on returning to work.[18,19,20,21]

The use of intensive physical rehabilitation methods in athletes with musculoskeletal sports injuries (including back injuries) have demonstrated good responses to these intensive programs of physical treatment.[23] The extension of this approach to nonathletes with chronic low back pain has proved successful, with evidence of long-term success in a variety of studies.[18,19,20,21] The use of aerobic exercise in the rehabilitation of individuals with chronic low back pain was reviewed by Protas.[24] She clearly demonstrated the link between increased aerobic status, enhanced physical activity, and the likelihood of a decline in back pain. However, she emphasized that future research should be directed toward a more standardized approach, with multicenter trials and sufficiently large numbers to permit critical judgement of the outcomes in regard to the long-term influence of exercise on chronic low back pain.

NEUROMUSCULAR CONTROL OF THE LUMBAR MOTION SEGMENT

The first chapters of this book describe the anatomy, biomechanics, and pathology of the lumbar spine based mainly on numerous experiments on cadaver specimens, whether on individual motion segments or on whole lumbar columns. The authors have investigated the relative roles of the bones, joints, ligaments, and muscles in the normal function of the lumbar spine, but cadaver experiments are inadequate to determine the role of muscles and the nervous system in motion segment support and control. Partial answers can be obtained from the anatomic studies of Bogduk and Macintosh (Chapter 4), but the complex patterns of neuromuscular control can only be studied in living individuals. It has long been known that the column cannot remain stable in the absence of proper neuromuscular support. The collapsing forms of paralytic scoliosis have been well documented.[25]

Recent studies by physical therapists (Chapters 7 and 8) have greatly improved our understanding of the role of muscles in the control and stability of the lumbar motion segment and the interplay between chronic pain mechanisms and a breakdown in this essential control. In particular, it is the segmental muscles that control individual motion segments, rather than the global muscles that control the lumbar column as a whole, that have become the focus of attention. Our previous, rather vague appreciation that abdominal muscles were important in supporting the lumbar spine led to the advocacy of sit-ups and subsequently to various modifications of these crude exercises to develop rectus abdominis and external oblique in rehabilitation of the back-injured worker. These global muscles bridge from pelvis to thorax and are important, with the gluteal muscles, in controlling pelvic posture, but they do not exercise the fine control that may be required over individual injured segments.

VERTEBRAL DESIGN FOR SEGMENTAL CONTROL

The structure of the long vertebral transverse and spinous processes plus the prominent mamillary tubercles at the posterior extremity of the superior articular processes should give us clues to a better understanding of how vertebral design and muscle attachments can best control individual segments in the varied dynamic situations of everyday life. The muscles that gain attachments to these levers are best placed to exercise segmental control. The layered thoracolumbar fascia owes a part of its functional importance to the muscles that attach through these layers to individual transverse and spinous processes.

It has been well noted that the "rotator cuff–like" deepest fascicles of multifidus, which attach to the mamillary processes, are the parts that atrophy in chronic LBP states. These muscles are in the best position to control the zygapophyseal joints of the motion segments.

RETRAINING DISORDERED NEUROMUSCULAR CIRCUITS

Loss of control and atrophy of the transversus, internal oblique, and multifidus has been recognized as an important feature of many chronic LBP conditions, particularly in segmental instability associated with injury to the disc and Z joints. This is not merely a matter of muscle loss; it is also a matter of loss of neuromuscular control. The mechanisms leading to these specific atrophies are ill-understood and require further research, but it is a matter of record (Chapter 7) that individuals with this loss of function can be retrained to use the segmental muscles to regain a measure of control over the injured segment and thus over their chronic or recurrent pain. Segmental instability in chronic low back syndromes is much more common than is generally appreciated, and the condition remains frequently undiagnosed. Many years ago, Kirkaldy-Willis[26] described how instability could eventually be spontaneously resolved over the years by processes of stabilization—particularly by overgrowth of facet margins and loss of disc thickness or bony fusion across incompetent discs. A better and more functional method of stabilization is now available to us, even though it may not be universally effective. Spinal fusion has been a traditional treatment for segmental instability with chronic pain, but this operation has been widely discredited as a panacea for chronic segmental pain. It may be the only solution for gross instability in a few patients, but any conservative means of achieving control without surgery is a major step forward. The complementary work recorded in Chapters 7 and 8 will almost certainly prove to be major breakthroughs in this field.

REFERENCES

1. Kirkaldy-Willis WH, Cassidy J: Spinal manipulation in the treatment of low back pain. Can Fam Physician 31:535, 1985
2. Jayson MIV: The inflammatory component of mechanical back problems. Br J Rheumatol 25:210, 1986
3. Walsh K, Cruddas M, Coggon D: Low back pain in eight areas of Britain. J Epidemiol Commun Health 46:227, 1992
4. Deyo RA, Tsui-Wu YJ: Descriptive epidemiology of low back pain and its related medical care in the United States. Spine 12:264, 1987
5. Reisbord LS, Greeenland S: Factors associated with self reported back pain prevalence: a population based study. J Chron Dis 38:691, 1985
6. Laslett M, Crothers C, Beattie P, et al: The frequency and incidence of low back pain/sciatica in an urban population. NZ Med J 104:424, 1991
7. Dodd T: The prevalence of low back pain in Great Britain in 1996: A report on research for the Department of Health using the ONS Omnibus Survey. The Stationary Office, London, 1997.

8. Hart LG, Deyo RA, Cherkin DC: Physician office visits for low back pain: Frequency, clinical evaluation and treatment patterns from a US national survey. Spine 20:11, 1995

9. Waddell G, Low back pain: a twentieth century health care enigma. Spine 21:2820, 1996

10. Spitzer WO, Leblanc FE, Dupuis M: Scientific approach to the assessment and management of activity related spinal disorders. Report of the Quebec Task Force on Spinal Disorders. Spine 12:(Suppl 7):1, 1987

11. Schwatzer AC, Aprill CN, Derby R, et al: The relative contributions of the disc and zygapophyseal joints in chronic low back pain. Spine 19:801, 1994

12. Phillips D, Twomey LT: A comparison of manual diagnosis with a diagnosis established by a uni-level lumbar spinal block procedure. Man Therapy 1:82, 1995

13. Jull G, Bogduk N, Marsland A: The accuracy of manual diagnosis for cervical zygapophyseal joint pain syndromes. Med J Austral 148:233, 1988

14. Melzack R, Wall PD: Pain mechanisms: a new theory. Science 150:971, 1965

15. Boden S, Davis DO, Dina TS, et al: Abnormal magnetic resonance scans of the lumbar spine in asymptomatic subjects. J Bone Joint Surg 72A:403, 1990

16. Wallis BJ, Lord SM, Barnsley L, Bogduk N: Pain and psychological symptoms of Australian patients with whiplash. Spine 21:804, 1996

17. Aprill C, Bogduk N: High intensity zone: a pathognomonic sign of a painful lumbar disc on MRI. Br J Radiol 65:361, 1992

18. Waddell G: Clinical assessment of lumbar improvement. Clin Orthop Related Res 179:77, 1983

19. Mayer TG, Gatchell RJ, Kishino N, et al: A prospective short-term study of chronic low back pain patients utilising novel objective functional measurement. Pain 25:53, 1986

20. Bendix AF, Bendix T, Labriola M, et al: Functional restoration for chronic back pain. Spine 23:717, 1998

21. Mayer TG, Polatin PB, Gatchell RJ: Functional restoration and other rehabilitation approaches to chronic musculoskeletal pain disability syndromes. Crit Rev Phys Rehab Med 10:209, 1998

22. Deyo RA, Diehl AK, Rosenthal M: How many days of bed rest for acute low back pain. New Eng J Med 315:1064, 1986

23. Cinque C: Back pain prescription: out of bed and into the gym. Phys Sports Med 17:185, 1989

24. Protas EJ: Aerobic exercise in the rehabilitation of individuals with chronic low back pain: A review. Crit Rev Phys Rehab Med 8:283, 1996

25. Taylor JR, Liston CB, Twomey LT: Scoliosis: A review. Austral J Physio 28:20, 1982

26. Kirkaldy-Willis WH: Managing Low Back Pain: Churchill Livingstone, New York, 1983

Note: Page numbers in *italics* refer to illustrations; page numbers followed by t refer to tables.

Spondylolisthesis, 32, 78, 150
  braces in, 292
  degenerative, 205
  extension pattern of, *227*
  in children and adolescents, 361, 370, 371
  intersegmental motion levels in, 220
  lateral shift pattern in, *228*
  lumbar instability related to, 202, 203, 204, *204*
  lumbar segmental instability management of,
      238
Spondylolysis, 32, 51, 81
  in children and adolescents, 361, 364
  intersegmental motion levels in, 220
  lifting in, 350, 353
  lumbar instability related to, 204, *204*
  lumbar segmental instability management of,
      238
  occurrence of, 204
  segmental instability with, 215
  stress fractures in athletes with, 204
Spondylometer, lumbar, 71–72, *72,* 278
Sports, rehabilitation methods of, 389
  spondylolysis in athletes and, 204
Sports activities, and low back pain, in children and
      adolescents, 361, 362, 363–365
      management of, 370–371
      risk factors in, 363–365, 369
Squat position, double-leg, 330
  in lifting, 341–342, 343–344
    electromyography in, 341–342
    vs. to stoop lifting, 343–344, 349–350
  single-leg, 330
    loss of spinal control in, 330
Stabilization, active, 253–255
  categories of, 250
  in quadruped position, 341, *341–342*
  neuromuscular control in, 391
  of transversus abdominus, 332–333
Stabilizing muscles, 251–271, 338
  assessment of, 253–256, *256*
  dynamic stabilization in, 332
  dysfunction of, 252–256
  holding capacity or fatigability of, 255–256,
      258, 260
  in high-speed and skilled movements, 268–270
  in slow and controlled movements, 267–268,
      268
  isolation and facilitation of, 257–261
    in four-point kneeling position, 258, *259*
    pressure sensor in, 258, 259
    resistance applied in, 259, *260*
    verbal cues in, 257–258

spinal stabilization in, 332
static training of, 261–267
  at home, 265
  in different positions, 265, *266*
  with different resistance to trunk, 264–265,
      265
  with leg loading, 262–264
Stature, 59, 66–67
  age-related changes in, 67, 86
  definition of, 59
  diurnal variation in, 66–67
  creep in, 25, 67, 79
Stenosis, spinal, 20, 50, 279–294, *282*
  central, 279, 281
    computed tomography of, 289–290, *290*
    degenerative, 281, *282,* 285–286
    in hypertrophy of ligamenta flava, 283
    morphologic analysis of, 289
    size of dural sac in, 284–285, *285*
    surgery in, 294
  computed tomography of, 289–290, *290*
  congenital, 279
  degenerative, 279, 280
    anatomy in, 281, *282*
    computed tomography of, 289–290, *290*
    dynamic concept of, 283–284, 286–287
  developmental, 279, 281
  effect of pressure on nerve roots in, 285–286
  encroachment on nerve roots of cauda equina
      in, 286–287
  history of patient with, 289
  iatrogenic, 280, 283
  in children and adolescents, 370
  lateral, 279, 281
    degenerative, 282, *283*
    morphologic analysis of, 290
    surgery in, 294
  magnetic resonance imaging of, 289–290
  metabolic, 280, 282–283
  morphologic examination of, 289–290
  myelography of, 289
  pathophysiology of, 283–287
  physical examination of, 288
  postoperative recurrence of, 294
  posttraumatic, 280
  size of spinal canal and cauda equina in,
      284–285, *284*
    posture and load affecting, 283, 287
  treatment of, 291–294
    conservative, 291–294
    manipulative therapy in, 192–195
    surgical, 20, 293–294